Smart Patient

Journey Road Map

increasing your odds for success

Kathryn Alexander

Published in 2014 by Annexus Pty Ltd

PO Box 259, Maleny QLD 4552 Australia

Book design & layout: Kathryn Alexander

Cartoon characters: iclipart.com (royalty-free)

National Library of Australia Cataloguing-in-Publication data:

Alexander, Kathryn, 1954- author

Smart patient journey road map: increasing your odds for success/Kathryn Alexander

ISBN: 9780980376296 (paperback)

Patient self-monitoring.

Self-care, Health.

Medicine, popular.

Therapeutics.

613

Disclaimer

Smart Patient Journey Road Map does not constitute medical advice. If you require advice on any medical or related matter, the author and publishers of *Smart Patient Journey Road Map* suggest you seek that advice from a qualified professional. As far as the law allows, all people connected with the writing, editing and publishing of this book disclaim all liability arising from the negligence of writer and publisher of *Smart Patient Journey Road Map*.

Contents

My end point   51

How to find out who can help me   75

Rating each treatment   178

Monitoring 193

Templates & Charts 221

Case Studies 239

The story of the Journey Road Map

One afternoon in the summer of 2005 I came up from my office to the kitchen to find it in its usual state - taken over by Stephen's paperwork. I peered over his shoulder and saw some interesting diagrams and asked him what he was working on. He said it was a value framework, a collaborative model for multiple parties, either individuals or groups who may hold different criteria and aspirational end points but share areas of common ground where they can collaborate and find solutions for mutual benefit.

I got it in one. I was so excited as the potential for my work and for my patients was enormous. Imagine if a patient was able to manage multiple parties where the common ground was their health, where the platform for discussion was how to best help them achieve their aspirational end point. And all this within a system where patients may not seem to matter, where consultation times are often no longer than 15 minutes, just enough time to prescribe a drug and then get shown the door, where the pressure is on to make decisions where the patient takes all the risks, and in an environment that appears hostile to the individual patient's aspirations.

Over my previous 20 years of practice I had increasingly found myself in an advocacy role. Most patients that I attracted had come after they had tried everything else and were endeavouring to manage their chronic condition while balancing both conventional care with alternative or complementary medicine. They were usually at a cross roads where nothing was seeming to work, everyone had a different take on their case and how it should be managed, even practitioners from the same modality may not even seem to agree on the cause or the treatment. So it was either suppress with conventional medicine and slowly deteriorate, or pursue an expensive, time-consuming and costly hit and miss approach.

Perhaps the greatest frustration was not knowing how to get the best from the system and how to get meaningful answers in order to make informed decisions without being medically trained. Patients were quick to discover that medical professionals from both sides of the camp are not paid to teach but to present you with options from which you are supposed to make an informed decision within a short time frame, decisions that often carry risks. With the advent of the internet one could assume that patients have greater capacity to inform themselves but this has added yet another complexity, that of information overload with no capacity to apply this knowledge to the individual case.

For myself, a vital aspect of my work was to make sure that each one of my patients could move forward with confidence in their decision. We had to find the best pathway even in situations where we couldn't foretell the future, where the diagnosis wasn't clear and often in an environment where the patient could easily feel prejudiced if they didn't follow medical advice. Of importance to my patients was that the choices they were making were their choices that had been arrived at through careful consideration where they could be satisfied that they were doing the best for themselves, even if they arrived back at the original advice received from their medical specialist. The important thing was that it was their decision, and as such they had more confidence, less fear and less regrets.

Starting the journey of discovery by trying to extract even the minimum amount of information required to make a decision was the biggest stumbling block. Many patients weren't properly diagnosed, others didn't understand what their condition would mean to them both in the short and long term, others were more informed but were grappling to find someone or some treatment that would work.

For each of these patients I started constructing simple lines of enquiry, three or four questions that could easily be asked at any consultation without taking too much time or brain power that would extract just enough information to get to the next step. I found that if I advised my patients to stay on their side of the fence without trying to address the benefits and risks of treatment or even the mechanics of their condition they could make much more headway and not get locked in combat with a professional who could only advise according to their medical criteria.

I started to compile questions, questions that covered many eventualities, many different patient concerns for so many different conditions at different stages, and I started to see generic patterns emerge for each of the stages of a patient's journey. But perhaps the most sobering reality was having to go through the system myself with a close family member, where your vulnerability makes it difficult to think straight and even though you may be medically trained you find that it is of little help in getting the treatment you need nor does it change the culture that you suddenly find yourself navigating through. I found that unless I could be detached and portray the situation in a specific way, then we stood little to no chance. It's true that it meant seeing many different specialists, but after two years we got there. I can honestly say that we wouldn't have been able to do this without the journey road map, where it was tested and developed to its maximum, and enabled my close relative (who ultimately had to make all the very painful decisions) to do this with as much assurity as she could. Eventually she was supported by a medical team which was, for the most part, on her side. Today she is healthy and has a full life, which is pain-free and without major health risks.

All I can say is that the road map is a brilliant tool and methodology that has already transformed the lives of all my patients that have tried and tested it. It is agnostic in that it doesn't matter whether you choose conventional or alternative treatment and it doesn't require that you are medically trained to understand and plot a way forward, but it does require you to have an enquiring mind, a desire to take the reins and a sincere desire to improve your health outcome.

I am so grateful to Stephen for helping me perfect and apply his model for patients who are endeavouring to get the best from a fractured and at times broken health system, and where the system is often more important than the patient. It has taken nine years to develop and has been put on the top shelf three times where I couldn't stand to look at it anymore having realized that my logic was broken which meant going back to the drawing board and starting yet again.

We fixed the logic twice and eventually when it came together it was so simple and so eloquent that I couldn't believe that it had taken so long or had appeared so complicated. I commented on this to Stephen and he explained that the model itself is simple, but the complexities of working within an eco-world with multiple parties who hold different and sometimes opposing criteria required one to make sense of that world and tease out the various threads dispassionately in order to apply the model. Of course the model itself enabled me to tease out the logic - but this is something that you, the reader, do not have to worry about. You can just enjoy the fruits of this labour.

So thank you Stephen for your value road map, for your encouragement, for your patience and for all your help.

For myself, this work could never have been accomplished without almost 30 years of clinical experience assisting patients take the reins and seeing that reversal of chronic disease is possible when you make the right treatment choices. And so this model was born, tried and tested over and over again, in each case facilitating the patient's journey enabling them to filter through treatment options quickly and effectively and arrive at an informed decision with confidence.

As we move towards health rationing and reduced healthcare, I hope that this methodology will assist you in opening up your options on your journey to wellness.

Kathryn Alexander

April 2014

Stephen Alexander is an industry expert advising national and regional governments and health provider organizations on a range of strategic planning issues, including critical drivers for change, such as the emerging role of health consumers who take self-responsibility and play an active role in the management of their own health or on behalf of a family member.

"The framework that is embedded in Kathryn's book has been warmly received by many of these senior leaders and managers on the basis that its adoption will not only dramatically reduce the cost of healthcare but, based upon their own observations, that a smart patient also generates better clinical outcomes."

Stephen Alexander 2014

Your say ....

"We are going through the questions to ask tonight and my husband says he wishes that we had had all this information at the beginning of the journey, but better late than never. We have a tough decision to make, but now that we can clearly see our options and what these may mean to me I feel more prepared and more resolved to make the best decision for me." HG, WA

"It was so lovely to meet a health care professional who genuinely cares about helping people. Thank you for yesterday, it was fantastic. I was so scared, but now I feel so much hope. Your road map has changed everything for me and now I feel that I can make the right decision." KB, VIC

"The road map teaches you how to make informed decisions about your health with confidence. It allows you to take a step back and look at all your options and their outcomes to see if they match up with your personal desired end point. It gives you the courage to ask your practitioner questions so that you can take the reins of your life and no longer live in the dark. By weighing up the pros and cons of each treatment, it makes it easier to choose which one suits you and enables you to tailor your own pathway dependent on your lifestyle and values." ER, QLD, Australia

"The clinician was the driving force in the 20th century, [but] the patient will be the driving force in the 21st century."

"Knowledge [of what works] will become the enemy of disease."

Sir Muir Gray, Director of Clinical Knowledge of the UK's NHS

5 steps

1   My starting point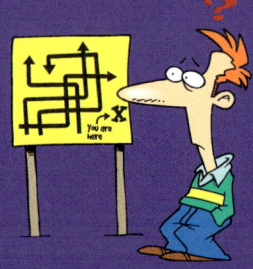

2   My end point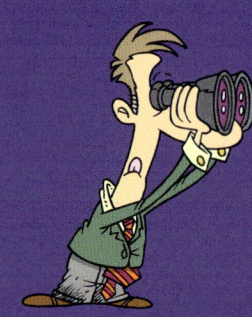

3   Who can help me?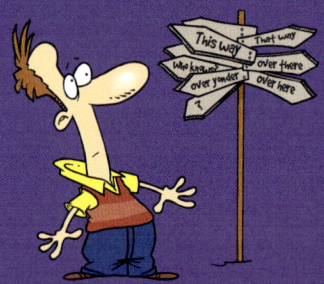

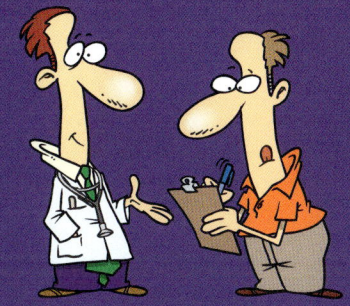
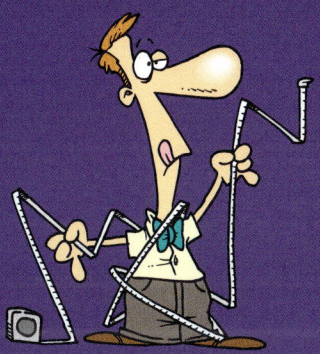

"The clinician was the driving force in the 20th century, [but] the patient will be the driving force in the 21st century.....

Knowledge [of what works] will become the enemy of disease. "

Sir Muir Gray, Director of Clinical Knowledge of the UK's NHS

My starting point

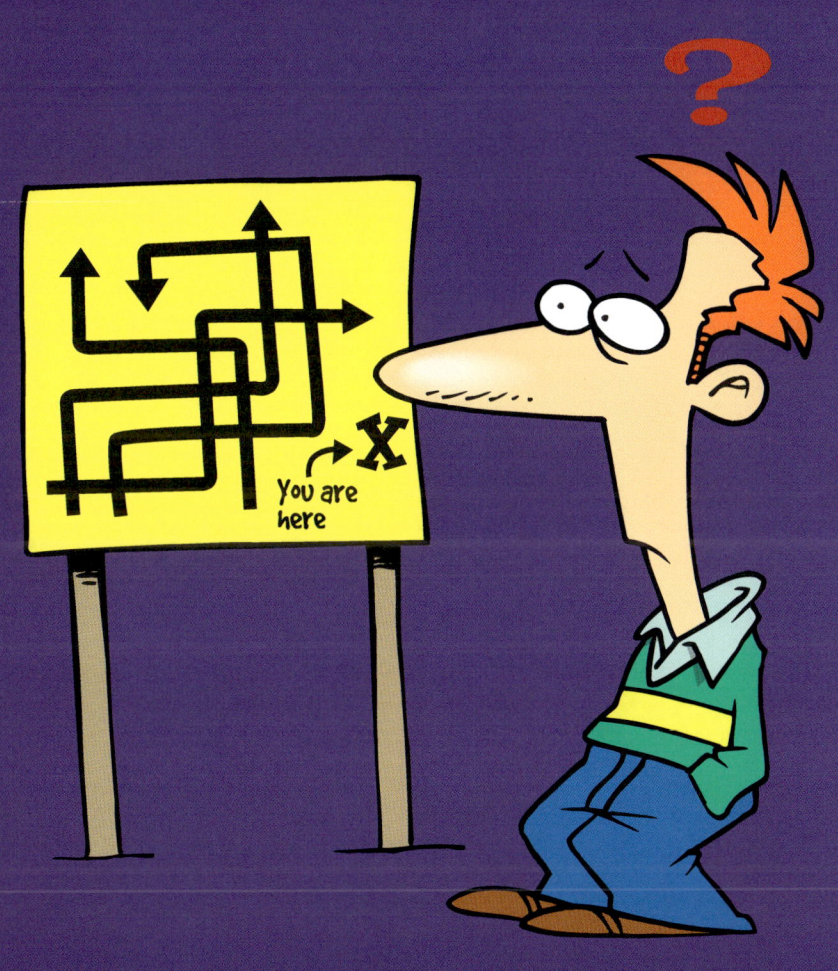

To do

1 Get your diagnosis

Follow the *Diagnosis pathway*

Collect your test results

2 Understand your diagnosis

Choose your questions from *Understanding my diagnosis: a conversational approach*

Research your diagnosis

3 Define your starting point

Follow the statement guide in *My Health Statement - My Starting Point*

Why do I need an accurate diagnosis?

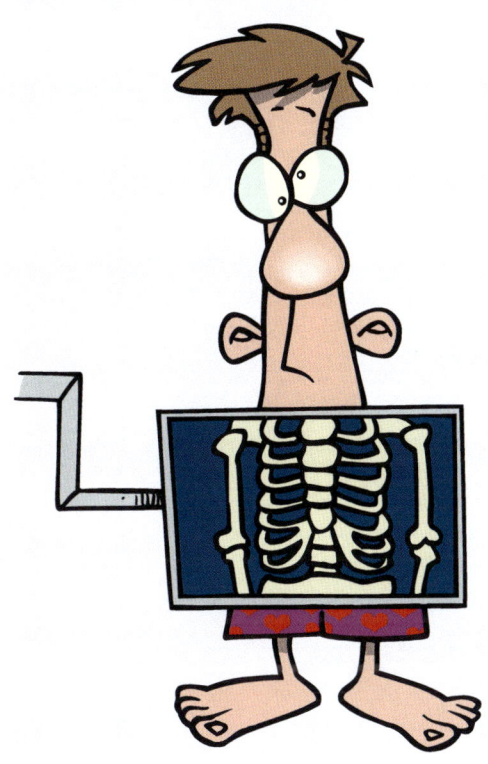

Because no-one will know what you need to do, what to treat & how to monitor in order to make sure you get to your end point.

My Journey Road Map: my starting point

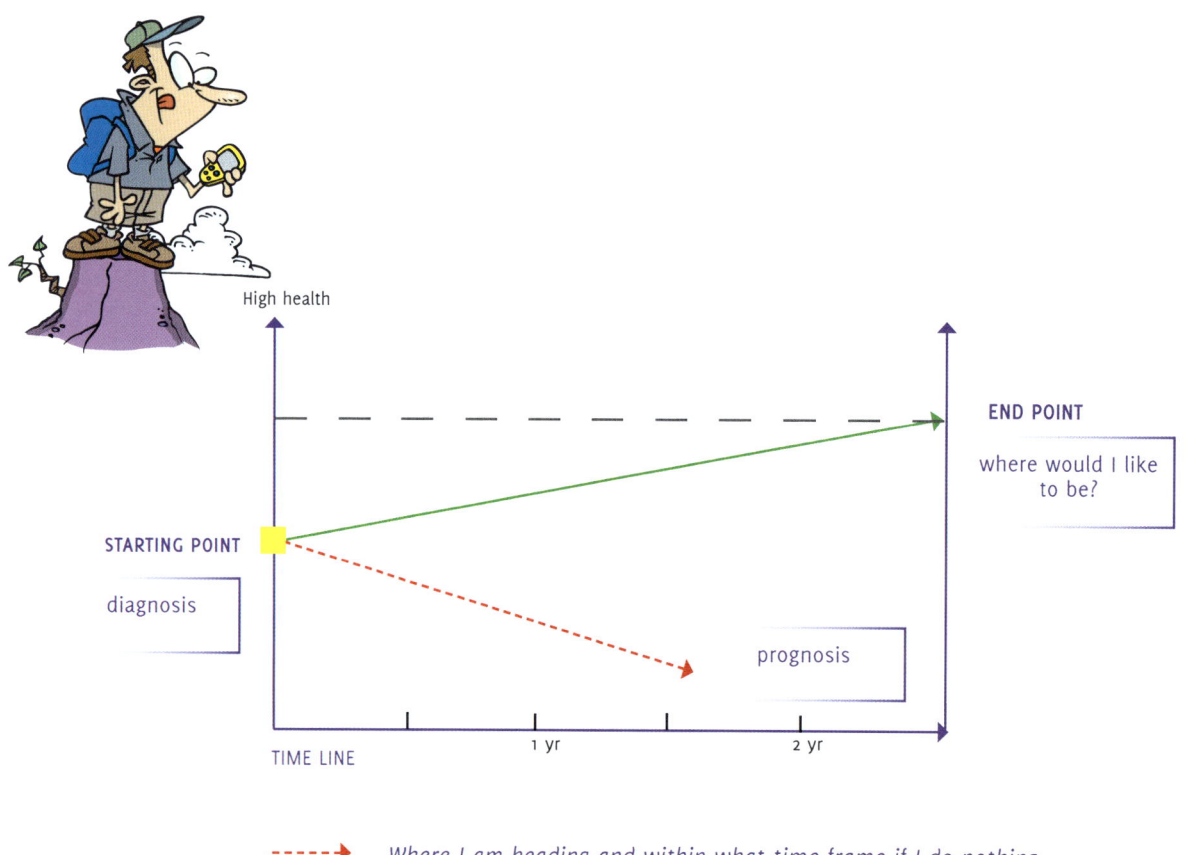

High health

END POINT

where would I like
to be?

STARTING POINT

diagnosis

prognosis

TIME LINE   1 yr   2 yr

- - - - ▶   *Where I am heading and within what time frame if I do nothing*

My starting point is where I am now (diagnosis),
where I am currently heading (prognosis) and how fast.

1 Getting your diagnosis

Before you attend your initial appointment I would recommend that you make some notes about your health in order to give enough detail to your GP or specialist to facilitate more informed decision making on the possible diagnosis. Use the following as a guide.

The appointment

1. List your current symptoms along with any factors that make your condition better or worse, and indicate the length of time you have been suffering from these.

2. Make a note of your past history which may be relevant to the doctor:

Remember to take copies of any past medical records that you may have with you.

- previous diagnoses & dates of diagnoses;
- previous treatments for the conditions (medication, surgery etc.);
- length of time of each treatment, and dates; and
- outcome of treatment (did it work, is it ongoing?).

3. Make a note of any relevant family history

Family members, such as grand-parents, parents and siblings, that have been diagnosed with chronic conditions or conditions similar to yours.

Before the appointment familiarize yourself with the *Diagnosis Pathway* (p24) so that you know what to expect. From your description of your symptoms and other relevant information that the doctor may ask about he may have formed a fairly good idea of what is wrong with you and may simply prescribe a drug, and if the symptoms abate then this would confirm the diagnosis. Alternatively, he may run some routine examinations and send you off for a blood test or a scan, or make a referral for you to see a specialist if your condition or its diagnosis is outside his scope of expertise.

Before the end of the appointment it's a good idea to ask about the strategy using whichever of the following questions apply:

- Tests/scans: what is the test/scan for and what will it indicate?
- Treatment: what is the treatment and what will it address?

The diagnosis

Make sure that you obtain copies of your results. Write down the name of your tests along with the results that confirm the diagnosis.

Test	Result	Diagnosis
Blood test		
Endoscopy		
CT scan		
Ultrasound		

Once you have your diagnosis fill in the **Now** column on the *Full Alignment Template* (p20) with the tests you have undertaken, your diagnosis and your list of symptoms. If you do not have a medical diagnosis, or are unable to get one, then you may need to start by filling in the symptoms and any test results. If you are seeing other practitioners (allied &/or alternative) complete the non-medical section by adding the therapy type (i.e. naturopathy, TCM [Traditional Chinese Medicine], homoeopathy etc.) and their diagnosis/es.

It's a good idea to research your diagnosed condition on the internet to make sure that you have had all the appropriate tests for the diagnosis. (See p23, p30 and p223 for useful websites.)

Full Alignment Template

WHY	NOW			FUTURE HEALTH RISKS
Causes/Risks	Tests	Diagnosis	Prognosis	
	Medical			
	Non-medical			
End Point				
Symptoms &/or diagnostics	Prioritized list of Goals	End point alignment	THERAPY	TREATMENTS	MONITORING

The Full Alignment Template chart will enable you to cross reference what's on offer (therapies and treatments) against what you are trying to achieve and where you hope to end up.

As we go through the 5 steps you will be filling in the various sections so that you have all the basic information on one page making it easy to see where practitioners fit into your strategy, and who and what treatments are mission critical in getting you to your endpoint. Putting your findings on this one page will help you stay on track and less likely to head down cul-de-sacs which could be detrimental particularly if time is not on your side.

Pauline, whom we will meet later, has filled in her symptoms, or what she would like addressing, along with her various diagnoses and the tests that determined these. Later she will research her condition and find out about the possible causes and also any future health risks.

WHY	NOW			FUTURE HEALTH RISKS		
Causes/ Risks		Tests	Diagnosis	Prognosis		
	Medical	▶ blood test ▶ eye test ▶ X-rays ▶ Bone densitometry	▶ rheumatoid arthritis ▶ iritis ▶ osteopaenia, vit D deficiency ▶ anaemia (iron deficiency) ▶ amenorrhoea ▶ psoriasis			
	Non-medical					
	End Point					
	Symptoms &/or diagnostics		Prioritized list of Goals	End point alignment		
	▶ pain & stiffness in joints ▶ inflammation in eyes & skin ▶ no periods ▶ underweight ▶ fatigue, anaemic ▶ low bone density ▶ mineral & vitamin deficiencies					

The Cancer Diagnosis

The cancer diagnosis requires various tests and imaging scans. Diagnosis often follows this path:

- an initial appointment/physical examination with your GP;

- a blood test looking for cancer indicators (cancer markers such as PSA, CEA, CA 15-3), liver function, kidney function, complete cell count etc.;

- imaging scans: CAT/CT scan, PET scan, mammogram, ultrasound or MRI (to determine the location, size and spread of the cancer); and

- a biopsy of the cancer tissue following surgical removal or fine needle aspiration (FNA) or punch biopsy. The microscopic examination (histology report) determines the type of cancer, its behaviour and its potential rate of growth (degree of differentiation).

From this information the cancer can be named, staged and graded. These are the criteria upon which your specialist bases his diagnosis, prognosis and recommended treatment.

So if you have been diagnosed with cancer then it is important to ask for:

- the name of the cancer;

- the stage of the cancer; and

- the grade of the cancer.

It's a good idea to keep a copy of all the scan and histology reports since the date of diagnosis so that you and others have something to refer to when monitoring your progress.

Name of cancer

The histology report will tell you the organ and tissue of origin and its sub-type. For example, brain cancer may either be a glioma or an astrocytoma. Similarly, breast cancer may be ductal or lobular, or lung cancer may be small cell lung cancer or non-small cell lung cancer.

Staging

The imaging scan will indicate the staging. The basic staging is stage 1 to stage 4.

The higher the staging, the greater the spread and the poorer the prognosis. Staging can be summarized thus:

- Stage 1: the disease is local and has not spread

- Stage 2: there is local spread to the lymph nodes

- Stage 3: there is spread to distant lymph nodes

- Stage 4: there is distant spread to other organs

The staging classification is based on the **TNM** system. **T** refers to **T**umour size; **N**, regional or local lymph **N**ode involvement; **M**, evidence of **M**etastases. Staging enables the specialist to estimate survival time and compare treatment results in similar groups entered in clinical trials. Each cancer type has its own classification system, so letters and numbers don't always mean the same for every type of cancer.

Grading

The histology report will tell you how the cancer will behave, how quickly it is likely it is to grow and spread. The basic grading is usually from grade 1 to grade 3, with grade 1 being the least aggressive and slower growing, and grade 3 being fast growing. When looking at the cancer cells through the microscope there are various features that may display which will show how fast the cancer cells are dividing. This is known as the degree of *differentiation* of malignant cells, or the extent to which the tumour cells differ from their normal tissue counterpart. A fully differentiated cell is a normal cell that has reached maturity and does not divide; the further the cell departs from the normal differentiated state, the more rapidly it divides and the more aggressive the cancer. Therefore an undifferentiated or poorly differentiated malignant tumour has a greater rate of growth than a moderately differentiated tumour and is said to be more aggressive. A grade 3 cancer has a poorer prognosis than a grade 1 cancer.

Fully differentiated	Normal, does not divide
Well differentiated	
Moderately differentiated	
Poorly differentiated	
Undifferentiated	Malignant, divides rapidly

Scoring

Sometimes a score is applied to the grade. For example, in prostate cancer the Gleason score is used and in breast cancer the Bloom and Richardson score is used. The grade is based on the score and will give the specialist further information about how the grading has been established.

Some useful websites for investigating your cancer diagnosis:

- ▸ http://www.nhs.uk/conditions/Cancer/Pages/Introduction.aspx
- ▸ http://www.patient.co.uk/
- ▸ http://www.cancer.net
- ▸ http://netdoctor.co.uk/cancer/index.shtml
- ▸ http://www.cancer.gov/cancertopics/alphalist/
- ▸ http://www.medicinenet.com/
- ▸ http://www.macmillan.org.uk/Cancerinformation/ http://news.cancerconnect.com/
- ▸ http://www.cancernetwork.com/
- ▸ http://www.cancerhelp.org.uk/index.htm
- ▸ http://www.upmccancercenter.com/cainformation/alltypes.cfm
- ▸ Http://www.uptodate.com

The Diagnosis Pathway

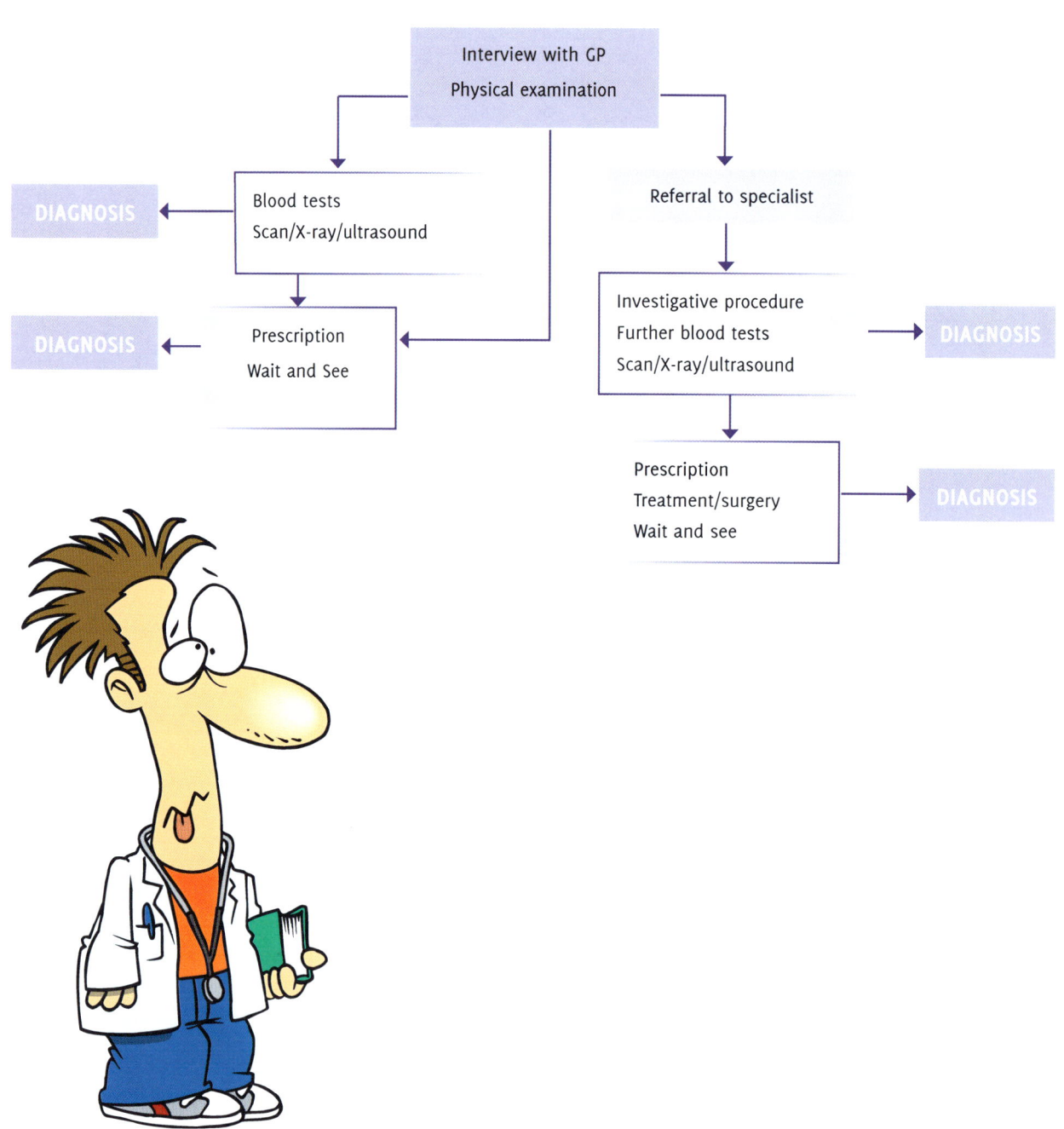

Interview with GP
Physical examination

DIAGNOSIS ← Blood tests
Scan/X-ray/ultrasound

Referral to specialist

DIAGNOSIS ← Prescription
Wait and See

Investigative procedure
Further blood tests
Scan/X-ray/ultrasound → DIAGNOSIS

Prescription
Treatment/surgery
Wait and see → DIAGNOSIS

Why do I need to collect my medical records?

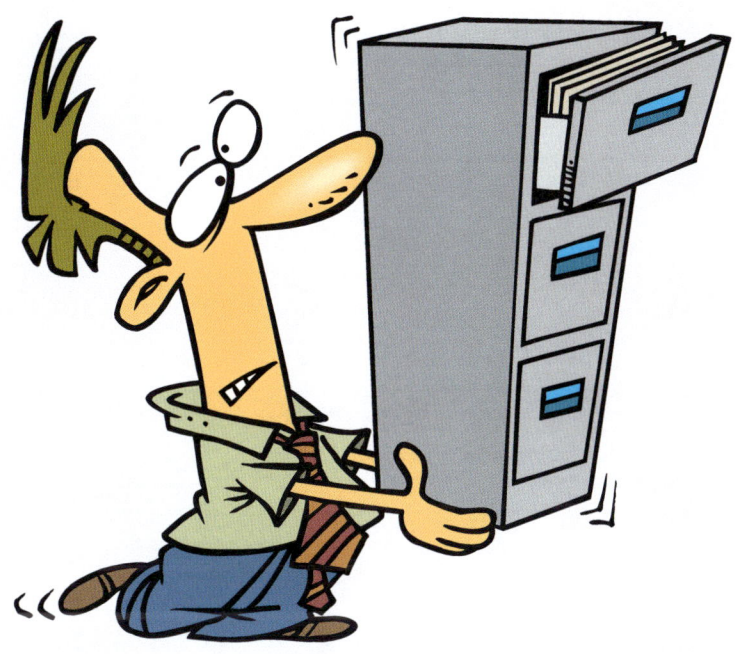

Because nobody else will and you need to refer to a full medical record to make an informed clinical decision.

Keep all your medical records because:

- no one person or medical establishment will have all your records;
- your records are the trusted proof of your condition;
- access to your records will reduce the risk of medical error in diagnosis & treatment;
- you will reduce duplication of tests & facilitate appropriate treatment; and
- it will enable you to monitor your progress by comparing your results with previous records.

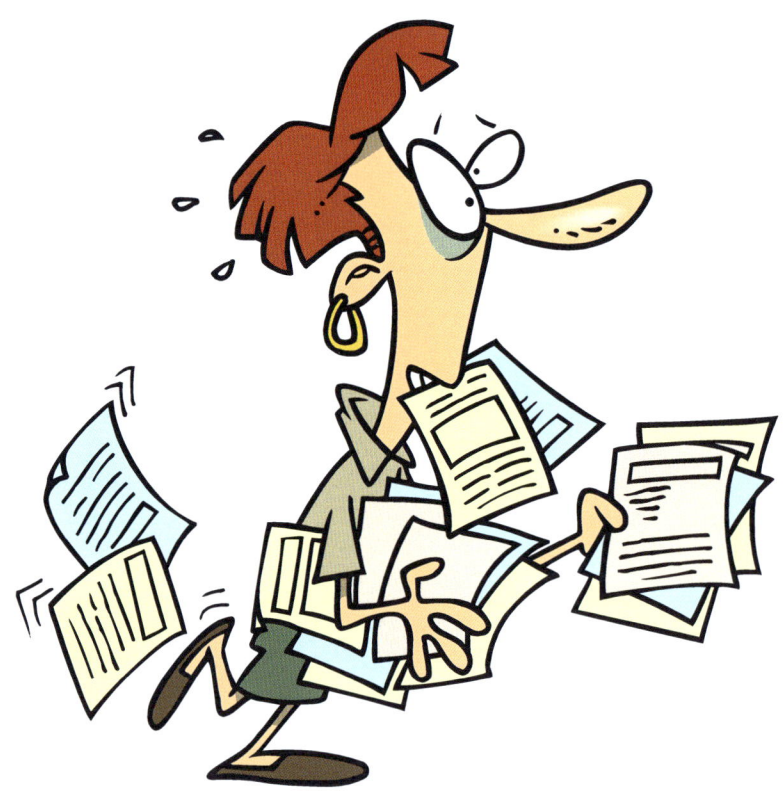

Why do I need to understand my diagnosis?

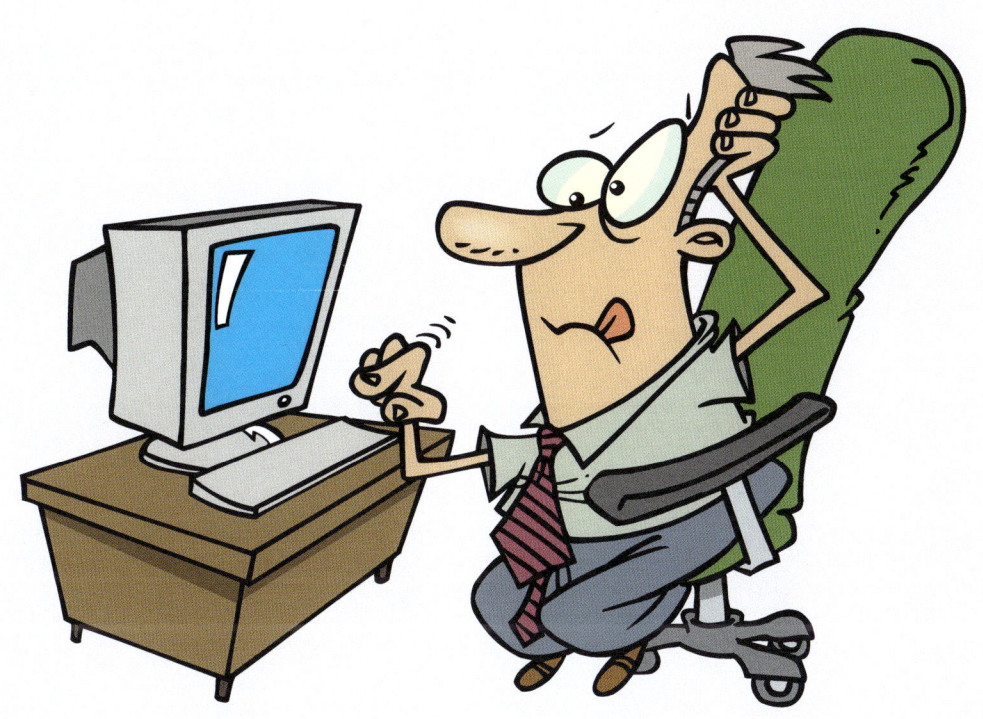

Because you need to assess whether other people do & whether their treatments are core to getting you to your end point.

2 Understand your diagnosis

Once you have a diagnosis, or if not a set of symptoms, you will need to find out as much as you can about your condition. The reason that you need to understand your condition is simple: the diagnosis tells you very little - it tells you what's wrong but not what has caused the problem or what will make it worse, nor does it tell you what you can expect in the future. So the diagnosis tells you what's wrong, and the prognosis tells you what may lie ahead, particularly if you do nothing.

Once you understand your condition, in particular the reasons why you may have the condition, you will be in a better position to find someone who can help you fix your problem and be more discriminative about the treatments that may help.

Start your research by asking the practitioner who has made the diagnosis some simple questions (follow the question guide *A conversational approach: understanding my diagnosis and prognosis, p29*), then follow-up with your own research on the internet or from the library. There are many good on-line sites where you can research everything about your condition, its diagnosis and treatment, and you may even join various internet-based common interest groups to find out the experience of others with a condition similar to yours.

To fast track your research narrow it down by selecting pivotal information on your condition's potential causes and risk factors (things that increase the risk for the development of a condition). Use the check-list from *Common causes and risk factors* (p31) as a guide, but remember that this list is not exhaustive, so you would still need to do your own research. Your list will need to highlight where you can and can't help yourself, and where you may need to seek additional help.

It pays to do your research as problems can occur when two practitioners on the same case have different interpretations on the cause of the condition. When this happens you run the risk of becoming piggy-in-the-middle as each practitioner may be advocating a different treatment for the same diagnosis. Problems arise when a recommended treatment is in direct conflict with another recommended treatment. When all the practitioners over-seeing the case are not on the same page (or on the same page as the patient), then the journey can become exhausting for the patient. However, if a patient has enough information to understand their diagnosis and its likely causes, then they are able to discriminate between treatments that are more likely to get them to their end point from those which may send them in the opposite direction or be a waste of time and money.

Sharon is seeking treatment for unexplained infertility. She has had the normal medical tests and investigative procedures but they can find nothing wrong. She decides to go to a natural fertility clinic where the naturopath runs a range of tests and find that she is sub-clinically hypothyroid. Sharon is told that this is the cause and that once her thyroid is fixed, her chances of falling pregnant will increase. She recommends a range of herbs and nutritional supplements, including iodine. Sharon is also seeing another naturopath who specializes in dietary healing. This naturopath says that the cause of the thyroid problem is oestrogen dominance, and that when this is resolved not only will the thyroid rebalance, but she will start to ovulate regularly which will improve her chances of becoming pregnant. Sharon does her own research and by checking through all her symptoms and looking at her family history, which has a high incidence of breast cancer, she realizes that she does indeed have oestrogen dominance, and therefore decides to follow the second naturopath's advice.

A conversational approach:
understanding my diagnosis & prognosis

QUESTIONS	About my diagnosis	About my prognosis (How will my condition affect me?)
Why ask these questions?	You need an accurate diagnosis in order for you and others to know what needs to be fixed.	You need to know where you are heading (what to expect) in the short & long-term in order to set goals and time frames.
Questionnaire Guide	▸ What is my condition/diagnosis? ▸ Which of my symptoms relate to this condition? ▸ What are the causes of my condition? ▸ What things may worsen my condition or are associated with a poorer prognosis? (risk factors) ▸ Is my condition reversible/curable with your treatment; or ▸ Is my condition reversible/curable without your treatment? *If you don't have a proper diagnosis then you need to ask:* ▸ What tests could I have or which person should I see in order to get a diagnosis? ▸ What will these tests tell me?	▸ What could happen to me and within what time frame if I do nothing? (Complications of disease; acute events.) ▸ How great is this risk? (What are the odds of this happening to me?) ▸ What are the health risks for my condition if left untreated and when could these occur? (Related health risks.) ▸ If I take treatment am I likely to experience any adverse or medical events related to my condition? If so, what are these and when, in your opinion, could these occur? (Events against a time line. This will give me my time frame/s.) ▸ Could I narrow my options on treatment if I leave my decision for too long?
What the answers mean to me	▸ How advanced my condition is (how far away am I from where I would like to be?); ▸ How quickly it may progress (how quickly am I going in the opposite direction?); ▸ If there are any immediate, medium or long-term health risks (where could I end up if I do nothing?); and ▸ What I need to do, and how quickly I need to act in order to make sure that I am heading in the right direction without narrowing my treatment options.	

Researching my diagnosis & prognosis

Diagnosis: common causes & risk factors

Causes
- genetic
- environmental exposure (toxins/allergens)
- iatrogenic (caused by drugs)
- primary nutrient deficiencies
- lifestyle (diet, smoking, alcohol, sedentary, stress)

Your Risk factors
increases the risk for the development of a condition, worsens the prognosis or compounds the problem
- age
- gender
- ethnicity
- inherited susceptibility
- initiating factors (infection, sunlight, surgery, pregnancy)
- weight
- lifestyle (diet, smoking, alcohol, sedentary life, stress)
- correlative factors (nutrient deficiency, exposure to toxins, specific disease markers, age at menopause/menarche)
- other health conditions
- specific drug medications

Exacerbating factors
aggravates an existing condition
- exposure to toxins/allergens
- lifestyle (as above)
- hormonal shifts

Prognosis: what could happen and when

How serious is my condition?
- How much time do I have to address my condition?
- What are my future health risks in the short, medium and long-term?

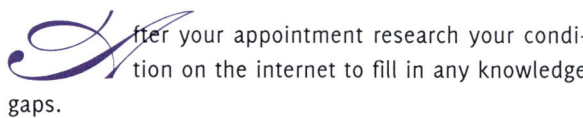 fter your appointment research your condition on the internet to fill in any knowledge gaps.

Some useful sites include (also see p23 and p223):

- http://health.usnews.com/health-conditions
- http://www.omnimedicalsearch.com/conditions-diseases/index.htm
- http://www.omnimedicalsearch.com/forumsearch.html
- http://www.uptodate.com
- http://www.nhs.uk/
- http://www.netdoctor.co.uk/
- http://www.medicinenet.com/

Once you have all the facts complete the first and third sections of the *Full Alignment Template* placing the information about causes and risk factors in the **WHY** column and future health risks (prognosis) in the **FUTURE** column. There may be a cross over for some of the causes, risks and exacerbating factors. For example, exposure to an allergen may be a cause and an exacerbating factor, or excess weight may be a cause for hypertension, a risk factor for heart disease and an exacerbating factor. Don't worry about this just list them all in the **WHY** column.

Full Alignment Template: the WHY and FUTURE columns

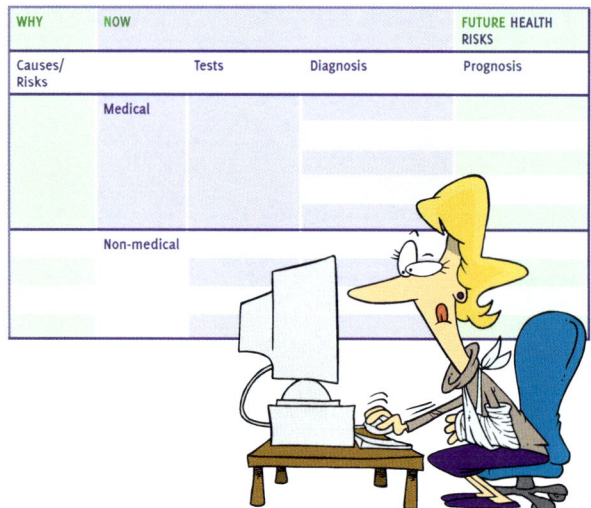

WHY	NOW				FUTURE HEALTH RISKS
Causes/ Risks		Tests	Diagnosis		Prognosis
	Medical				
	Non-medical				

Common causes & risk factors

Causes may include:

▸ genetic: congenital (you were born with the condition), or you are genetically predisposed;

▸ exposure to chemicals and toxins: these can induce genetic change (both before and after birth) and lead to various conditions including cancer;

▸ iatrogenic: conditions caused by drug medication;

▸ lifestyle factors: too much alcohol, over-eating, stress, insufficient exercise, indoor living etc; and

▸ primary nutrient deficiencies.

Treatments that address the cause will have the best outcome and can lead to cure. In many cases the cause may be unknown or treating the cause may prove difficult or impossible if inherited or due to genetic mutation.

Risk factors or things that will increase the risk for the development of a condition:

▸ age: some diseases tend to occur in specific age groups and in older populations;

▸ gender: some diseases tend to occur predominantly in females, while others occur in males;

▸ ethnicity: some races are more predisposed to certain conditions and diseases;

▸ genetic susceptibility: genetic variance may increase susceptibility to various health conditions which may run in the family;

▸ initiating factors: factors that are known to trigger the development of a disease or condition, such as pregnancy, sunlight, infection;

▸ correlative factors: a common factor that is associated with increased risk/poorer prognosis of a disease/ condition within a specific group;

▸ lifestyle: smoking, alcohol, over-eating, sedentary lifestyle, stress;

▸ other health conditions that predispose to the worsening or development of the condition; and

▸ medical drugs: drugs taken for one condition may cause another condition.

Several risk factors together may worsen the prognosis. The more risk factors you can address, then the better your prognosis will be.

Exacerbating factors: factors that aggravate but don't cause your existing condition, such as:

▸ lifestyle factors: diet, weight, smoking, alcohol, stress; and

▸ toxin/allergen exposure.

It may be possible to alleviate your condition by addressing these factors, but if they haven't caused the problem then you will not see cure but you may improve your outcome. It is generally at this level that you can help yourself.

Future health risks for the condition

These will alert you to:

▸ the possible direction your condition may take you;

▸ the symptoms *or* events to watch out for; and

▸ indicate areas for preventive treatment.

Time frame: what medical events are likely to occur and when

This will indicate:

▸ how much time you may have (or your window of opportunity) to address your condition before you require medical treatment; and

▸ ensure that you don't narrow your options by leaving things too late.

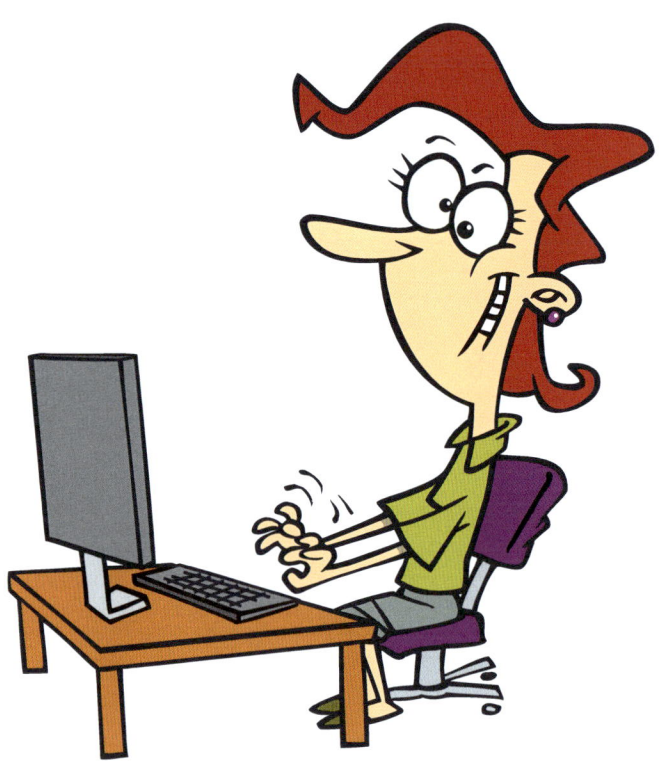

Strategy Flow Chart

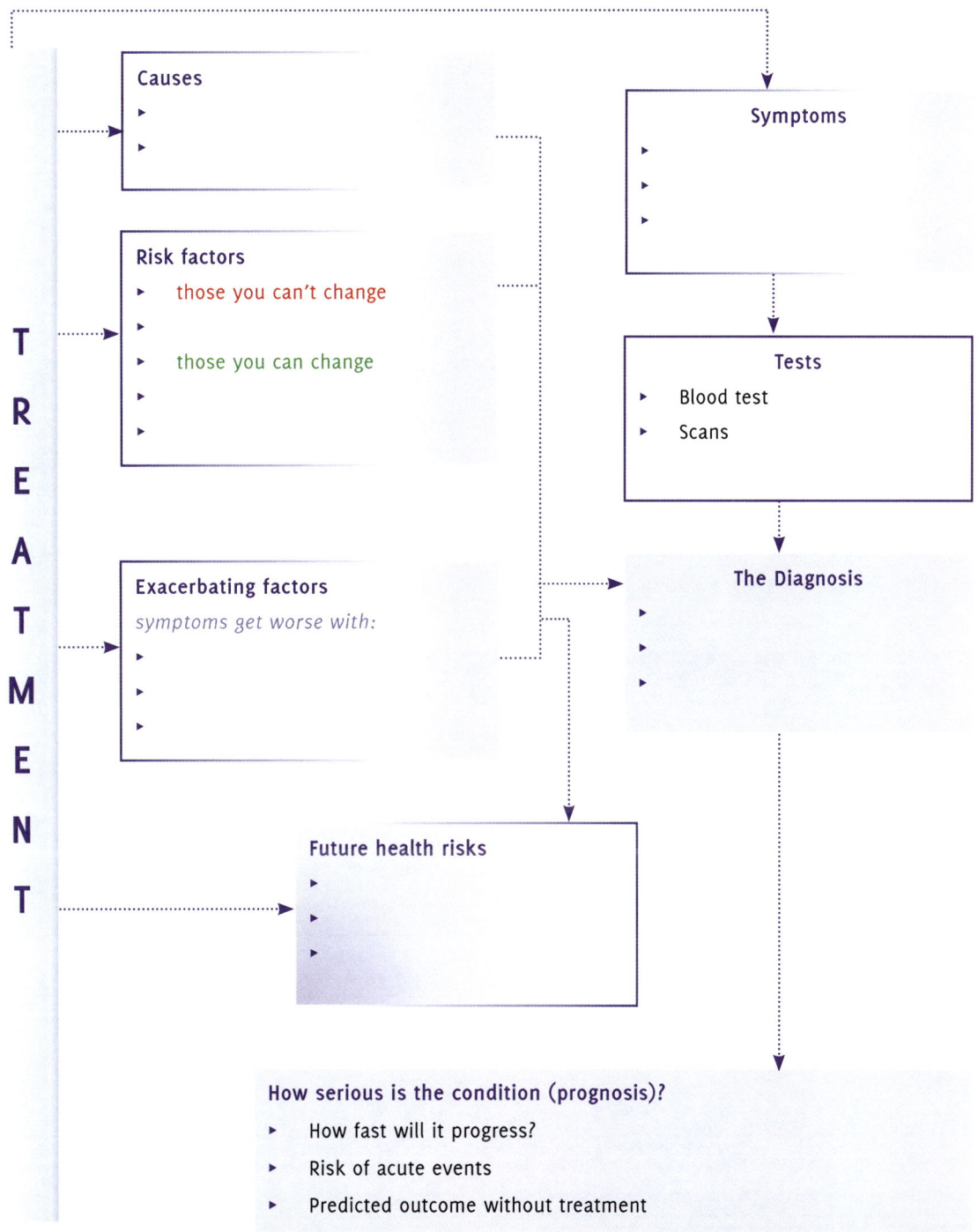

Causes
- ▸
- ▸

Risk factors
- ▸ those you can't change
- ▸
- ▸ those you can change
- ▸
- ▸

Exacerbating factors
symptoms get worse with:
- ▸
- ▸
- ▸

Future health risks
- ▸
- ▸
- ▸

TREATMENT

Symptoms
- ▸
- ▸
- ▸

Tests
- ▸ Blood test
- ▸ Scans

The Diagnosis
- ▸
- ▸
- ▸

How serious is the condition (prognosis)?
- ▸ How fast will it progress?
- ▸ Risk of acute events
- ▸ Predicted outcome without treatment

Strategy Flow Chart for the cancer patient

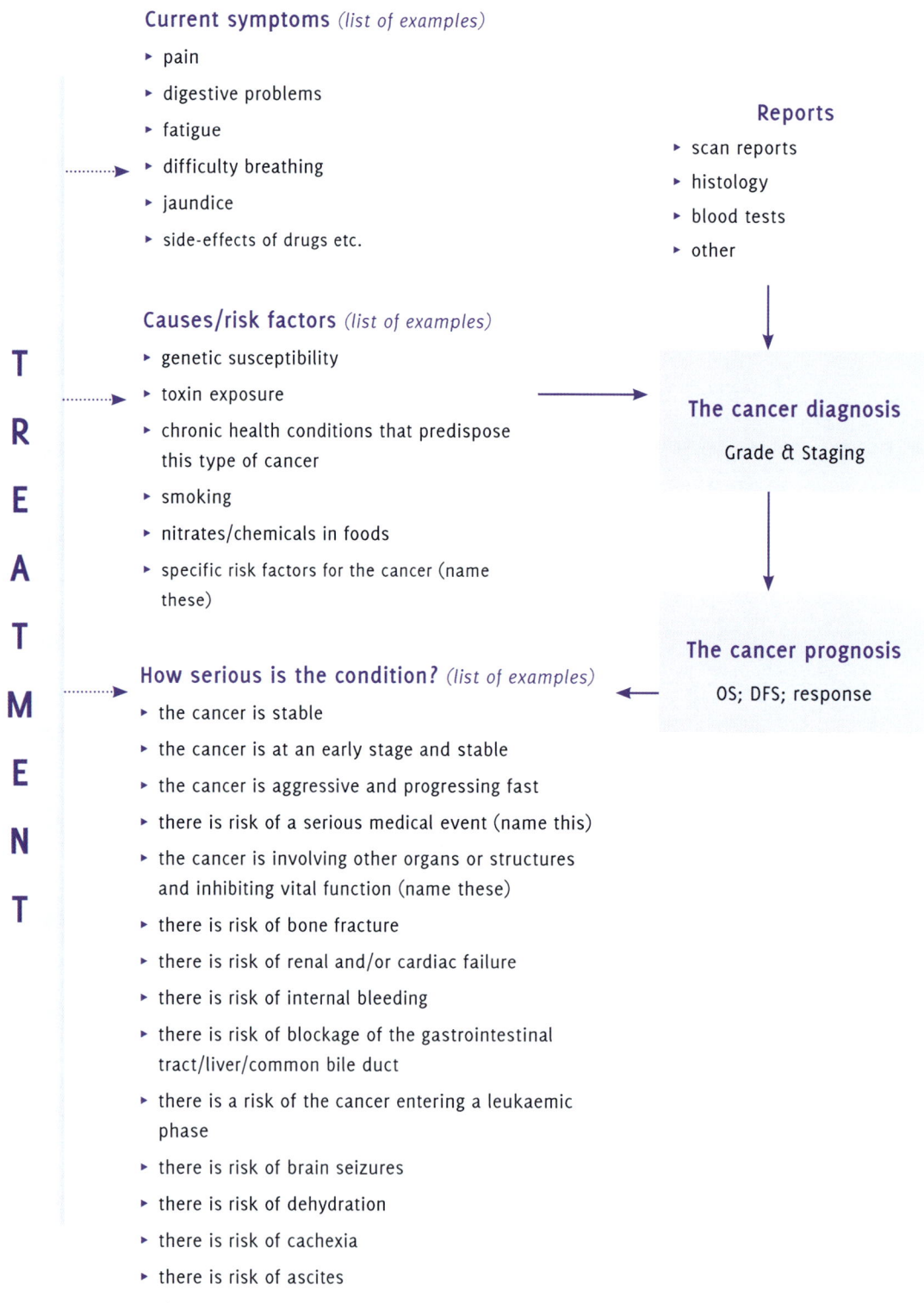

Current symptoms *(list of examples)*

- ‣ pain
- ‣ digestive problems
- ‣ fatigue
- ‣ difficulty breathing
- ‣ jaundice
- ‣ side-effects of drugs etc.

Causes/risk factors *(list of examples)*

- ‣ genetic susceptibility
- ‣ toxin exposure
- ‣ chronic health conditions that predispose this type of cancer
- ‣ smoking
- ‣ nitrates/chemicals in foods
- ‣ specific risk factors for the cancer (name these)

How serious is the condition? *(list of examples)*

- ‣ the cancer is stable
- ‣ the cancer is at an early stage and stable
- ‣ the cancer is aggressive and progressing fast
- ‣ there is risk of a serious medical event (name this)
- ‣ the cancer is involving other organs or structures and inhibiting vital function (name these)
- ‣ there is risk of bone fracture
- ‣ there is risk of renal and/or cardiac failure
- ‣ there is risk of internal bleeding
- ‣ there is risk of blockage of the gastrointestinal tract/liver/common bile duct
- ‣ there is a risk of the cancer entering a leukaemic phase
- ‣ there is risk of brain seizures
- ‣ there is risk of dehydration
- ‣ there is risk of cachexia
- ‣ there is risk of ascites
- ‣ there is risk of pleural effusion

Reports

- ‣ scan reports
- ‣ histology
- ‣ blood tests
- ‣ other

The cancer diagnosis

Grade & Staging

The cancer prognosis

OS; DFS; response

T R E A T M E N T

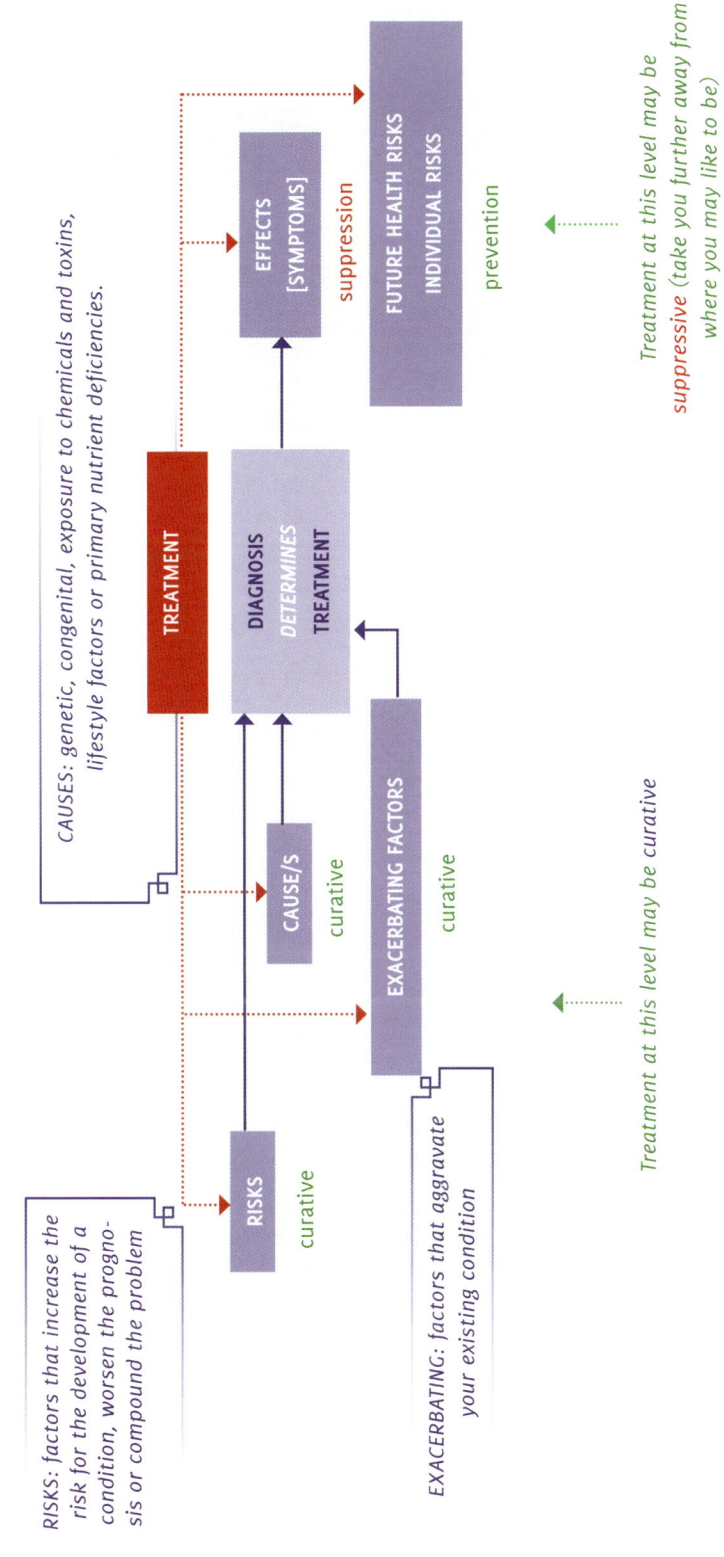

Diagnosis determines treatment

CAUSES: genetic, congenital, exposure to chemicals and toxins, lifestyle factors or primary nutrient deficiencies.

RISKS: factors that increase the risk for the development of a condition, worsen the prognosis or compound the problem

EXACERBATING: factors that aggravate your existing condition

TREATMENT

DIAGNOSIS *DETERMINES* TREATMENT

EFFECTS [SYMPTOMS]

suppression

FUTURE HEALTH RISKS INDIVIDUAL RISKS

prevention

CAUSE/S

curative

EXACERBATING FACTORS

curative

RISKS

curative

Treatment at this level may be suppressive (take you further away from where you may like to be) or preventive

Treatment at this level may be curative

No diagnosis = hit & miss approach

Troubleshooting the diagnosis

*Y*ou need to feel comfortable that you have the right diagnosis. A wrong diagnosis can lead to inappropriate treatment that could have dire consequences. It is quite common for doctors to prescribe a drug to determine the diagnosis. The doctor may have a good idea of what is wrong with you, prescribe a drug and if the symptoms abate then this confirms the diagnosis. However, sometimes drugs can alleviate the symptoms but the actual disease goes unchecked. The same is true when the doctor or specialist applies a best guess scenario. This may occur when there is no firm diagnosis, or if tests are not undertaken that would confirm the diagnosis. If the best guess is not the correct guess then treatment may be inappropriate and the patient may lose valuable time, suffering the consequences.

If in doubt, seek a second opinion.

By doing your research you are more likely to be able to determine if you have been given the right diagnosis and received the right diagnostic tests, the correct medical information for your condition and the correct advice on recommended treatments.

Similarly, if a definitive diagnosis cannot be reached then having a greater understanding of your symptoms and what they may indicate would allow you to monitor your condition appropriately.

Trouble shooting the diagnosis

- Use the Diagnosis Pathway (p24) as an overview of typical pathways.
- Use the various internet health sites to find the information you need about your condition, its diagnosis and prognosis, and its treatment.
- Make sure that you have been given all the appropriate tests and that the diagnosis is accurate.
- Cross check against *Troubleshooting the diagnosis* (facing page) to be aware of any pitfalls that can occur when making a diagnosis.

*T*racey has digestive problems with bloating, flatulence and irregular, loose stools. She has been diagnosed with irritable bowel by her GP and leaky gut by her naturopath. The drugs from her GP have alleviated some of the painful spasms, but the digestive enzymes, probiotics and dietary changes recommended by her naturopath have not helped. Tracey has two different diagnoses which simply means that two different labels have been fixed on her group of symptoms. Neither treatment is working. This is because the cause of her symptoms is due to an allergy to sulphur dioxide, a common preservative. Once foods containing this were removed, Tracey's digestive problems resolved. By addressing the cause Tracey needed no other treatment. The diagnosis should have been allergy to sulphur dioxide.

Symptoms are not the diagnosis: the same symptoms may have different causes.

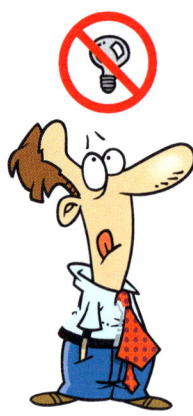

Unless you know the cause of the symptoms, you will be unable to treat the condition.

Troubleshooting the diagnosis

When treatment determines diagnosis *try this and see*	▸ You may suppress the symptoms but the underlying condition continues to deteriorate *(treating the symptoms, not the cause)*; ▸ If the real condition is ignored, then you may not be treated or monitored appropriately until it may be too late; ▸ You may have more than one condition, or two related conditions, but if the medication resolves symptoms and normalizes any blood results then this may give you a "false-positive" result for treatment *(treating blood results rather than the patient)*.
A best guess	▸ This occurs when there is either insufficient data to make an accurate assessment because the appropriate tests are not requested, or relevant data is ignored. This may lead to misdiagnosis, under-diagnosis or "wait and see" - all of which may increase your risks.
Unable to get a diagnosis	▸ This may occur when the physician doesn't have enough skill or expertise to make a diagnosis, when appropriate tests are not undertaken (due to cost or unavailability of equipment, lack of expertise), or when tests have failed to indicate a diagnosis. You may need to seek alternative referrals, but without a diagnosis your starting point will be based on your symptoms and your journey will involve the monitoring of those symptoms.
Wait and see	▸ This occurs when no treatment can be offered until the symptoms worsen or until the condition deteriorates; ▸ When the doctor is unsure of the diagnosis and needs to evaluate to see how the patient progresses; or ▸ If the doctor feels that the condition will resolve by itself.

If in doubt, seek a second opinion

Why do I need to understand my prognosis?

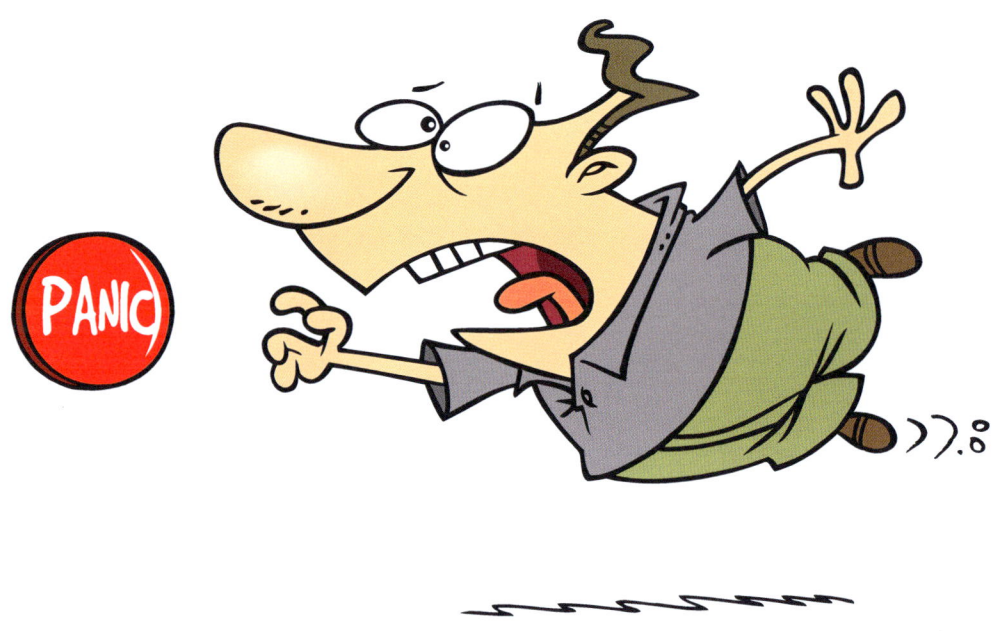

Because you need to know how fast you may be heading in the wrong direction so that you don't miss opportunities or narrow your treatment options.

The prognosis - what could happen and when

Once you are satisfied that you have the right diagnosis, you will need to understand the prognosis, or where you are heading and how fast; in other words *"what could happen to me if I don't take treatment, and how soon?"* The answer to this question will tell you how quickly you need to start treatment, whether there is a window of opportunity to make a difference to your condition before you absolutely have to have medical treatment, and what clinical events may occur and when. This information governs key decisions on time frames for treatment and monitoring (to make sure you are heading in the right direction and within a specific time frame).

Use the questions from the chart *A conversational approach: understanding my diagnosis and prognosis (p29)* in the about my prognosis column. Answers to these questions will give you enough information about what your condition could mean to you, how it could behave, what might happen - and how quickly.

When you ask these questions your doctor or specialist may factor in your individual risk factors, if they know your case. These risk factors are what make you different to others with the same diagnosis in-so-much as how the disease may affect you and how you may respond to treatment. These individual risk factors are generally linked to genetic variance (hereditary factors), your age and any other condition you have which may negatively impact the case and its treatment.

When these individual risks are not factored into the treatment, patients may be prescribed a treatment that could worsen their overall health and take them in the opposite direction. If you know your individual risk factors it means that you can check any contraindications for treatments/drugs and match these against your individual risks.

Knowing these things will give you a clue as to why certain treatments may produce adverse reactions in your case. Factoring this knowledge into your strategy means that you can tailor your treatment to meet your individual case.

Natalie was 21 years old when she sought help for endometriosis, polycystic ovarian syndrome and haemorrhagic ovarian cysts. She was offered a progesterone cream to slow the progression of her condition. Natalie applied the cream without realizing that it could worsen the nausea, vomiting and jaundice that she experienced with each cycle. She did some research on synthetic hormones in relation to her symptoms and found that they could cause gallstones in those predisposed. As her father had his gallbladder removed, and as she herself would get sick if she ate fatty food, she concluded that she had probably inherited this predisposition and that maybe synthetic hormones were not the most appropriate treatment for her condition. Natalie also discovered that hormonal imbalances often aggravated gallstone formation - so her condition was also putting her at risk for gallstones.

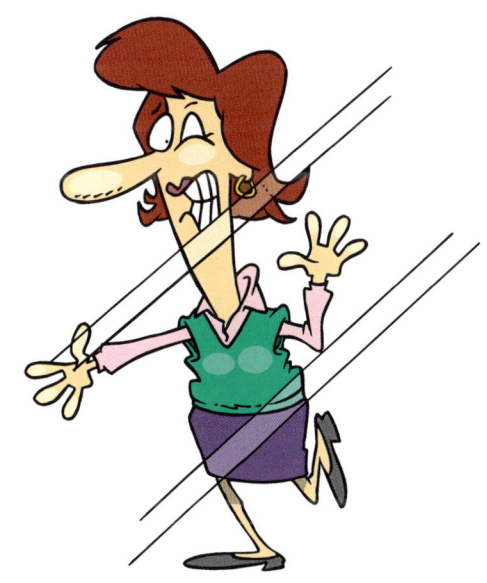

The Cancer Prognosis

*D*etermining the prognosis in cancer relies heavily on survival statistics for the type of cancer, its stage and grade and other features, such as receptor status. For example, the outcome with conventional treatment for a breast cancer that is oestrogen receptor positive may be better than for a breast cancer with a receptor negative status, even though the staging and grade may be the same.

As the prognosis is dependent upon an accurate staging and grading it is important that you obtain both so that you understand your starting point and can make an informed decision on treatment.

Making a decision on treatment without all this information has many pitfalls:

▸ you won't have a realistic benchmark (starting point) against which to measure your progress;

▸ if your condition is worse than you believe it to be then you could deteriorate more rapidly than expected; and

▸ if the rate of deterioration is rapid then you could narrow your options on treatment. What may have been offered at the outset, such as a simple treatment/procedure, may no longer be appropriate and a more invasive and systemic treatment is offered which may carry additional risks and complications.

Getting the prognosis

Once you have your diagnosis you simply need to ask two questions:

▸ What is my overall survival if I take your recommended treatment?

▸ What is my overall survival if I do nothing?

Overall survival is the percentage of people with the same diagnosis, on the same treatment, who are still alive after a specified period of time. You need to make sure you have figures for the percentage of people and the period of time they survived, both with and without treatment. Once you have these figures you can make a graph to show the survival rate against time. You can see in the example on the opposite page that the prognosis for this lady was very poor should she not opt for con-

ventional treatment as her cancer, although only stage 2, was aggressive and receptor positive for oestrogen, progesterone and HER2.

Using the same graph you can add projection lines for different combinations of treatments where you can see at a glance how the statistics stack up. For example, you may be recommended the "best" combination of treatments which fits your specialist's criteria but you then discover that if you have a lesser treatment, or a different combination of treatments, that the overall survival may only be reduced by a few percent. On review you may feel that the benefits of a less toxic treatment on your overall health may outweigh the risks of dropping a few percent particularly if well over 75 percent from both groups make it to 5 years.

Once you have the overall survival statistics, make sure you ask fundamental questions about your condition. Use *A conversational approach: understanding my diagnosis and prognosis (p29)* to formulate these questions and then follow-up with your own research on the internet or from the library. Use the internet links (p23 & p223) to learn everything about your cancer, its staging and grading, its prognosis, its causes and risk factors and even its treatment. By becoming informed you will be able to factor in any inherent health risks which may contraindicate some treatment recommendations.

Overall survival, disease-free survival & response rate

It's a good idea to familiarise yourself with other terminology, such as disease-free survival, progression-free survival and response, so that you do not become confused over what treatments can offer you.

Overall survival (OS) simply means still being alive. It does not indicate whether these patients are well or disease-free. *"This treatment gives a 93 percent, 4 year OS time for patients with your condition."* This means that 93 percent of patients were still alive at 4 years following treatment.

Disease-free survival (DFS) only applies when the treatment delivers a complete response, that is no sign of cancer following treatment. The disease-free period is the length of time before the cancer is likely to recur. *"This treatment gives a DFS of 4 years for 86 percent of* *patients with your condition."* So 86 percent of patients were still disease-free at 4 years following treatment.

Progression-free survival (PFS) only measures the effect of treatment on tumours, or by how far it can stabilize the disease and stop it from progressing. This may not have any bearing on overall survival or any associated benefits for the patient especially if the side-effects of the treatment worsen the general condition. In many cases stabilization may only be months. *"This treatment gives an PFS time of 9 months for 60 percent of patients with your condition."* From this example 60 percent of patients were stable for 9 months before the cancer started growing again.

Response is a term where you may need to qualify what is being measured: is it the percentage of people who responded to the treatment (response rate) or is it the percentage of shrinkage of the tumoural masses? When measuring shrinkage, a complete response (CR) means that there is no evidence of the cancer after treatment, and a partial response (PR) is at least a 50 percent reduc-

tion in the tumoral masses. So if your specialist says that they expect a 50 percent response with treatment you would need to clarify whether that means a 50 percent response rate (50 percent of people responded) or a 50 percent shrinkage (partial response).

At the appointment you may wish to ask your specialist for their own clinical opinion of how well they would expect you to do given your individual case. Sometimes this differs from the statistical evidence. It is useful to try and determine your odds at the outset as this may become an important factor in your choice of treatments.

Medical events

You also need to ask if there are any health risks for your condition in the short to medium term (with and without treatment) and whether there is risk of an acute medical event. Being prepared means that you know what to watch out for and what action to take. You will also be able to investigate other therapies to find out whether they could help reduce or prevent these risks.

Breast cancer: stage 2, grade 3, triple positive

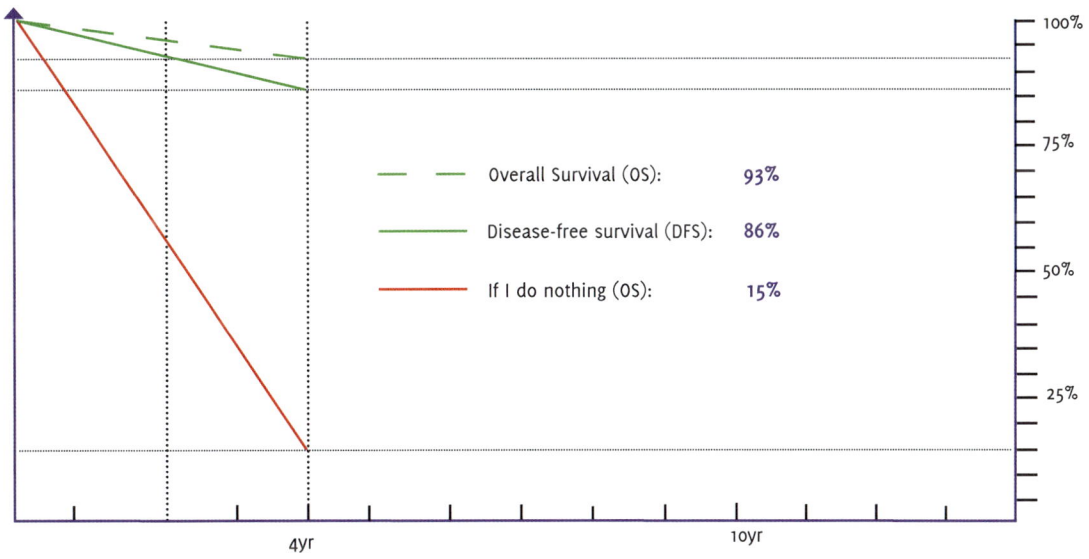

— — Overall Survival (OS):	**93%**
—— Disease-free survival (DFS):	**86%**
—— If I do nothing (OS):	**15%**

4yr   10yr

100% / 75% / 50% / 25%

These statistics are the clinical trial results for patients with stage 2, triple positive breast cancer treated with a combination of surgery, ACT chemotherapy, radiotherapy, Tamoxifen & Herceptin. They show that there was a 93 percent overall survival (7 percent died) at four years with 86 percent remaining disease-free. This means that of those that survived only a small percentage relapsed. Of those patients who did nothing only 15 percent were alive at 4 years.

To Recap

- ▸ Research your condition thoroughly

- ▸ Understand the procedure for diagnosis and treatment and make sure that the diagnostic tests are appropriate for your condition

- ▸ Make sure the advice you are receiving is the right advice

- ▸ Understand all your risk factors, your individual ones and the general risks for your condition

- ▸ Understand the causes and any factors that could worsen your condition

- ▸ Understand the time frame you have to make a difference.

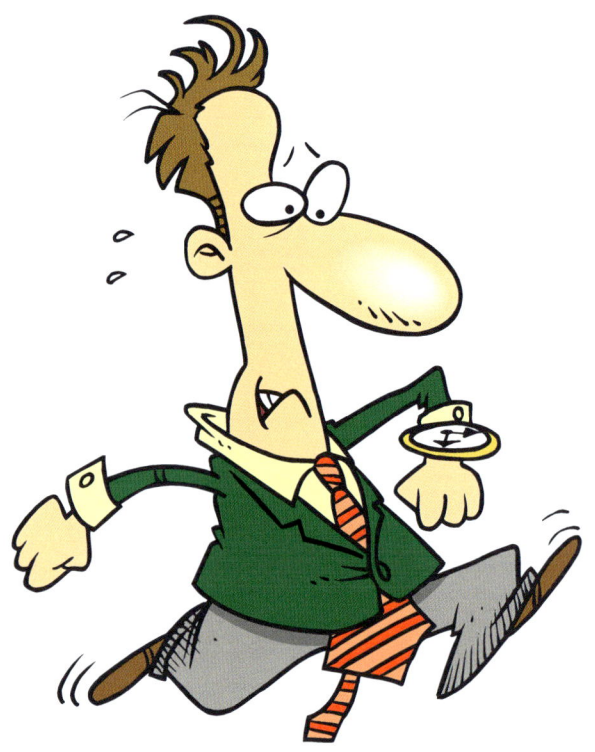

Pauline is 35 years old and has been diagnosed with a couple of autoimmune conditions, rheumatoid arthritis and iritis. After a recent relapse of her condition her specialist recommended corticosteroids to resolve the inflammation and bring her into remission. It was her specialist's opinion that the condition would continue to deteriorate and that if she didn't take treatment now then her joints would become increasingly swollen and painful and harder to move. She said that the condition was incurable and that if she left treatment too long then the damage would become permanent. There was a family history of autoimmune conditions and diabetes, and Pauline had a history of anorexia in her teens and early 20s, had not menstruated since her mid-20s, she was in a lot of pain, had low energy, digestive problems with many food intolerances, suffered psoriasis, she was underweight and a recent bone density scan indicated osteopaenia in the spine and hip, and her blood test indicated vitamin D deficiency and anaemia. Although she already has one child one of her main goals is to become pregnant and she is seeking further help to increase her fertility whilst deciding at the same time to try and resolve all her other health issues.

WHY	NOW		FUTURE HEALTH RISKS
Causes/Risks			**Prognosis**
▴ gender	**Medical**		▴ Lose mobility
▴ age	**Tests**	**Diagnosis**	▴ Impaired eyesight
▴ inherited predisposition	▴ blood test	▴ rheumatoid arthritis	▴ Osteoporosis
▴ inflammatory condition can cause anaemia	▴ eye test	▴ iritis	▴ General deterioration of health
▴ low weight can cause amenorrhoea/infertility	▴ X-rays	▴ osteopaenia, vit D deficiency	▴ Infertility
	▴ bone densitometry	▴ anaemia (iron deficiency)	▴ Develop other autoimmune conditions
		▴ amenorrhoea	
		▴ psoriasis	
	Non-medical		
	End Point		
	Symptoms &/or diagnostics	**Prioritized list of Goals (measurables)**	**End point alignment**
	▴ pain & stiffness in joints		
	▴ inflammation in eyes, skin		
	▴ no periods		
	▴ underweight		
	▴ fatigue, anaemic		**THERAPY**
	▴ low bone density		
	▴ mineral & vitamin deficiencies		**TREATMENTS**

Why do I need to define my starting point?

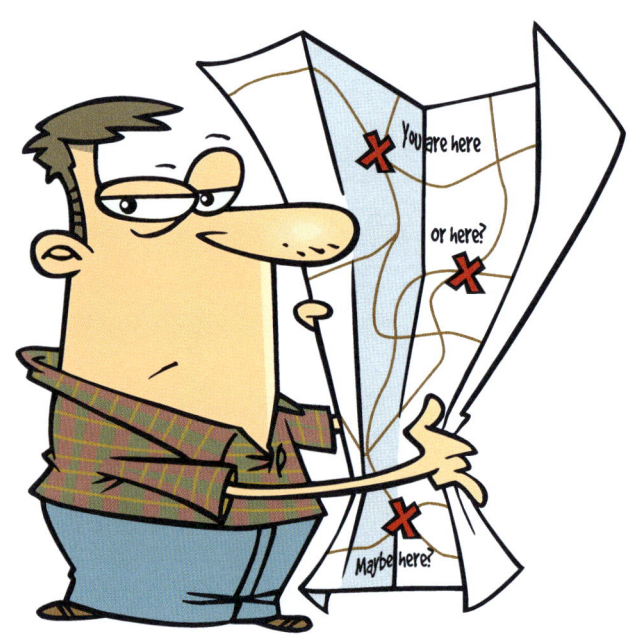

Because you need to make sure that you and others
are starting from the same place.

3 Define your starting point

At the moment all the facts you have amassed may seem confusing, so your job is to simplify your starting point in order to be able to make a concise statement that you and others can understand. Remember, your starting point is your diagnosis, your prognosis and your individual risk factors.

When you are making an initial enquiry to see if a practitioner can help you, you need to convey your condition within 15-30 seconds so that an immediate assessment can be made. This may seem a tall order, but it's not that difficult to put the key points into a nutshell.

If you follow *My Health Statement*, column one My Starting Point (p46) you will see that there are only 4 key points (5 points if you have known allergies/risks) that you need to cover in this first part of your health statement:

▸ your diagnosis and most pressing symptoms (if you have more than one diagnosis then mention all your diagnoses);

▸ when you were diagnosed and/or how long you have had these symptoms;

▸ what medical treatment you have had for your condition/s; and

▸ if you have a time frame before your condition becomes serious.

At the outset you do not need to mention other individual risk factors, but you will keep a reference to these in your own notes.

Your Health Statement

includes the points that every practitioner on your case should know at the outset

Here is Pauline's statement. She is suffering from two autoimmune conditions and has been given a time frame within which to make a difference.

" I was diagnosed with rheumatoid arthritis 5 years ago and iritis this year and have recently had an acute episode. I have had corticosteroids in the past which brought me into remission, but I have been off drugs for 3 years. My rheumatologist has said that if the inflammation doesn't reduce within 3 months I will need to take medications. "

In this very short statement you can see that Pauline is able to convey sufficient information for any practitioner to make an assessment as to whether they feel they can help her with her core problem and within the required time frame.

From this statement Pauline is able to tell others:

▸ what needs to be treated

▸ what needs to be monitored

▸ how fast she is heading in the wrong direction

▸ where she could end up if she does nothing

▸ the time frame she has to make a difference

▸ a time line for monitoring

We know that Pauline has a lot of other symptoms that she would also like addressing but this statement simply represents the points that every practitioner on her case should know (and factor in) at the outset.

Review *My Health Statement* and use the examples from My Starting Point to formulate this first part of your statement. Only add existing risk factors that you know about if they directly apply to your current condition. There's no need to worry about giving more information as a practitioner should ask you to fill in any gaps they require to make an assessment, such as your age and other risk factors.

My Health Statement: part 1 - my starting point

	My starting point	My end point	My criteria
Why state this	You need to give a concise account of your diagnosis and treatment to date to allow the practitioner to make a judgement on whether they feel they can help you.	You need to tell the practitioner where you want to get to and then match where the practitioner can take you against your own aspirations.	You need to measure how much synergy the practitioner and their treatments share with your values, convictions and criteria.
Statement Guide	▲ I have been diagnosed with_____ and I have _____ (symptoms) ▲ I have had this condition for _____ (length of time) ▲ I have received medical treatment/am not on medication (indicate treatment, when you received it & length of time on treatment) ▲ I have been given a time frame (months/years) before my condition becomes serious ▲ I have these known allergies/inherited risks	▲ I would like to achieve _____ (remission/cure, improved outcome/slow progression) ▲ I would like to reduce my drug/product/treatment dependency ▲ I would like to reduce the risk factors for my condition (name these) ▲ I would like to reduce my future risk/s of _____ associated with this condition ▲ I need help in addressing _____ (symptoms) ▲ I would like to see improvement in _____ (within a specific time frame)	▲ Do you have *experience & success* in treating people with similar conditions to myself? (i.e. can you help me and with what aspect of my case?) ▲ Can you tell me *how long* the therapy/treatment will last? ▲ What *lifestyle changes* may I need to make? ▲ Can you give any indication of the *costs* involved? ▲ Are you open to working with me if I use *a mix of conventional and alternative treatments?* ▲ Are you open to *collaboration or liaising with other practitioners?* ▲ Are you open to working with me if I *refuse any medical intervention?* ▲ My religion/culture *forbids specific treatments,* can you still work with me?

What the answers mean to me

▲ If the practitioner can help me;

▲ What, specifically, the practitioner may be able to help me with;

▲ How far they can take me and within what time frame I can expect improvement;

▲ Whether I can undertake the treatment (afford it, lifestyle limitations); and

▲ Whether I will "get on" with the practitioner.

Journey Road Map

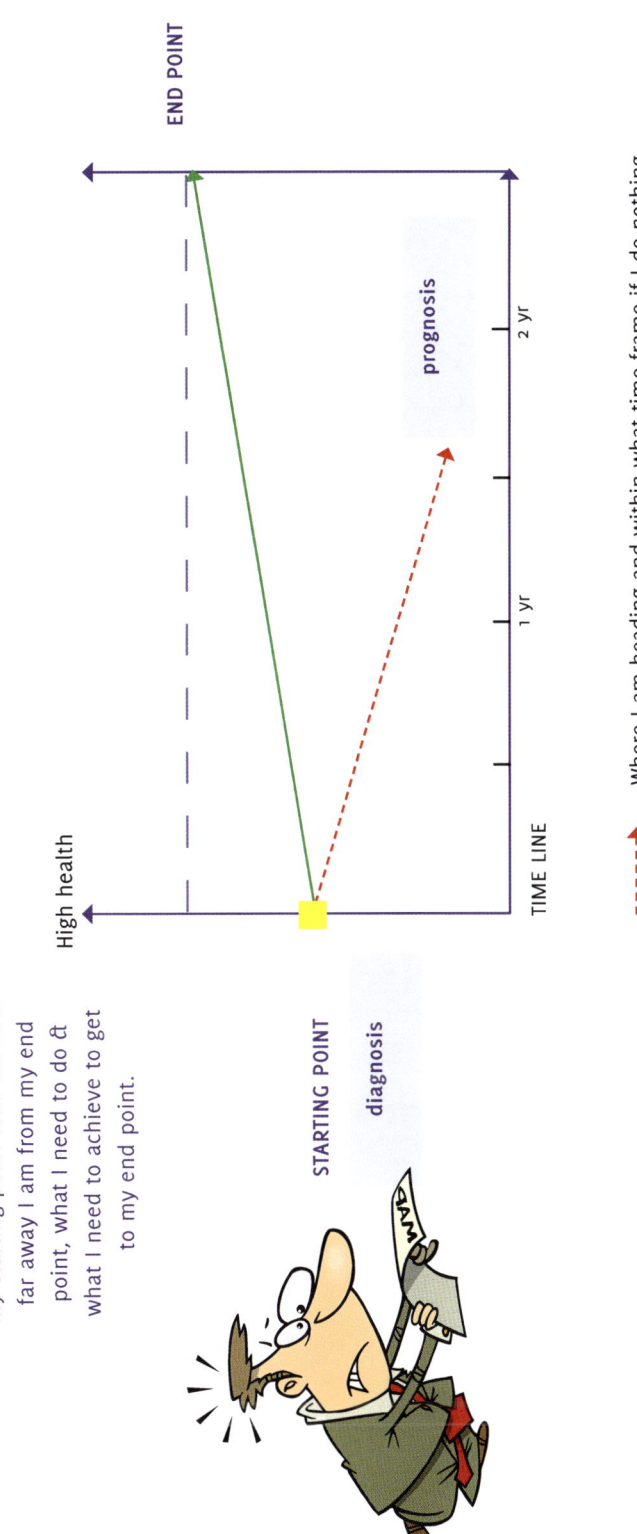

My starting point tells me how far away I am from my end point, what I need to do & what I need to achieve to get to my end point.

END POINT

High health

STARTING POINT

diagnosis

prognosis

TIME LINE

1 yr

2 yr

Where I am heading and within what time frame if I do nothing

Your journey road map will help you & others stay on track & monitor progress.

The Journey Road Map

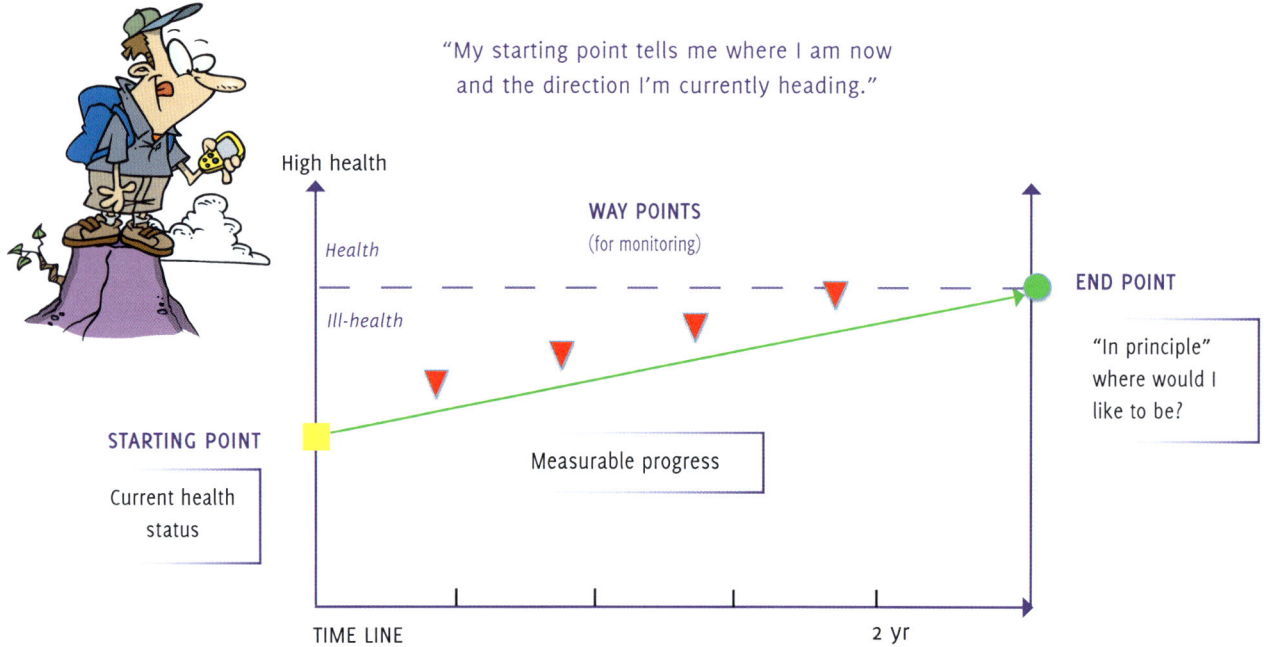

"My starting point tells me where I am now and the direction I'm currently heading."

High health

WAY POINTS
(for monitoring)

Health

Ill-health

END POINT

"In principle" where would I like to be?

STARTING POINT

Current health status

Measurable progress

TIME LINE

2 yr

As you can see from the diagram above the journey road map is a simple graph where you can plot and measure your progress (improvement or deterioration) over time. Progress is monitored at specific way points either from objective reports (scan reports, blood tests, weight loss) or subjectively (how much improvement do I feel/by what percentage have my symptoms improved). When you are heading in the right direction, your line will move upwards towards your destination end point.

At this stage, you will simply be entering your starting point, a time line and way points where you will monitor progress. So, for example, if you have been given a time frame to make improvements, or if you have been told that within a certain time you will deteriorate and may have an acute event, then these predictions need to be entered on your map as they become the benchmark for monitoring improvement or deterioration over time.

Let's take a moment to familiarize ourselves with the Journey road map.

— — **The threshold line** is the dotted line across the graph. On or above this line is where you would like to be and should ideally represent what is realistically achievable.

The starting point is a point below the threshold line on the vertical start line. This point is arbitrary and simply represents your current health condition or the point from which you are starting. At this moment in time you may not have a diagnosis, but just a list of symptoms, or you may have more than one diagnosis. This does not matter for the purposes of setting up the road map. If you feel that you have a long way to go in order to get to your end point, then this will influence your time line.

The end point is where you wish to end up. Your end point acts as your compass and will form the basis of any working relationship that you have with your health partners. It represents the general direction of where you are heading. For example, imagine you are travelling to Paris. You may need to plan a route where you change flights or take different modes of transport at specific way points (locations) of the journey. As long as you know where you are heading you can navigate your way forward even if you have to take a detour due to bad weather. So the end point represents where you wish to end up and not necessarily where others will take you. Other practitioners may be integral in getting you to specific way points, but you need to make sure that all the practitioners on your case are heading in the same direction so that you can easily match and validate their claims and monitor your progress against your aspirational end point.

▼ **Time line & way points** are determined when you have found out what may be possible for you to achieve within a given time frame. You will need to determine the time frame for monitoring progress (way points) based on where others say they can take you. This becomes important when you have a condition where you can't afford to slip backwards so it is vital that you monitor progress to make sure that the chosen treatment is living up to its expectations.

By understanding my starting point I will:

▸ be able to judge whether others understand my case;

▸ know what can be medically treated and what can't;

▸ know what I may need help with;

▸ know how I may be able to help myself;

▸ know how to protect against or reduce my risk factors;

▸ know what to expect on my journey (associated health risks, potential medical events and future health risks);

▸ know how long it may take for my condition to become serious; and

▸ know what to monitor and how to monitor progress.

Steps

Step 1: Get your starting point (diagnosis and prognosis)

Step 2: Draw in your time line

Step 3: Enter way points against the time line for monitoring progress

Step 4: Enter predicted events against the time line

Once you have completed these steps, then your chosen practitioners can understand your starting point, where you are currently heading, events that could occur (and when), and how and what to monitor.

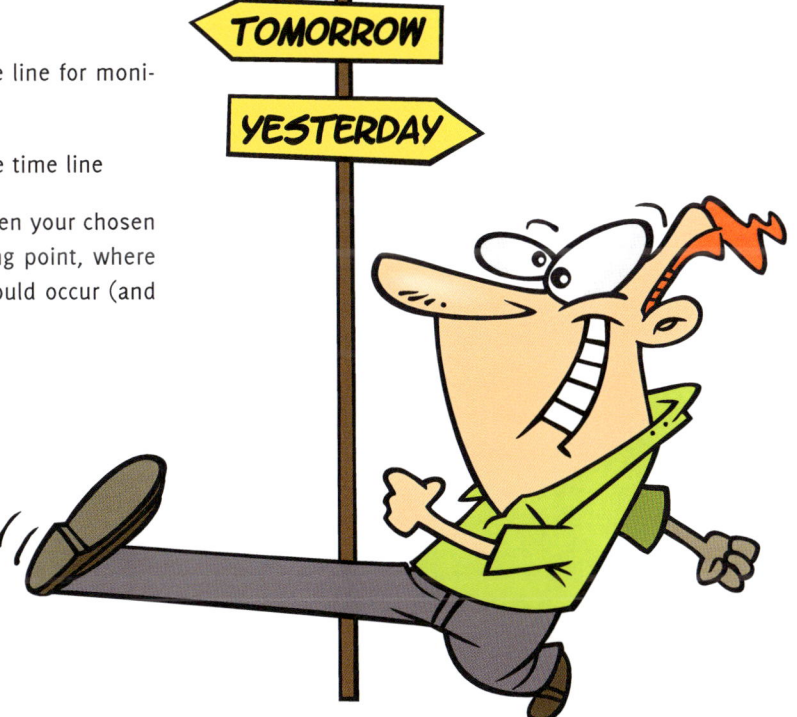

My Journey Road Map: my starting point

START

END

- - - → Where I could end up if I do nothing (predicted progress line)

My starting point is my **diagnosis** (what's wrong now) and **prognosis** (what will happen and how fast if I do nothing).

enter way points for monitoring progress

event 1

event 2

event 3

plot when future events/complications are likely to occur with or without treatment (name them)

Time line

My end point

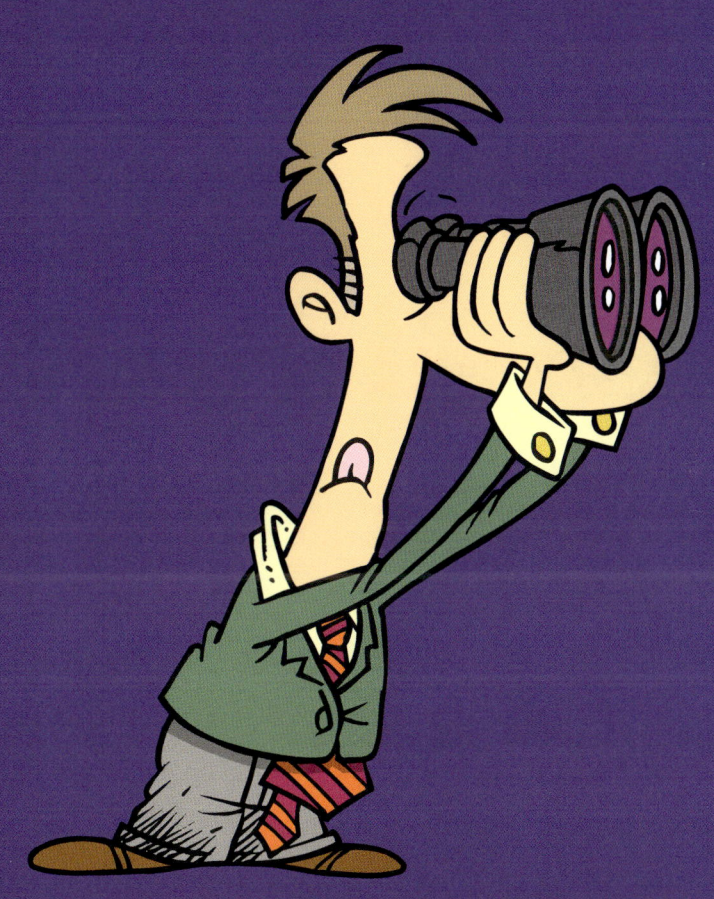

To do

1 Work out where you'd like to end up

Select your criteria for your end point & goals

Use *My Value Template* to establish these

2 Prioritize your goals

Complete the *Full Alignment Template*

- ▸ determine what you can & can't change
- ▸ prioritize your risks
- ▸ match each goal to a destination end point

3 Redefine your end point

Revisit the *Full Alignment Template* to determine your realistic end point

Why do I need to work out where I'd like to end up?

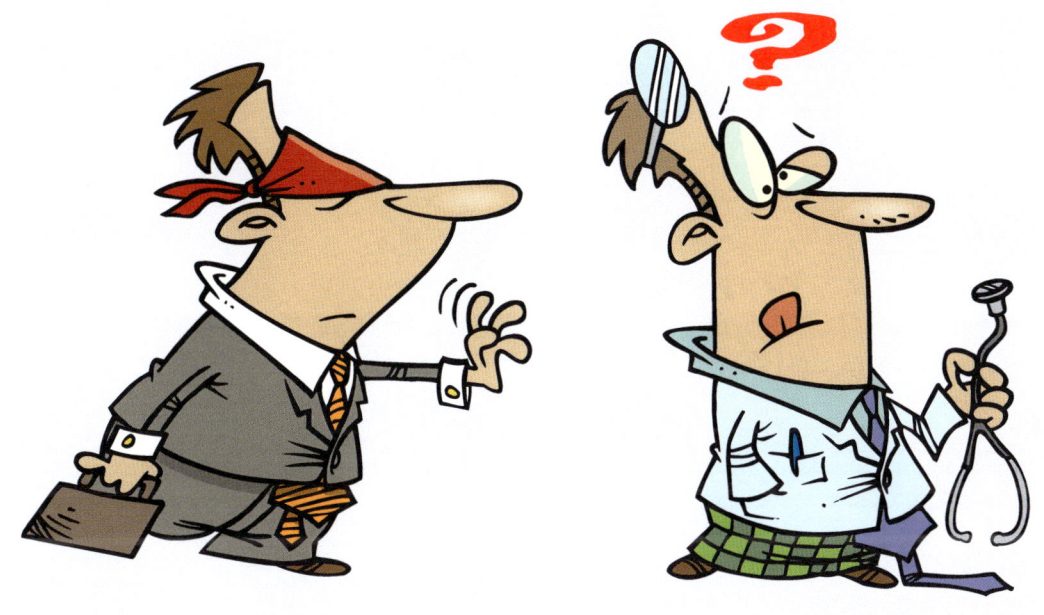

Because if you don't know where you're heading then how will you know if others are taking you in the right direction?

1 Work out where you'd like to end up

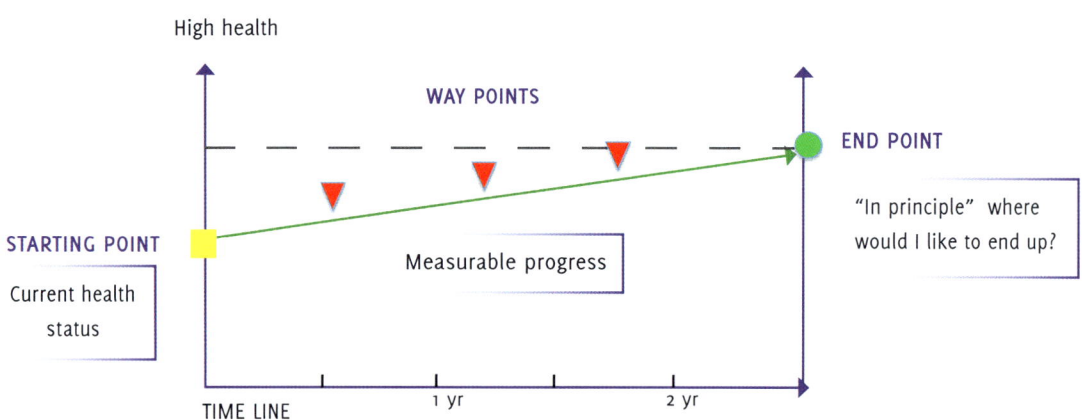

Your **end point** is "due north", or the compass point against which you can rapidly match the direction of the practitioner's therapy, their treatment and your progress to make sure you are on track. Unlike goals, which are specific, your end point is governed by the "in principle" rule. If, in principle, you wish to end up with better health and be drug-free, then any treatment or practitioner that is not aligned to your end point would quickly be filtered from the equation. Having a defined end point keeps the focus and ensures that all practitioners working on your case are heading in the same direction.

Your **goals** are the specifics of what you need to achieve on your journey, or the *means* to the *end*. They are measurable and are used for monitoring progress, like passing through each town on a journey where each town represents a leg of the journey, but not the destination.

The end point also determines *how* you travel. For example, on your journey weight loss may be a specific goal, but if the end point is to maintain long-term weight loss and become healthy, then *how* you achieve the end

point should be through a healthy sustainable dietary weight loss program that incorporates lifestyle changes. Simply losing weight may take you in the opposite direction if you regain all the weight lost *and* lose your health in the process!

My defined end point will:

▸ Form the basis of any enquiry

▸ Be the focus for collaboration

▸ Allow me to rapidly filter through options that support my fundamental aspirations

▸ Give me direction on whom to approach

▸ Give me direction on which treatments may help

▸ Give me a barometer against which to evaluate claims of help

▸ Give me direction on monitoring my progress

Selection criteria for defining the end point & goals

Examples of destination end points

Section 1: Overall outcome

- Cure
- Reversal of condition
- Remission/arrest the disease process
- Slow progression of the disease process
- Longer survival
- Improved health/recovery potential
- Maintain my current health status
- Better quality of life

Section 2: Products & treatments

- Become drug-free &/or product-free (restore the natural balance)
- Reduce drug-dependency
- Reduce treatment dependency

Section 3: Risk factors

- Reduce risks for my condition (list these)
- Reduce exacerbating factors for my condition (list these)
- Reduce future health risks associated with my condition (list these)

*Y*ou will need to draw your aspirations from the list provided under the four section headings and then separate these into two sections: your **end point** (overall aspirations) and your **goals** (what you need to achieve to get to your end point). Be *realistic* rather than *idealistic* to avoid narrowing your treatment options. Imagine if you had, what was regarded by most medical professionals, an incurable condition but your end point was cure, you would be hard pushed to find a practitioner or treatment that was aligned with this. But if you changed this to long-term remission or slow the disease process it would open up a greater range of options. Your **end point** ideally should have no more than 2-3 key criteria. If this list is any longer then you run the risk of diffusing your focus and the capacity to rapidly filter through treatment options. Your list of goals may be longer and be drawn from sections 3 and 4. Sometimes goals can become an end point, but this is dependent upon where you wish to get to and your criteria.

Section 1 represents your desired overall health outcome, or your aspirations in a nutshell. Try to choose just *one* key criterion from this section.

Section 2 relates to product & treatment dependency. If applicable, choose *one* key criterion from this section. If reduction of drug dependency is an end point, then any proposed strategy must factor this in and if you are already on drugs then you will need to monitor your progress in reducing drug-dependency. By having this as an aspirational end point it will govern *how* you get to your end point.

Section 3 relates to your risk factors: **causes** and **exacerbating factors** (ones that aggravate an existing condition, which often relate to lifestyle issues that can be resolved independently or with professional help), **individual risk factors** and **future health risks**. This list will give you the clarity on what you **can** and **can't** change, what you need help with and whom to approach. You may be able to save yourself time and money by assessing what you can do for yourself and where you may need help in treatment and monitoring.

Don't be tempted to gloss over this section and be sure to factor in all your individual risks. By being aware of your health risks you are forewarned of likely adverse reactions to treatments. Factoring this knowledge into your strategy means that you can tailor your treatment to meet your individual case. It may also reduce any future risk of medical error.

Section 4: Specific goals (measurables)

▸ Improvement within a specific time frame (give time frame)

▸ Symptom-free (name symptoms)

▸ Improved symptom management/ symptom relief (name symptoms)

▸ Improve my response to treatment

▸ Reduce side-effects of treatment

▸ Specific outcome: e.g. to increase my fertility, reduce weight/cholesterol

Section 4 relates to **specific goals**. These are usually the barometer whereby you can measure the outcome or success of any treatment and they are the essential way points for getting you to your end point. They usually relate to your symptoms and/or your diagnosis/ test results. For example, you may have determined that you need to reduce your weight and your blood pressure in order to achieve better health and so that you don't end up on long-term medication. Your doctor may have given you a time frame of six months to see if you can achieve this. So your end point may be to improve your health and come off drugs, while your goals in achieving this will include losing a specific amount of weight and reducing your blood pressure within a specific time frame. Alternatively, you may wish to improve your response and/or reduce the side-effects of your existing treatment with a complementary approach. *All these goals are measurable.*

▸ Present your end point to every practitioner, but not all your goals;

▸ Present specific goals to practitioners who have the required expertise to help you with these;

▸ Remember that a practitioner's end point may simply be one leg of your journey. Different practitioners will help you on different legs of your journey;

▸ Remain focused on the end point so that you don't end up going where others want to take you; and

▸ Use the defined end point as a reference to match all claims, products and treatments. This is the single-most important mechanism to filter through any of your options.

The Strategy Health Flow Chart

Pauline's strategy health flow chart illustrates how she has separated the causes, risk factors and exacerbating factors for her condition. Laying it out like this can be useful in determining your end point and goals. In Pauline's case, the causes for her condtion are unknown, but she has discovered her main risk factors and what will worsen her condition, some of which she can change, and some of which she can't. If Pauline's end point is to improve her overall health, then she will need a strategy that takes into account all the risk factors for her health issues. Pauline knows that her symptoms worsen with various foods, alcohol and stress; she knows that risk factors for her osteopaenia are lack of ovulation (early menopause), vitamin D deficiency and being unable to exercise; she knows that unless she can gain weight then resuming menstruation is unlikely. She is beginning to build her own health picture; she can see where she is at right now, where she's heading and, more importantly, where she would like to be and what needs to be done to achieve this.

Pauline's Strategy Health Flow Chart

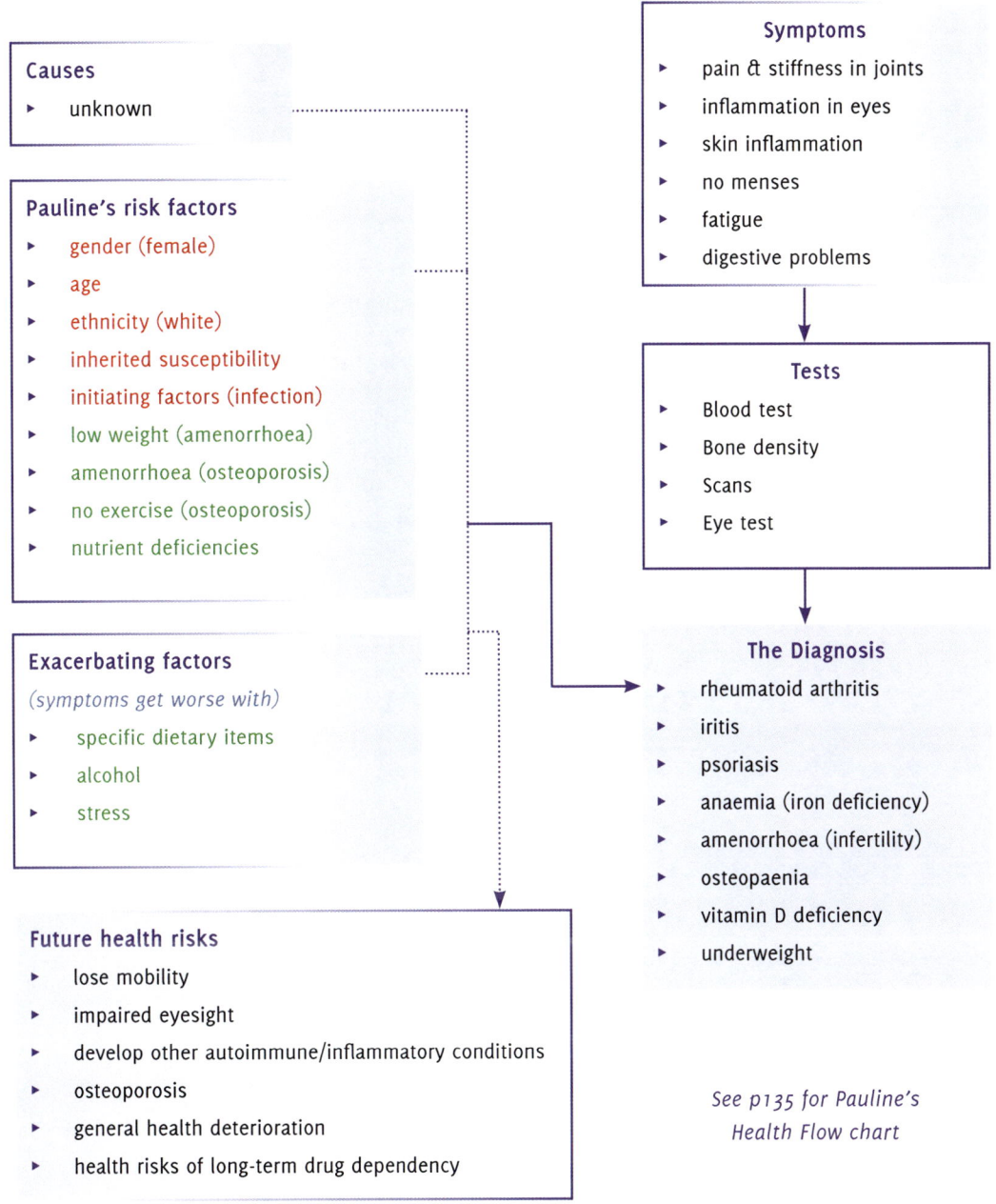

Causes

▸ unknown

Pauline's risk factors

▸ gender (female)
▸ age
▸ ethnicity (white)
▸ inherited susceptibility
▸ initiating factors (infection)
▸ low weight (amenorrhoea)
▸ amenorrhoea (osteoporosis)
▸ no exercise (osteoporosis)
▸ nutrient deficiencies

Exacerbating factors

(symptoms get worse with)

▸ specific dietary items
▸ alcohol
▸ stress

Future health risks

▸ lose mobility
▸ impaired eyesight
▸ develop other autoimmune/inflammatory conditions
▸ osteoporosis
▸ general health deterioration
▸ health risks of long-term drug dependency

Symptoms

▸ pain & stiffness in joints
▸ inflammation in eyes
▸ skin inflammation
▸ no menses
▸ fatigue
▸ digestive problems

Tests

▸ Blood test
▸ Bone density
▸ Scans
▸ Eye test

The Diagnosis

▸ rheumatoid arthritis
▸ iritis
▸ psoriasis
▸ anaemia (iron deficiency)
▸ amenorrhoea (infertility)
▸ osteopaenia
▸ vitamin D deficiency
▸ underweight

See p135 for Pauline's Health Flow chart

How serious is Pauline's condition?

▸ It will progress within 3 months without treatment
▸ She may prejudice her outcome or narrow her treatment options if she doesn't accept treatment
▸ It may become serious without treatment and appropriate monitoring

Introduction to My Value Template

My value template is a chart that covers a range of criteria that will form the backbone of your enquiries and a reference point for making sure that whatever options you choose will work for you. By doing the end point and goal exercise, you will have already determined the list for your first column *Any choice of treatment must work for me.*

If you review the template (facing page) you will see that there are four columns. The first column covers the selection criteria for defining your end point and goals, something you will be familiar with by now and is under the heading *Any choice of treatment must work for me*. The second column covers the selection criteria for lifestyle *Any choices must fit my lifestyle* which is about the feasibility of any program which includes its affordability.

The third column covers the selection criteria for your medical preferences *Any choice of treatment must fit with my own values and convictions.* This is important if you feel strongly about the type of treatment you prefer (say conventional or alternative) or if your culture or religion forbids specific treatments. It is far better to choose a health professional at the outset who is empathetic to your convictions as this will make for a more positive relationship and will smooth the road, particularly if you are having to make difficult and, at times, challenging decisions.

The fourth column covers the selection criteria for choosing practitioners and treatments *Any practitioner/product/service must demonstrate a value in helping me with my journey.* It is a set of qualifying criteria for both the practitioner (how much experience do you have) and the treatment (the type of proof you would require for the claims made). Some patients, if they have a good relationship with their practitioner and their risks are not too high will base their decision on trust, whereas others may require proof, such as clinical evidence or scientific proof, particularly when they may be heading down a path where the outcome is uncertain or if they have to make a choice between treatments.

My value template is about choice: it's about defining your own criteria for measuring the value of any option and it will help you to filter out choices that may not work for you so that you can focus on the ones or the people that could offer greater value. You will be returning to the template at various stages of your journey and it is useful to use it as your reference guide to help keep you on track.

Choice, for many, is a difficult concept in healthcare. We have choice in most areas of our lives but sadly choice in health is something we seem to have forfeited in exchange for the notion that it's "free" or that "doctor knows best". One could say that these notions have been the basis of our criteria for quite a few decades, but with chronic disease on the increase more and more questions are arising as to whether what's on offer is the right way forward and whether the doctor does know best.

Even if the doctor does know best, in a climate of escalating healthcare costs and dwindling government health budgets doctors may also become victims of an inevitable health service rationing and may be unable to offer the services they know you require.

My value template is a platform that I hope will help bring choice back into your lives and will enable you to approach professionals and their recommended treatments with the objectivity that is often required when making decisions that can seriously impact one's life.

My Value Template

will help me filter out all the things that will not work for me so I can look more closely at what might work best for me

Any choice of treatment
must work for me

Any choices
must fit my lifestyle

Any choices
**must fit with my own
values & convictions**

Any practitioner/product/service
must demonstrate a value
in helping me with my journey

Prerequisites

Clinical outcome

Time frame

Cost

**Capacity to embrace
lifestyle changes**

**My stance on medicinal
treatments**

Religion &/or culture

**Level of expertise in treating my
condition**

**Proof that it works/how far it will
take me**

Be able to monitor treatment

Criteria for measuring value

Cure
Reversal of condition
Remission/slow the disease
process
Longer survival
Improved health/recovery
potential
Maintain my health
Give me better quality of life
Reduce exacerbating factors (list
these)
Reduce risks associated with my
condition & prognosis (list these)
Reduce future health risks as-
sociated with my condition (list
these)
Reduce drug/product dependency
Be symptom-free (name these)
Improved symptom-management/
symptom relief (name these)
Specific goals: e.g. to increase my
fertility, reduce weight etc.

Must work within my time frame

Cost (within my specified budget)

I need to be able to do at home
It must fit with my family
I can travel for treatment
I must be able to carry on work-
ing/education
I can take time off work
I have no physical impairments
I have physical impairments
I require a specific diet
I can change my diet
I can make lifestyle changes
(name these)

---

natural/non-toxic only
conventional treatment only
integrative (both conven-
tional & alternative)

my religion &/or culture
forbids specific treatments
(name these)

Must be experienced in my condition
Must have success in treating my condition
Must be able to collaborate with other
practitioners

clinical proof
scientific proof
anecdotal
faith-based

makes sense that it could help
indicate how far it will it take me
be core to my case
the benefits must outweigh the risks

Must be able to monitor results objectively
(what my tests say)
Must be able to monitor results subjectively
(how I feel)

Summarize your end point & list your goals

Now we need to make a distinction between your end point and your goals. Remember your end point is your destination, and your goals are the measurable way points. Create two lists: your end point list and your goals.

If you remember Pauline has recently relapsed with two autoimmune conditions, rheumatoid arthritis and iritis, and has been told that if the condition doesn't resolve in 3 months then she will need to take drugs. However, Pauline has many health issues. The diagram below shows Pauline's end point and her goals, or what she needs to achieve in order to get to her end point. You can see from this example that although getting pregnant could be a goal, she has made it one of her end points, but in order to achieve this she must resolve her fertility issues.

My end point (predominantly sections 1 & 2)

Choose one statement from each of the sections 1 & 2. Identify other aspirations that could also qualify as an end point from sections 3 &/or 4.

1.

2.

3.

4.

My goals (sections 3 & 4)

List all your goals which may range from specific symptoms to reducing related health risks or known risk factors.

Your goals are the way points by which you measure your progress. At this stage this list may be as long as you like.

1.

2.

3.

4.

5.

6.

7.

END POINT

remission, reduce future health risks
become drug-free, get pregnant

SPECIFIC GOALS

reduce inflammation (pain-free) within 3 months,
increase mobility
restore menses, gain weight, improve energy
restore digestion, increase bone density

END POINT

"In principle" where I would like to be

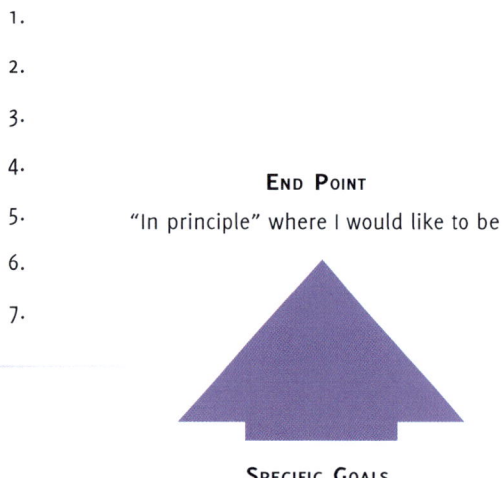

SPECIFIC GOALS

measurables

Full Alignment Template: end point and prioritized list of goals

WHY	NOW			FUTURE HEALTH RISKS	
Causes/ Risks		Tests	Diagnosis	Prognosis	
	Medical				
	Non-medical				
	End Point		remission		
			become drug-free		
			reduce future health risks		
			get pregnant		
	Symptoms &/or diagnostics		Prioritized list of goals/ measurables	End point alignment	
	pain & stiffness in joints		reduce inflammation (be pain-free)	remission, reduce future health risks	
	inflammation in eyes, skin		restore mobility	reduce future health risks (osteoporosis)	
	digestive problems		resolve digestive problems	remission, reduce future health risks	
	underweight		gain weight	fertility, reduce future health risks	
	low bone density		restore menses	fertility (get pregnant), reduce future health risks	
	no periods		improve bone density	reduce future health risks	
	fatigue, anaemia		improve energy	reduce future health risks	
	mineral & vitamin deficiencies (vitamin D and Iron)		restore nutritional status	reduce future health risks	

*U*se the chart and fill in your aspirational end point which should be no more than three key criteria (four at a pinch).

By now you will also have a list of goals, or what you need to achieve in order to reach your end point. Although these goals may relate to your symptoms, risk factors or diagnoses, the difference is that goals have to be measurable targets.

▸ So your symptoms and the diagnosis indicate what is wrong: *I feel......, I have......, I am......*

▸ and the goals are what you need to fix in order to get to your end point: *I need to...... in order to.......*

▸ and each goal should be matched against a destination end point: *by reaching this goal I will achieve.....*

Pauline may say "I am *underweight*. I need to *gain weight* in order to *improve my bone density* and *restore my menstrual cycle*. By reaching these goals I will have a chance of *getting pregnant* and *reduce my future risk of osteoporosis*."

Why do I need to prioritize my risks?

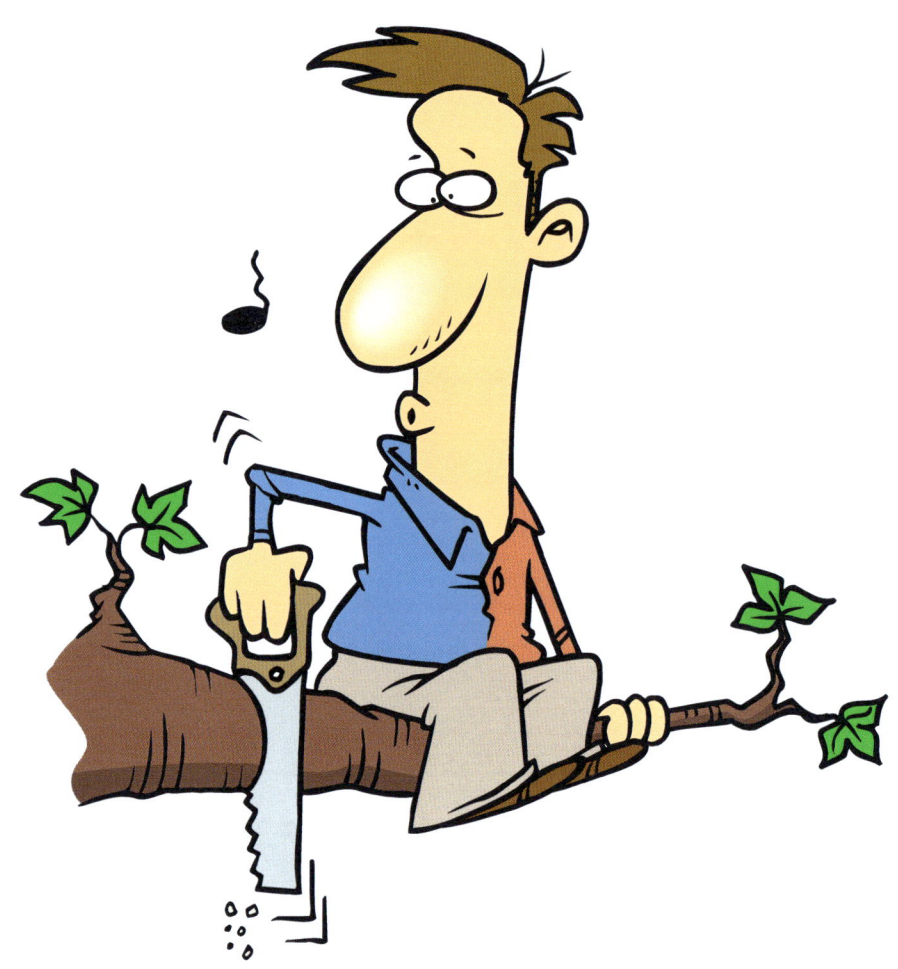

Because symptoms that carry the greatest health risks, if ignored, will land you in the most trouble and could take you in the opposite direction.

2 Prioritize your risks & goals

As you can imagine not all symptoms carry the same health risks. For example, a reduction of blood pressure in a patient at risk from heart attack will take them closer to their end point than a reduction in their arthritis which may be chronic, but not as life-threatening. This is where a strategy comes in: to make sure that you are dealing with the most important risks and any initiating causes, without which you may end up heading in the opposite direction. In order to plan your strategy we need to revisit your *Full Alignment Template*.

Re-visit your Full Alignment Template

Take the information in the **WHY** column (causes, risks, exacerbating factors) and colour code the risks into risks

you *can* change and risks you *can't* change. Risks you can't change will be things like age, gender, ethnicity, inherited susceptibility, past toxic exposure; and the things you can change will more likely be related to lifestyle issues. Then review your diagnosis/es and list of symptoms in the **NOW** column and try to prioritize these according to which of these symptoms pose the most risk - or those that if left untreated would take you backwards. Then put them as goals in order of importance, or categorize and colour code them into high, medium and low risk:

1: high risk (not much time on your side);

2: medium risk (some time on your side, symptoms that could eventually lead to chronic health); and

3: low risk (time on your side, or minor symptoms).

WHY	NOW			FUTURE HEALTH RISKS		
Causes/ Risks		Tests	Diagnosis	Prognosis		
risks you can't change	Medical					
risks you can change						
	Non-medical					
	End Point					
	Symptoms &/or diagnostics		Prioritized list of goals	End point alignment	THERAPY	TREATMENTS
			High Risk			
			Medium Risk			
			Low Risk			

Link the potential cause/s of your problems to specific goals; the more causes you can address the further you will get to your end point.

Risks that fall into the high/medium risk bracket will determine core treatments, or those that have the most value in getting you to your end point.

You may need additional help in prioritizing your goals, so bear this in mind when you have a consultation. You can ask each practitioner to confirm what your risks are, whether they are high, medium or low, and short or long-term. These answers will guide you in your prioritization.

You can appreciate that not all your goals carry the same weighting. A 50 percent improvement in a symptom or condition that carries a greater health risk will be a greater achievement than a 75 percent improvement in a lesser complaint, and it will be more core to your end point. So it's important not to lose focus on your biggest health risks.

Try to link the causes/risks of your condition to your goals. The more associations you can make, the more discriminative you will be in choosing key treatments as through addressing the cause or risk factors you will achieve your goal. Sometimes you will not know the cause of a symptom or a diagnosis, and this is where you might seek further clarification. The risks or causes you *can't* resolve are the areas where you may need help.

Next you will need to align each goal to a specific end point criterion. By doing this you will see how far each goal can take you in relation to your end point.

You may need help in completing your strategy, but it is worthwhile having a go by yourself as you will be clearer on whom to approach for help and what information you need to acquire in order to fill the gaps in your knowledge. Having done this exercise you will be in a position to frame your questions and make sense of the answers.

The immediate benefit of this exercise is that you will be able to see what you can do to help yourself and have a good idea of what you'll need help with.

In many instances there is a core focus to the case which, if addressed, could lead to the resolution of most, if not all, of the health issues. So if the stated end point is cure, then unless the core issue (usually a cause) can be resolved one would be unlikely to achieve cure and the focus may have to be redirected at managing lesser risk factors or even the symptoms themselves in order to prevent or reduce future health risks and preserve the quality of life. This exercise will help you determine a realistic end point through realizing what may or may not be possible.

Check out Andrew's end point (p66). This is a simple case where you can follow his alignments, his "in principle" end point and the goals he needs to achieve to reach his end point. His entire strategy depended on on weight reduction as its core focus. Andrew did need help on his strategy health flow chart, and input from both his doctor and his naturopath assisted him with his understanding.

The monitoring of goals is essential either through tests (objective) or by "how do I feel?" (subjective). If you can't monitor a treatment then you won't know if you are going in the right direction.

This is Pauline's end point alignment. You can see that she has prioritized her goals and has indicated where these goals will take her. By reducing the inflammation she will achieve remission, and by restoring her mobility she will be able to exercise and improve her bone density thereby reducing her future health risks.

End Point	
▸ remission	
▸ become drug-free	
▸ reduce future health risks	

Prioritized list of goals (measurables)	End point alignment
reduce inflammation	▸ remission, reduce future health risks
restore mobility	▸ reduce future health risks (osteoporosis)
resolve digestive problems	▸ remission, reduce future health risks
gain weight	▸ fertility, reduce future health risks
restore menses	▸ fertility (get pregnant), reduce future health risks
improve bone density	▸ reduce future health risks (osteoporosis)
improve energy	▸ reduce future health risks
restore nutritional status	▸ reduce future health risks

Why do I need to work out what I can change?

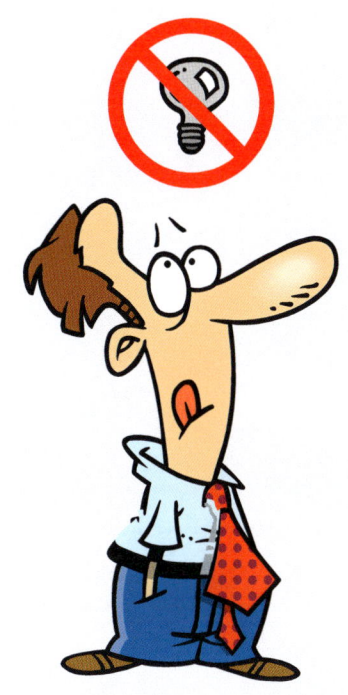

Because it will tell you how good your odds are on achieving your aspirational end point.

I now know

✓ What I can't change

✓ What I can change to resolve my symptoms and reduce my risks

✓ Where I should look for expert help

✓ What I should monitor, and how frequently

Andrew's end point

Andrew is 45 years old, is overweight and has high blood pressure, high cholesterol and early signs of diabetes (high blood glucose). His father suffered from *a heart attack in his 50s*, and also had *late onset diabetes*. Andrew is not given any specific advice other than he should try to reduce his weight and is offered cholesterol-lowering medication. You can see from Andrew's strategy flow chart that he can change most of his risks through good diet and exercise.

Andrew has added his diagnosis to the **NOW** column, has listed all the known risk factors for developing his various conditions in the **WHY** column, most of which he finds apply to him, and he has placed his **FUTURE** risks (i.e. if he does nothing) in the far right column and thinks about his ideal end point. Although he may be genetically predisposed to diabetes, he knows that with diet and exercise he will reduce this risk. So his ideal end point of being healthy and drug-free for the rest of his life *is realistic*, provided he can make all the lifestyle changes.

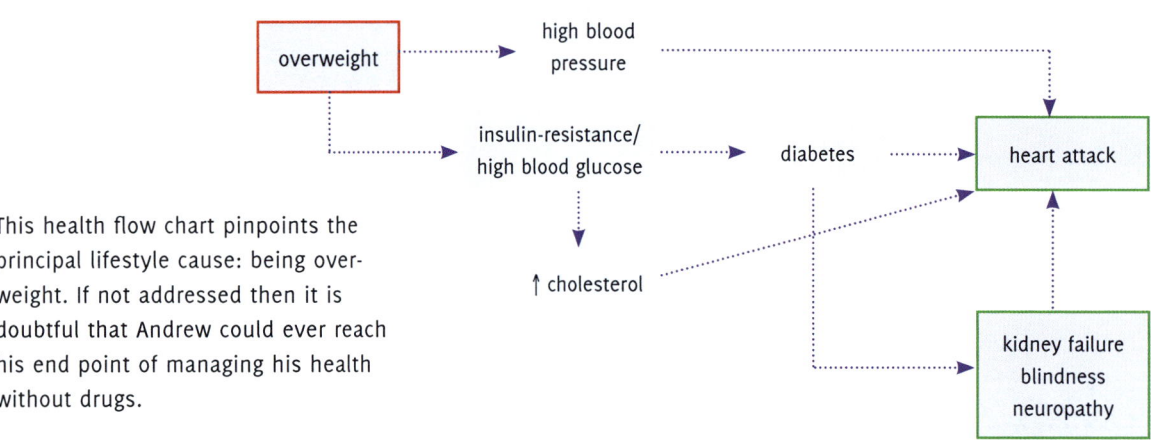

This health flow chart pinpoints the principal lifestyle cause: being overweight. If not addressed then it is doubtful that Andrew could ever reach his end point of managing his health without drugs.

WHY	NOW			FUTURE HEALTH RISKS
Causes/Risks		Tests	Diagnosis	Prognosis
▸ age	**Medical**	blood test	▸ overweight	▸ heart attack
▸ inheritance		blood pressure	▸ high blood pressure	▸ heart attack
▸ overweight			▸ high blood glucose	▸ diabetes, heart attack
▸ poor diet			▸ high cholesterol	▸ heart attack
▸ stress				
▸ sedentary life-style				
▸ alcohol				

Andrew's Full Alignment Template

WHY	NOW		FUTURE HEALTH RISKS		
Causes/Risks	Tests	Diagnosis	Prognosis	THERAPY	TREATMENTS
Medical	blood test, blood pressure	▲ overweight ▲ high blood pressure ▲ high blood glucose ▲ high cholesterol	▲ heart attack, diabetes ▲ heart attack, stroke ▲ diabetes, heart attack ▲ heart attack		
▲ age ▲ inheritance ▲ overweight ▲ poor diet ▲ stress ▲ sedentary lifestyle ▲ alcohol					
Non-medical					
End Point		▲ reduce future health risks ▲ improve general health ▲ be drug-free			

	Symptoms &/or diagnostics	Prioritized list of goals (measurables)	End point alignment	THERAPY	TREATMENTS
	no symptoms, routine check	reduce blood pressure	▲ reduce future health risks (heart attack), be drug-free		
		reduce weight	▲ reduce future health risks (heart, diabetes), be drug-free		
		reduce blood glucose	▲ reduce future health risks (diabetes), be drug-free		
		reduce cholesterol	▲ reduce future health risks (heart attack), be drug-free		

Andrew's dietician drew up the strategy chart and explained to Andrew that his major health risk was his high blood pressure, but that could be addressed by simply losing weight and doing some exercise. She explained that a reduction of blood glucose and cholesterol would probably follow as a consequence of weight loss and healthy eating options. Andrew has prioritized his goals and colour coded them. He can monitor and measure his progress through various tests and monthly weigh-ins.

Why do I need to characterize my end point?

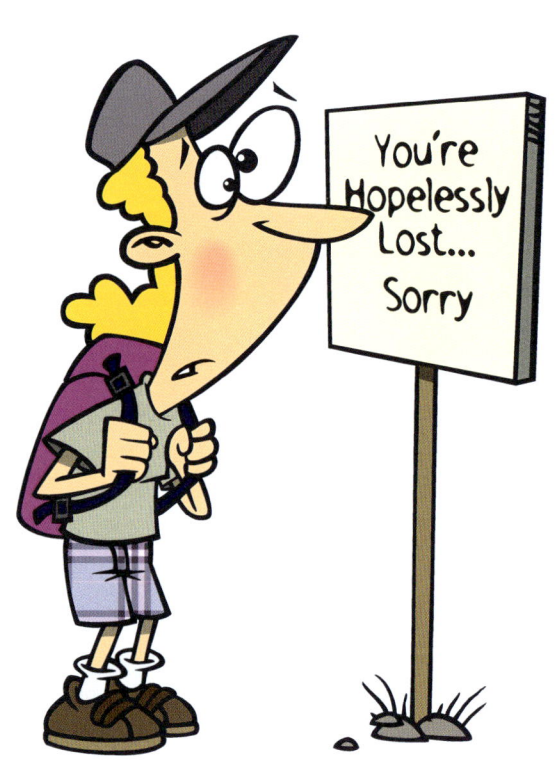

Because you need to have a sense of your general direction so that you can match where others claim they can take you with where you want to go.

3 Redefine your end point

Your end point is your homing device which allows you to match where others claim they can take you and measure how far treatments will take you against your end point. Your end point may also determine how you wish to get there. By having a defined end point you will be able to rapidly filter through treatment options, discarding those which will take you on a detour, and embracing others that may take you all or part of the way. By having a strategy you will also know which leg of the journey comes first, and be able to add treatments to your journey at the appropriate time. By sharing your journey road map and your end point with others, each party will see where they fit into the picture, what is expected from their treatment and how you will monitor to make sure their treatment is taking you in the right direction.

So it's important to characterize the end point, the purpose of which is to point in the general direction, much like a compass will point due north acting purely as a guide on direction. Your general direction may not make allowances for the fact that you may need to circumnavigate one leg of your journey by travelling east for a while, or take a different mode of transport when covering difficult terrain.

Your characterized end point needs to be simple and to the point. You will share this with every practitioner that you have on your case, regardless of which leg of the

I will share my end point with all my practitioners

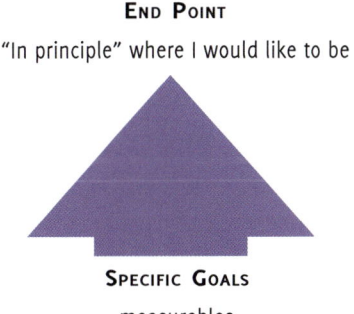

END POINT
"In principle" where I would like to be

SPECIFIC GOALS
measurables

I will share different goals with different practitioners

journey they are helping you with. It will focus all practitioners on your general direction. You will also have goals which you need to achieve in order to get to your end point, but you will only present these to the individual practitioners who have the necessary expertise to help you.

There are three points to remember:

▸ make your end point realistic rather than idealistic;

▸ your end point should be given to every practitioner; and

▸ different goals will be presented to different practitioners.

You may like to revisit your original statement to make any adjustments to ensure that your end point is realistic, particularly if you have many risk factors that you can't change, or if your condition is very advanced.

Redefining your end point will naturally pinpoint your key issues. In Andrew's case his weight problem was the key to resolving his problems and getting him to his end point. He could have taken the line "If I get my cholesterol down, then I reduce my risk for heart attack" and simply have taken drugs; but as the reduction of his cholesterol wasn't his main risk factor, then simply achieving this with drugs could lead him into greater drug-dependency and ultimately increase his risks for diabetes which, in turn, would increase his risk for heart attack. By defining his end point every practitioner can be clear that Andrew does not wish to end up product-dependent, and be confident that Andrew knows that he has to address the causes if he is to reverse his health.

Once you have done this exercise you will be ready to write the second part of *My Health Statement (p70)*. In order to help you, choose from the six guidelines in column 2: *My end point*. You will find that this exercise will give the clarity required to keep everyone, including yourself, on track. Once you have completed this you can write your end point criteria on *My Journey Road Map* to share with others.

My Health Statement: part 2 - my end point

	My starting point	My end point	My criteria
Why state this	You need to give a concise account of your diagnosis and treatment to date to allow the practitioner to make a judgement on whether they feel they can help you.	You need to tell the practitioner where you want to get to and then match where the practitioner can take you against your own aspirations.	You need to measure how much synergy the practitioner and their treatments share with your values, convictions and criteria.
Statement Guide	▲ I have been diagnosed with_____ and I have _____ (symptoms) ▲ I have had this condition for _____ (length of time) ▲ I have received medical treatment/am not on medication (indicate treatment, when you received it & length of time on treatment) ▲ I have been given a time frame (months/years) before my condition becomes serious. ▲ I have these known allergies/inherited risks	▲ I would like to achieve _____ (remission/cure, improved outcome/slow progression) ▲ I would like to reduce my drug/product/treatment dependency ▲ I would like to reduce the risk factors for my condition (name these) ▲ I would like to reduce my future risk/s of _____ associated with this condition ▲ I need help in addressing _____ (symptoms) ▲ I would like to see improvement in _____ (within a specific time frame)	▲ Do you have *experience & success* in treating people with similar conditions to myself? (i.e. can you help me and with what aspect of my case?) ▲ Can you tell me *how long* the therapy/treatment will last? ▲ What *lifestyle changes* may I need to make? ▲ Can you give any indication of the *costs* involved? ▲ Are you open to working with me if I use *a mix of conventional and alternative treatments?* ▲ Are you open to *collaboration or liaising with other practitioners?* ▲ Are you open to working with me if I *refuse any medical intervention?* ▲ My religion *forbids specific treatments*, can you still work with me?
What the answers mean to me	▲ If the practitioner can help me; ▲ What, specifically, the practitioner may be able to help me with; ▲ How far they can take me & how long can I expect improvement; ▲ Whether I can undertake the treatment (afford it, lifestyle limitations); and ▲ Whether I will "get on" with the practitioner.		

Pauline's Health Statement: end point

Pauline's aspirational end point

END POINT

remission, reduce future health risks
become drug-free, get pregnant

SPECIFIC GOALS

reduce inflammation (pain-free) in 3 months,
increase mobility
restore menses, gain weight, improve energy
restore digestion, increase bone density

Pauline's revised end point

END POINT

remission, reduce future health risks
eventually become drug-free

SPECIFIC GOALS

reduce inflammation (pain-free) in 3 months,
restore menses, gain weight, improve energy
restore digestion, increase bone density,
become pregnant

Group 1:

Pauline decides that getting *remission* from her autoimmune conditions is her chief end point.

Group 2:

She would like to be *drug-free,* however, if this is not possible in the immediate future, then this would be her long-term goal.

Group 3:

Her biggest and most immediate health risk is uncontrolled *inflammation* in the joints and eyes as so many future health risks will be exacerbated by this.

Group 4:

Her main objective is to become *pain-free.* Then she can exercise more and reduce the risks of *osteoporosis.* She would like to restore her *fertility,* improve her *energy* and *gain weight*.

Time frame: She needs to make an impact within *three months* - even if the benefits are small, she has to see results. She may prejudice her outcome if she doesn't achieve improvement within this time.

You can see that "getting pregnant" is no longer an aspirational end point as Pauline now views this simply as a goal which is not characteristic of her overall end point.

Health statement: Pauline's starting point

"

I was diagnosed with rheumatoid arthritis 5 years ago and iritis this year and have recently had an acute episode. I have had corticosteroids in the past which brought me into remission, but I have been off drugs for 3 years. My rheumatologist has said that if the inflammation doesn't reduce within 3 months I will need to take medications.

Health statement: Pauline's end point

I am looking to improve my condition and to try and get into remission, without using drugs, if possible. I need to reduce the pain and inflammation and I can use this as a marker for progress. "

Pauline's updated Full Alignment Template

WHY	NOW			FUTURE HEALTH RISKS
Causes/Risks	Medical			Prognosis
		Tests	Diagnosis	
▸ gender		▸ blood test	▸ rheumatoid arthritis	▸ Lose mobility
▸ age		▸ eye test	▸ iritis	▸ Impaired eyesight
▸ inherited predisposition		▸ X-rays	▸ osteopaenia, vit D deficiency	▸ Osteoporosis
▸ inflammatory condition can cause anaemia		▸ bone densitometry	▸ anaemia (iron deficiency)	▸ General deterioration of health
▸ low weight can cause amenor-rhoea			▸ amenorrhoea	▸ Infertility
▸ lack of exercise			▸ psoriasis	▸ Develop other autoimmune conditions
▸ stress				
▸ alcohol				
▸ nutrient deficiencies				
▸ dietary intolerance/allergy				

End Point			Diagnosis	
			▸ remission	
			▸ become drug-free	
			▸ reduce future health risks	

Symptoms &/or diagnostics	Prioritized list of goals (measurables)	End point alignment
▸ pain & stiffness in joints	reduce inflammation	▸ remission, reduce future health risks
▸ inflammation in eyes, skin	restore mobility	▸ reduce future health risks (osteoporosis)
▸ no periods	resolve digestive problems	▸ remission, reduce future health risks
▸ underweight	gain weight	▸ reduce future health risks - *also increase fertility*
▸ fatigue, anaemic	restore menses	▸ reduce future health risks (osteoporosis) - *also increase fertility*
▸ low bone density	improve bone density	▸ reduce future health risks (osteoporosis)
▸ mineral & vitamin deficiencies	improve energy	▸ reduce future health risks
	restore nutritional status	▸ reduce future health risks

Pauline's updated Full Alignment Template

Pauline has colour coded the risks that she *can* and *can't* change (first column). Through her research she has been able to identify other possible risks for her autoimmune conditions and other diagnosed conditions that her rheumatologist had not factored in or was unable to confirm. For example, Pauline knew that certain dietary items aggravated her condition and had found corroboration for this through an online community group where others experienced the same problems, so she was keen to explore this further. Pauline reviewed her list of symptoms and translated these into goals which she colour coded according to their degree of risk. Her top priority is to reduce the inflammation as this is "high risk" and is currently taking her in the wrong direction; her mobility and digestive problems are medium risk but if not resolved will lead to increased future health risks; and her weight, fertility problems, energy and nutritional status do not pose an immediate risk and can be resolved through improving her diet and digestion. Pauline's Health Flow Chart (p135) is another way of depicting the case that helps you appreciate the interactive influences on the case and what needs to be addressed and in what order.

Pauline's Journey Road Map

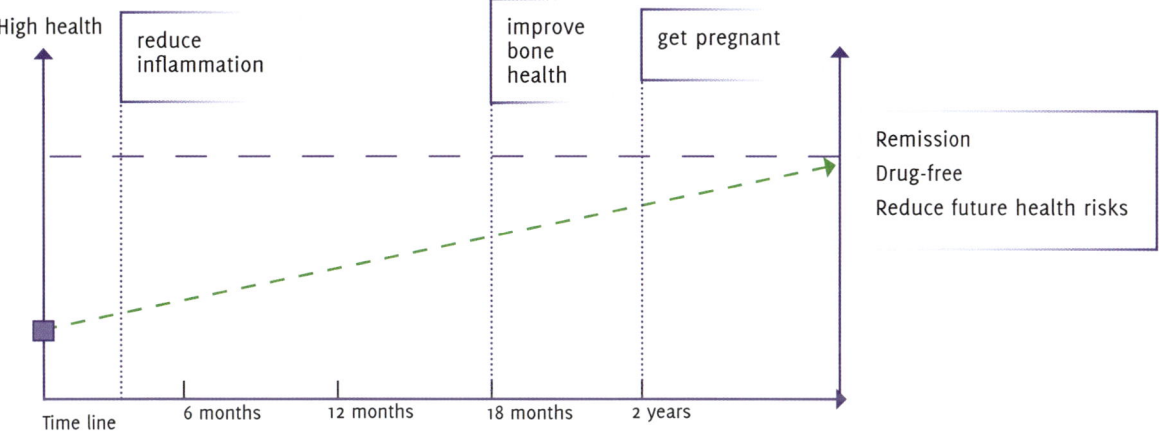

This is Pauline's Journey Road Map. You can see there is a three month goal for reducing inflammation as this is the time frame she has been given before she may narrow her options on treatment or prejudice her outcome. She is going to have a bone densitometry done in 18 months time as she has been told that she will not be able to monitor progress within this time as it takes 18 months to see an appreciable difference. She feels that if she works hard on her health by addressing all her risks, then it could be possible to become pregnant in 2 years.

You can see that she would like to be completely drug-free (and if possible product-free) at 15 months and go on to improve month by month. Are Pauline's aspirations realistic? Well, if she is right and her diet and digestion are playing a major role, and if this can be improved and any food intolerances resolved, then it should be possible to see these results. If she is wrong, and her condition does not respond to dietary changes, then she would have to go back to the drawing board and identify other potential risk factors and try to address these.

My Journey Road Map: My end point

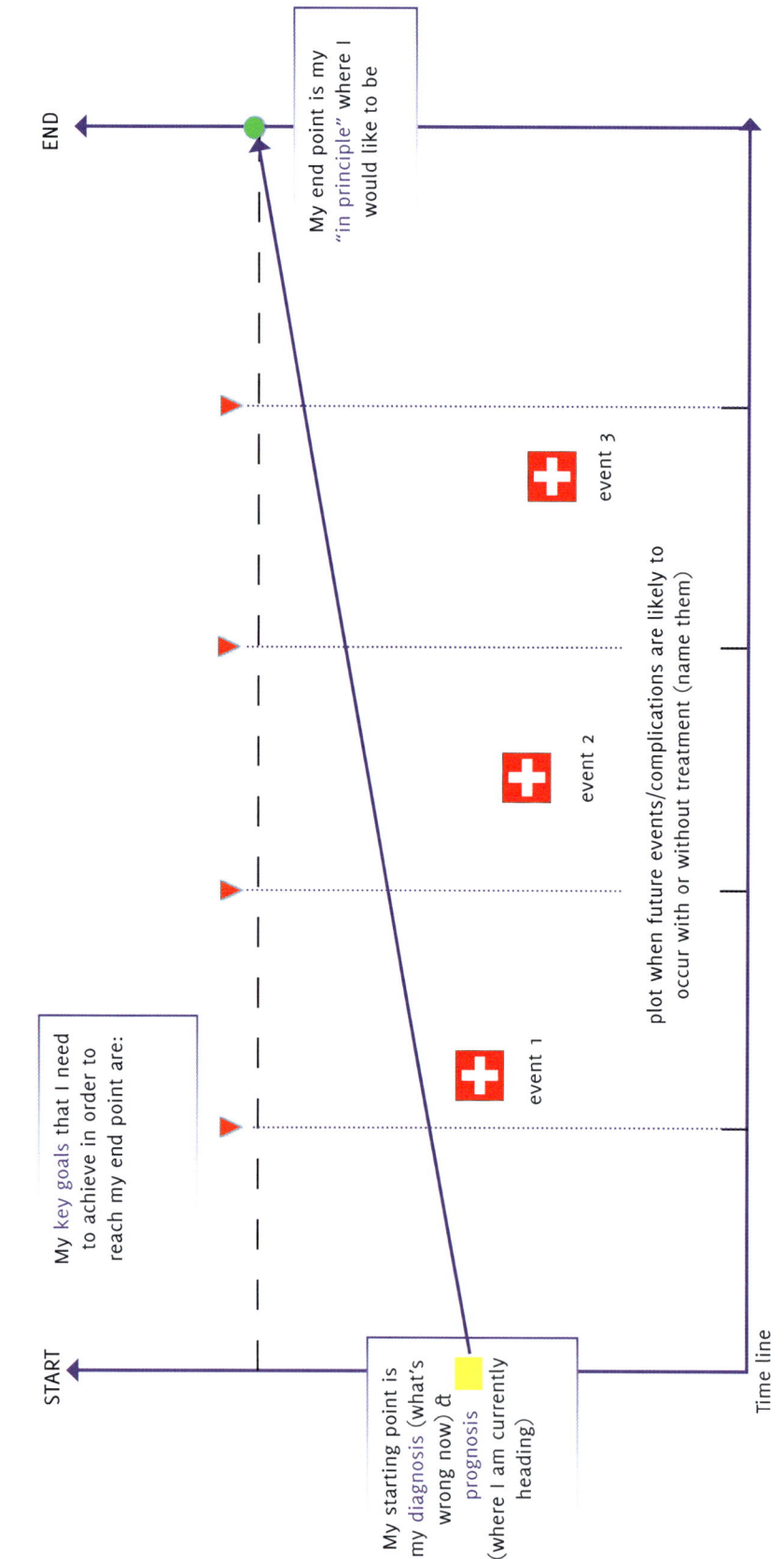

My key goals that I need to achieve in order to reach my end point are:

My end point is my "in principle" where I would like to be

My starting point is my diagnosis (what's wrong now) & prognosis (where I am currently heading)

event 1

event 2

event 3

plot when future events/complications are likely to occur with or without treatment (name them)

START

END

Time line

▶ Way points for monitoring progress

How to find out who can help me

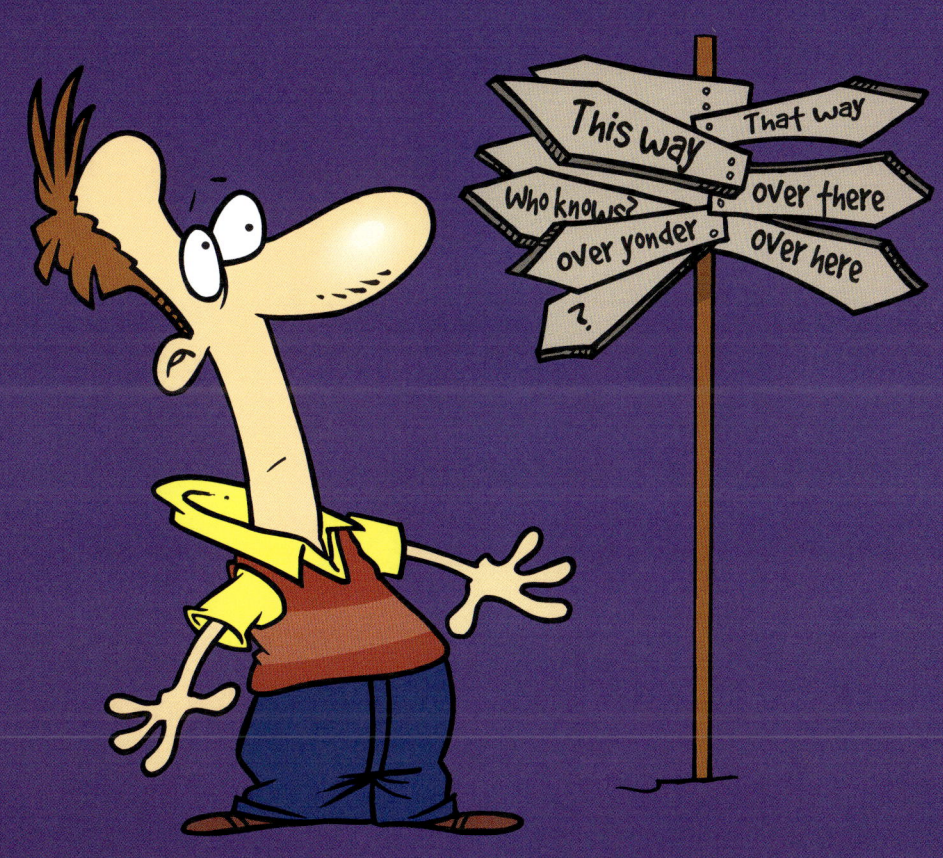

To do

1 Find out what type of therapy may help

Research therapies that could help you get to your end point.

Prioritize those that are core to getting you to your end point.

2 Find a practitioner who can help

Revisit *My Value Template* and select your measuring criteria.

Make your initial enquiries using your completed *My Health Statement*

3 Rate the value of each practitioner to your end point

Set up appointments with qualifying practitioners using your completed templates.

Rate each therapy as to how far you believe it will take you.

Why do I need to investigate
WHAT can help me?

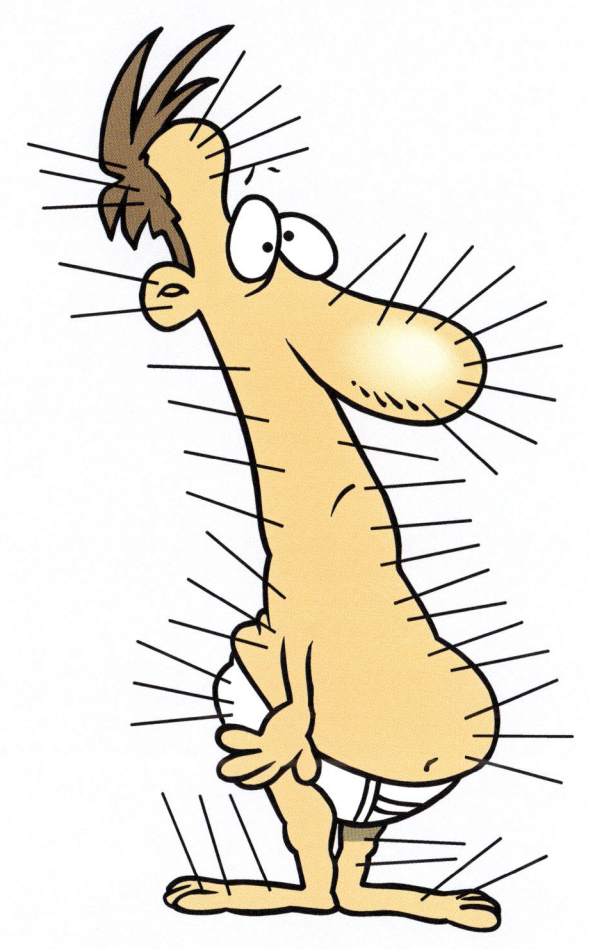

Because if you don't know "in principle" where a therapy could take
you, you won't know how relevant it is to
getting you to your end point.

1 Find out what type of therapy may help

Many patients make the mistake of not checking out what a practitioner can do for them before they embark on treatment, or not determining which type of health professionals they need on their team. Invariably a patient may need a range of therapies as each may offer specific advantages for the case, and combined treatments may offer an overall outcome that would be impossible to achieve with a single treatment.

Once you have understood your case you will have some idea of where you need help and how that should be prioritized. You then need to choose appropriate therapies that are aligned to your end point or with a specific goal. As you will be holding the reins of your case you will need to understand where each practitioner fits, how and where they are aligned to your case and which stretch of the journey they can take you on.

Don't assume that a practitioner of a chosen therapy is automatically aligned to your end point. In truth, the practitioner may not be able to take you where you wish to go.

By doing this module you will save yourself time and money and you will make sure that any practitioner you choose is aligned (to varying degrees) to your end point and meets most, if not all, of your criteria.

It's the same process as finding the right accountant or the right architect for the job. Imagine if you wanted to find an architect to design your house. If you had a good idea of the style of the building, the materials used, the size and number of the rooms, the direction they face, the fixtures and fittings, and your budget, then you are in a position to approach any architect and determine if they can deliver what you want within your budget and to your specifications.

Research the therapy

Before you approach any practitioner do some research on the therapy they offer to determine which key aspects of your case it could help and how core it is to the case.

If you have some knowledge of the therapy it will help you structure your questions and focus your enquiry around the practitioner's field of expertise and how they could help in your case.

In order to choose a therapy that may help you will need to find out:

▸ what it does (what it will treat);

▸ how it works; and

▸ how far it could take you.

Once you understand what the therapy does and what it can achieve you will avoid falling into the trap of waiting and hoping, going down a cul-de-sac, or even being taken in the wrong direction.

So to recap:

▸ match each therapy's end point against your own aspirational end point; (will it take me in the right direction?)

▸ match each therapy against your goals/symptoms; (what will it help me achieve and within what time frame?)

▸ prioritize the therapies that offer you the most promise in helping you to get to your end point (how far will it take me?).

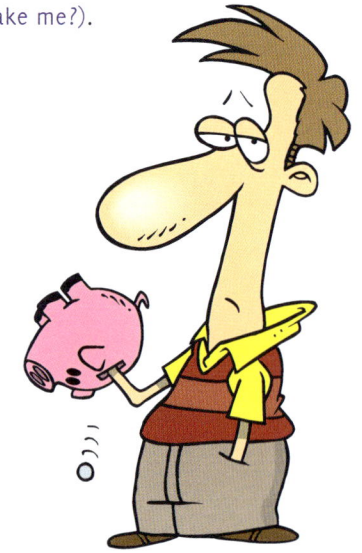

Characterizing therapy end points

*M*y advice to you when trying to define a therapy's end point (or where it will take me/what it can offer me) is to keep it really simple. Below are a few examples of the more common therapies to give you an idea of how to go about this. If you're not sure of a therapy, research it on the internet. Then try to define it in two sections: *what is it?* (a method to....) and *what does it achieve?* Try to keep your description down to a sentence.

General medicine

▸ *What is it:* a method to address conditions using pharmaceutical drugs; offers medical tests for diagnosis and monitoring.

▸ *What does it achieve:* it can alleviate/manage symptoms, it may control disease progression, it can resolve acute conditions, such as infection.

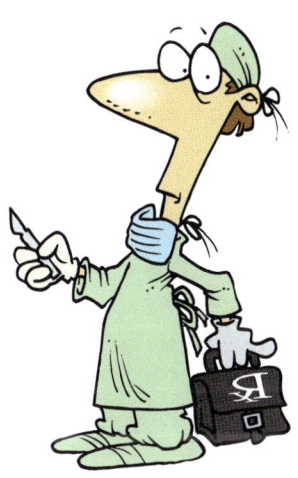

Acupuncture

▸ *What is it:* a method to stimulate and rectify the circulation of energy (qi) along the meridian lines, by applying fine needles at points which lie along the fourteen meridian lines running the length of your body. Diagnosis and monitoring are done through pulse and tongue signs.

▸ *What does it achieve:* it releases and redistributes the energy flow to alleviate symptoms and provide a better energy balance that supports natural healing. It may help reduce product-dependency.

Homeopathy

▸ *What is it:* a method to stimulate the body's natural healing capacity through the use of potentized homeopathic medications.

▸ *What does it achieve:* it stimulates the existing vital force which may help resolve the condition or alleviate symptoms and support healing. It will not rebuild the vital force. It may help reduce drug-dependency.

Classical Naturopathy

▸ *What is it:* a method to promote general health and address health conditions using diet and lifestyle to reduce the burden and address deficiencies.

▸ *What does it achieve:* if the condition is caused by poor diet and unhealthy lifestyle practices, then it will improve general health and create conditions for self-healing and help resolve physical complaints that are responsive to diet and lifestyle changes. It can also be used as preventive medicine. It may help reduce drug/product-dependency.

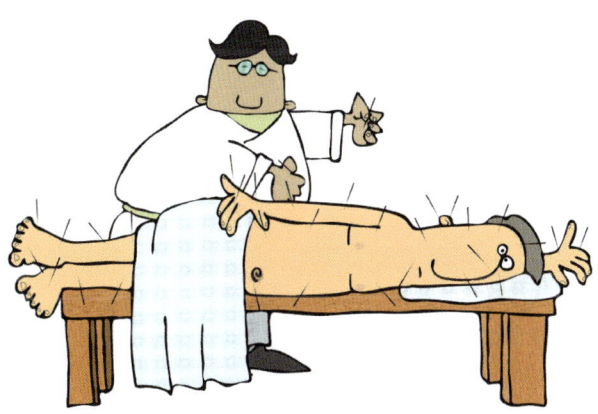

Modern Naturopathy

▸ *What is it:* a method to promote general health and address health conditions using non-toxic products, such as herbs, homeopathics, nutritional supplements and diet.

▸ *What does it achieve:* if the condition is caused by poor diet and unhealthy lifestyle practices, then it may improve general health and alleviate symptoms that are responsive to diet and specific products, such as herbs and nutritional supplements. It may help reduce drug-dependency and create conditions for self-healing.

Osteopathy

▸ *What is it:* a physical technique that makes subtle adjustments to the bones to free the flow of energy in the body.

▸ *What does it achieve:* if the condition is caused by disturbances in the alignment of bones then it will resolve the symptoms by releasing tension and restoring the energy flow.

Neuromusculoskeletal medicine

▸ *What is it:* a physical technique that makes subtle adjustments to the muscles and bones to free the flow of energy in the body.

▸ *What does it achieve:* if the condition is caused by an imbalance between the nervous system, blood vessels, musculature and skeletal framework then it will resolve the symptoms by releasing tension and restoring the energy flow.

Chiropractic

▸ *What is it:* a physical technique that focuses on realigning the spine and performing a series of adjustments to joints in the back.

▸ *What does it achieve:* if the condition is due to a misalignment of the spinal vertebrae then it will relieve pain and promote healing by releasing tension and restoring the energy flow.

Low level Laser Photonic Therapy

▸ *What is it:* a treatment that supplies energy to the body in the form of non-thermal "photons" of light.

▸ *What does it achieve:* it promotes healing by optimizing cellular activity and blood circulation. It may help reduce pain and inflammation.

Orthomolecular

▸ *What is it:* a method to prevent or treat chronic conditions using mega-doses of nutrients.

▸ *What does it achieve:* it may alleviate/manage symptoms, it may help control disease progression.

Herbalism

▸ *What is it:* a method to address system conditions using the pharmacological properties of plants as the primary agents.

▸ *What does it achieve:* if the condition is caused by disturbances in cell metabolism or infection it can alleviate these symptoms. Used as part of an holistic approach it can lend support in the management of chronic conditions, such as controlling disease progression. It can help resolve acute conditions, such as infection.

Traditional Chinese Medicine

▸ *What is it:* a method which addresses health conditions using acupuncture, herbs and dietary advice. Diagnosis and monitoring are done through pulse and tongue signs.

▸ *What does it achieve:* if the condition is caused by energetic imbalances (patterns of disharmony) which underpin disease, or disturbances in cell metabolism or infection it can alleviate/resolve symptoms. It can support in the management of chronic conditions, such as controlling disease progression; it can also be used as preventive medicine. It can help resolve acute conditions, such as infection. It may help to reduce drug-dependency.

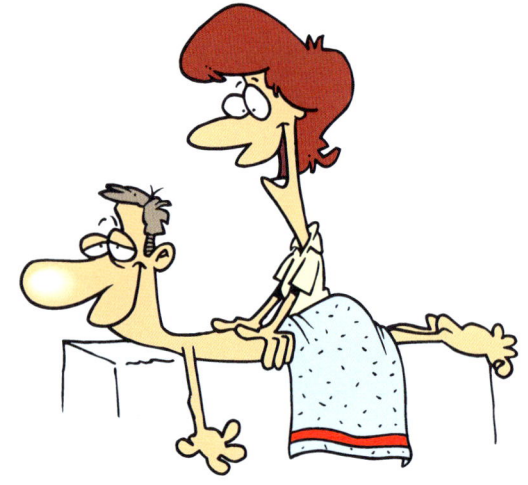

Shiatsu Massage

▸ *What is it:* a method to stimulate and rectify the circulation of energy along the meridian lines, by massaging specific pressure points which lie along the fourteen meridians running the length of your body.

▸ *What does it achieve:* if the condition is caused by poor circulation of energy it can unblock or re-divert energy flow by pressing specific pressure points. It may help alleviate symptoms.

Physiotherapy

▸ *What is it:* it uses physical techniques to restore functional ability to those with physical impairments or disabilities through physical exercises, massage, manipulation, or through the use of mechanical devices.

▸ *What does it achieve:* if the condition is caused by ageing, disease or injury that limits the ability to move and perform activities then it may help improve healing, mobility, quality of life and reduce pain.

Once you have determined which therapy end points most closely match your own end point then use the *Therapy Alignment Template* to cross check the alignments. You will be able to rate the therapy when you have spoken with the therapist who uses that modality to determine whether, or by how far, that therapy could get you to your destination end point.

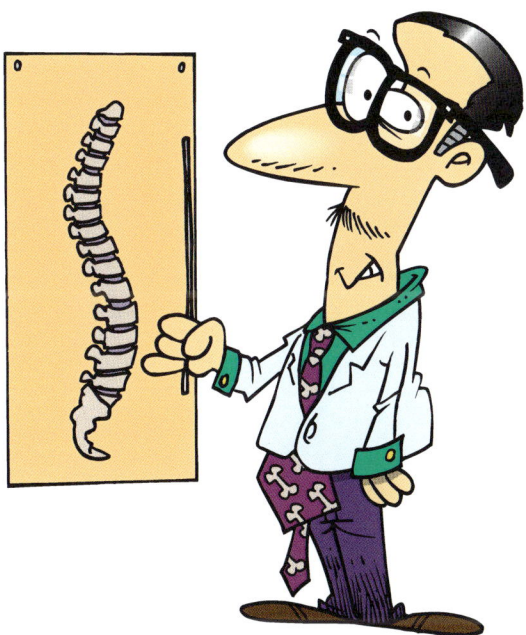

Troubleshooting therapies

Your end point	▸ Assess whether the therapy is aligned with the direction you are heading (your "in principle" end point) ▸ Work out what that alignment is
Your goals/symptoms	▸ Determine which of your goals/symptoms the therapy would address ▸ Find out how the therapy would address your goals/symptoms ▸ Match its claims of what it can achieve against your goals/specific symptoms and time frames (where it can take you and how fast)
Prioritized list	▸ Therapies that address the cause or reduce your risks/exacerbating factors will get you the furthest ▸ Therapies that treat the symptoms may slow the progression but may not get you to your end point

Tips

▸ Research how a therapy works & characterize its end point (what it does and how it works) before determining whether it could be of any value to you. Match the claims of where it will take you against your end point/goals/symptoms. For example, chiropractic treatment may claim to fix headaches, but if the headache is not caused by spinal misalignment then it may not help.

▸ Therapies that cannot deliver a measurable clinical improvement (what health improvements can I expect?) or cannot be monitored should be discarded. Many therapies rely more on science than clinical outcome and they may fail to further the patient's journey, or at worst take them backwards.

▸ Therapies that assist with symptoms may be important, but in isolation of addressing the cause, risks and exacerbating factors, may not get you to your end point.

▸ If you don't know the cause of the problem then you will need to identify a possible range of causes that could lead to the problem and then select a therapy on what you "think" the cause may be, or find a practitioner who may be able to help you identify the cause.

▸ Some therapists may offer testing and diagnostics, but not treatment. These may be just as critical in helping you to get to your end point as they will tell you if you are going in the right direction or not. (See pp201, 207.)

Therapy Alignment Template

THERAPY	TCM	GP	Naturopath	Homoeopath
My aspirational end point				
List of prioritized goals				
Tests for monitoring				

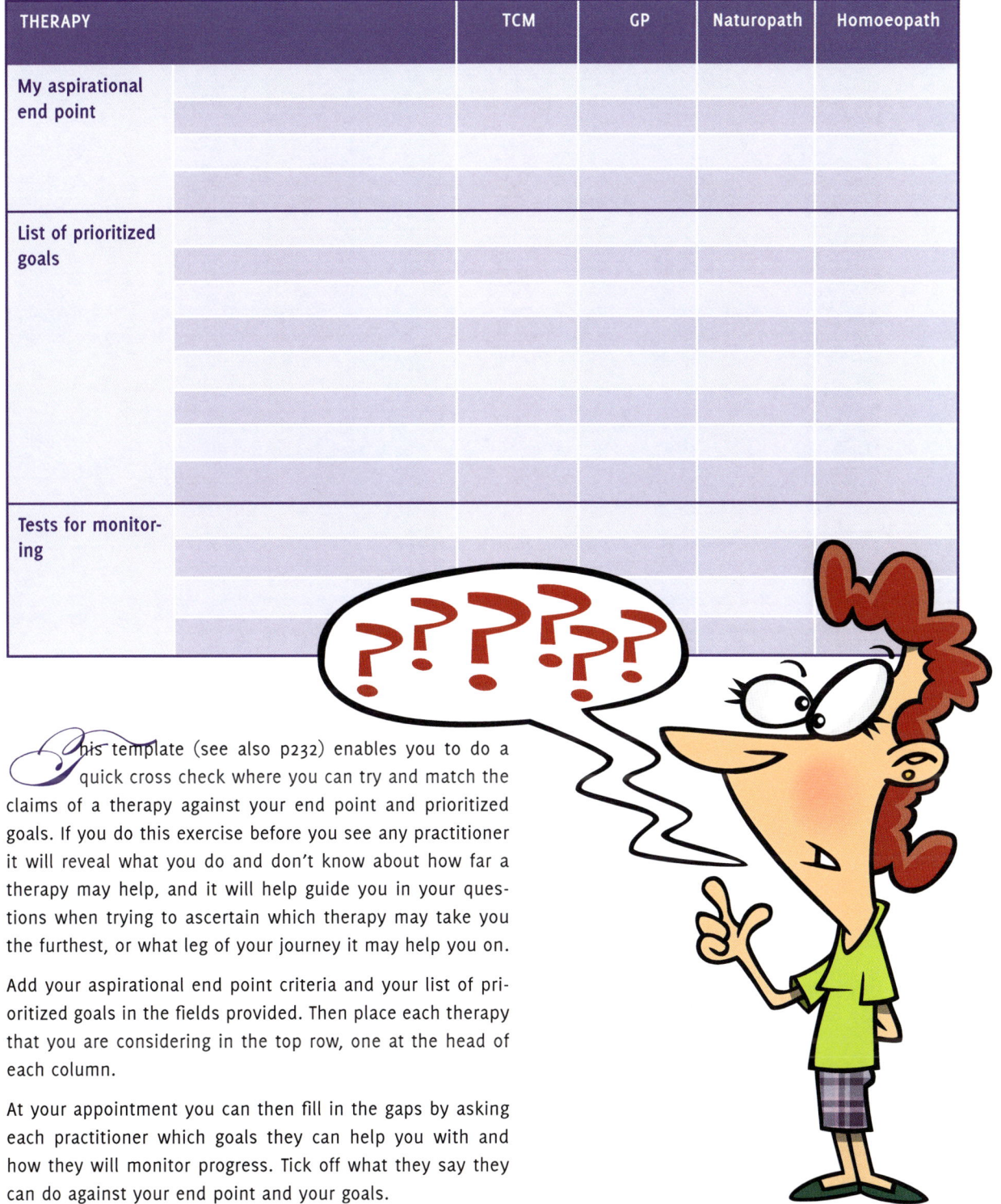

This template (see also p232) enables you to do a quick cross check where you can try and match the claims of a therapy against your end point and prioritized goals. If you do this exercise before you see any practitioner it will reveal what you do and don't know about how far a therapy may help, and it will help guide you in your questions when trying to ascertain which therapy may take you the furthest, or what leg of your journey it may help you on.

Add your aspirational end point criteria and your list of prioritized goals in the fields provided. Then place each therapy that you are considering in the top row, one at the head of each column.

At your appointment you can then fill in the gaps by asking each practitioner which goals they can help you with and how they will monitor progress. Tick off what they say they can do against your end point and your goals.

Pauline's Therapy Alignment Template

	GP	Diet therapy	TCM	Physiotherapy	Rheumatology
Pauline's end point					
▲ remission		?	?		√
▲ become drug-free		?	?		√
▲ reduce future health risks		?	?	√	?
List of prioritized goals					
reduce inflammation		?	?		√
restore mobility		√	?	√	√
resolve digestive problems		√	?		
gain weight		√			
restore menses		?	?		
improve bone density		√		√	
improve energy		√	?		
restore nutritional status		√			
Tests for monitoring					
▲ blood tests	√				√
▲ bone densitometry	√				√

Pauline has done her research and has found a number of therapy options that she will check out. She knows that she needs her GP and her rheumatologist on her team as they can monitor and treat her if her situation becomes acute. Pauline has found some potential risks for her case and is keen to explore these with other practitioners whom she feels may be able to help. She knows that she needs to fix her nutritional deficiencies and her digestion, and so a diet therapist would be worth a visit. She also knows that she will need an exercise plan to improve her mobility and restore her bone density, but at this early stage feels that some physiotherapy would be more helpful than a fitness instructor. Pauline will ask each practitioner if they can help and how they will monitor progress. She has provisionally filled in the chart and will confirm the areas that she is unsure of when she sees each practitioner.

Why do I need to find out WHO can help me?

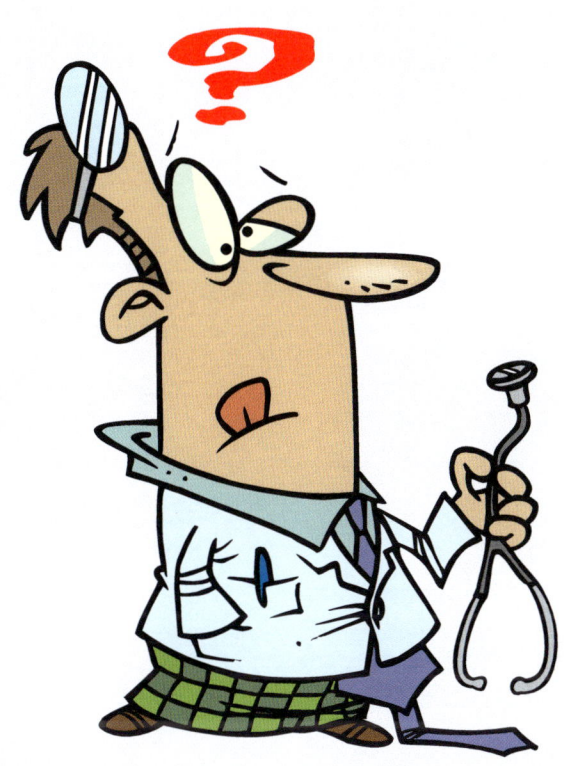

Because you have to make sure they are aligned with your journey and have the skills to get you there.

2 Find a practitioner who can help

As we all know, we may not select practitioners purely on their expertise, although this is a major consideration, but other important factors may come into play, such as the cost of treatment or lifestyle issues that may make compliance difficult. In addition, it can be very exhausting working with practitioners who cannot collaborate or take into account our individual criteria. We may waive a specialist's bedside manner if he is the best surgeon around for the job, but in the management of chronic disease when a practitioner is unyielding or prejudiced against other treatment modalities then this can become an obstacle for the patient who is aiming to get the best outcome. In principle, it is better to choose practitioners at the outset with whom you can work and communicate.

We need to return to *My Value Template* to draw up a list of criteria that we can use to measure how closely a practitioner is aligned to our criteria. We have used this template before to help define what we would like to achieve, but now we are using it to help determine the value of a practitioner. You will see at a glance that we will be drawing our list from the second column *Any choice must fit my lifestyle;* the third column *Any choice must fit with my own values and convictions;* and the fourth column *Any practitioner/product/service must demonstrate a value in helping me with my journey.*

The second column will reflect any limiting criteria regarding cost and feasibility. Obviously if you can't afford a treatment, or if you physically can't manage a treatment or if compliance would be an issue due to family or other commitments, then these criteria may rule out treatments that are too costly or too difficult. The third column reflects your own personal preferences and perhaps some cultural or religious criteria which may need to be accommodated. For example, if you were fundamentally opposed to conventional medicine you would need to make this known to any complementary health practitioner as if they felt your health risks to be too high without some conventional intervention, they would have the option of refusing to treat you on the basis of risk. The fourth column reflects the practitioner's own limiting criteria where you may ask them to qualify their experience of success, or their willingness to collaborate with other practitioners.

Draw up your list of criteria

The main criteria that will shape your choice of practitioners can be drawn from the lists presented in *My Value Template* and will broadly cover the following:

▸ whether the treatment they offer is aligned to your end point or goals;

▸ whether the treatment they offer can work within a specific time frame;

▸ their level of experience and success in treating patients with a similar condition;

▸ their capacity to work within your budget and/or lifestyle limitations; and

▸ how much synergy they share with your values and your convictions.

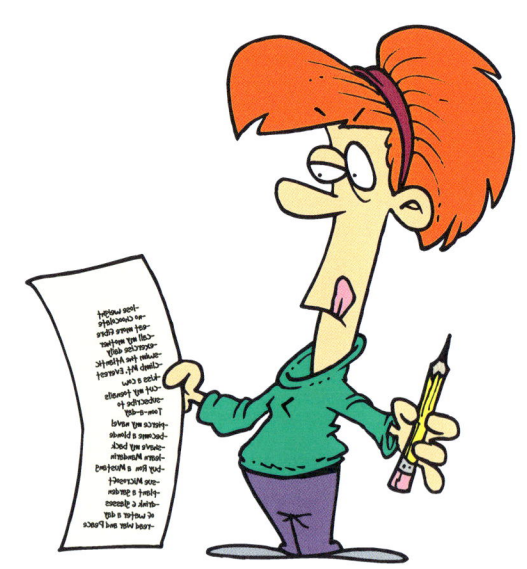

My Value Template

will help me filter out all the things that will not work for me so I can look more closely at what might work best for me

Any choice of treatment must work for me

Any choices must fit my lifestyle

Any choices must fit with my own values & convictions

Any practitioner/product/service must demonstrate a value in helping me with my journey

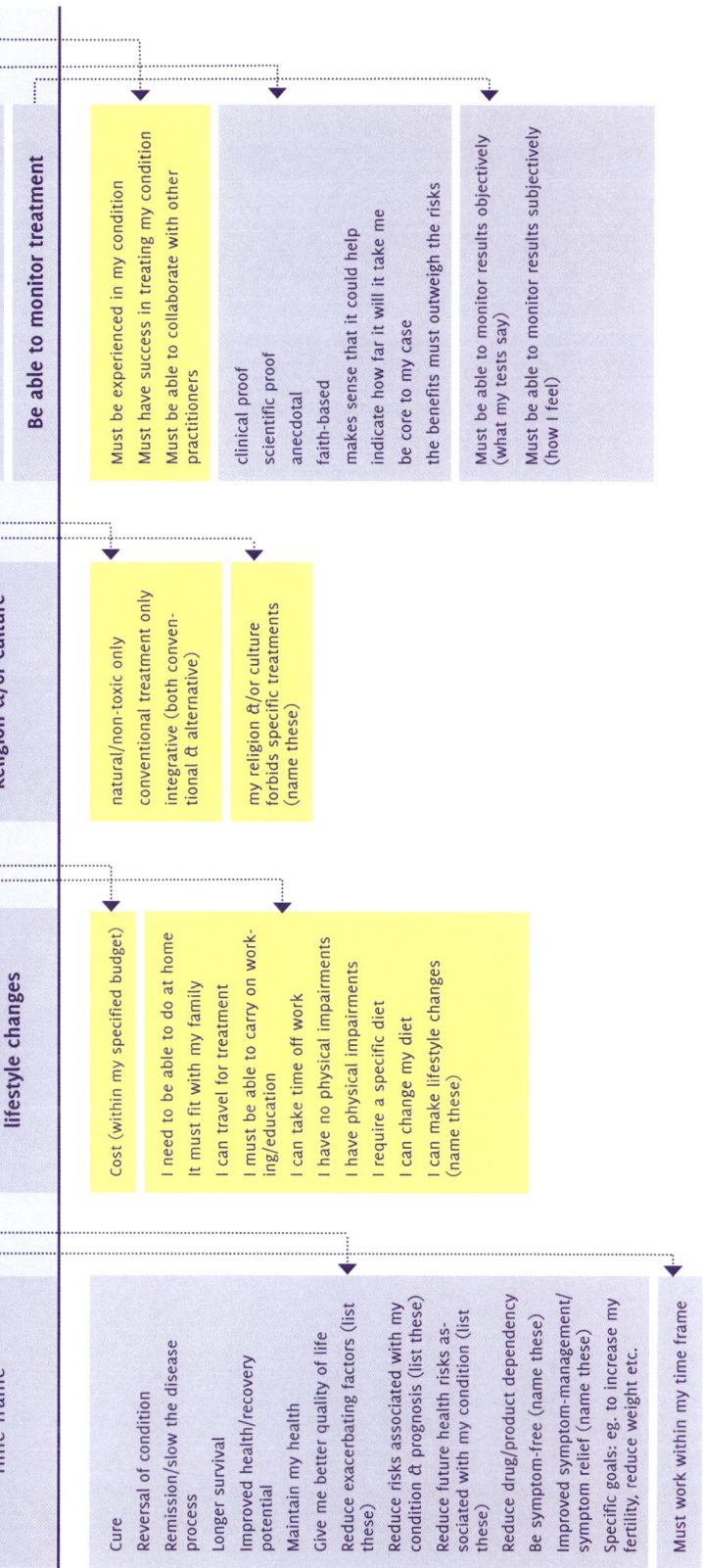

Prerequisites / Criteria for measuring value

Clinical outcome
- Cure
- Reversal of condition
- Remission/slow the disease process
- Longer survival
- Improved health/recovery potential
- Maintain my health
- Give me better quality of life
- Reduce exacerbating factors (list these)
- Reduce risks associated with my condition & prognosis (list these)
- Reduce future health risks associated with my condition (list these)
- Reduce drug/product dependency
- Be symptom-free (name these)
- Improved symptom-management/symptom relief (name these)
- Specific goals: eg. to increase my fertility, reduce weight etc.

Time frame
- Must work within my time frame

Cost
- Cost (within my specified budget)

Capacity to embrace lifestyle changes
- I need to be able to do at home
- It must fit with my family
- I can travel for treatment
- I must be able to carry on working/education
- I can take time off work
- I have no physical impairments
- I have physical impairments
- I require a specific diet
- I can change my diet
- I can make lifestyle changes (name these)

My stance on medicinal treatments
- natural/non-toxic only
- conventional treatment only
- integrative (both conventional & alternative)

Religion &/or culture
- my religion &/or culture forbids specific treatments (name these)

Level of expertise in treating my condition
- Must be experienced in my condition
- Must have success in treating my condition
- Must be able to collaborate with other practitioners

Proof that it works/how far it will take me
- clinical proof
- scientific proof
- anecdotal
- faith-based
- makes sense that it could help
- indicate how far it will take me
- be core to my case
- the benefits must outweigh the risks

Be able to monitor treatment
- Must be able to monitor results objectively (what my tests say)
- Must be able to monitor results subjectively (how I feel)

The initial contact

Now you are ready to complete the third section of My Health Statement: my criteria. These are the qualifying criteria which you can use to clarify whether the practitioner is suited and aligned with your journey before you make an appointment. The initial contact will be by telephone so remember that you may only have a couple of minutes to make your enquiry and ask the relevant questions: you need to make sure you are to the point. Being prepared in this way will facilitate your exchange and also focus you on what is relevant and what is not. Using your criteria from *My value template* work through the third column My Health Statement: My criteria (p89) making sure that you cover all your criteria when constructing the final part of your statement.

Pauline is ready to approach various practitioners to see if they can help her. Pauline has looked through *My Value Template* and has identified the criteria that most closely fit with her values. She uses the table *My Health Statement* and drafts her enquiry.

As each practitioner needs to know her diagnosis (starting point) and her general direction (end point) then the initial enquiry needs to cover this. She can then tailor this depending to whom she is speaking and include goals that are within their field of expertise.

Health statement: Pauline's goals

" I am looking to improve ....✐/ *or* I need help in addressing............in order to achieve..................without using drugs, if possible. "

You can appreciate that Pauline will seek expert help in a variety of therapies as she may need some nutritional support, advice on how she can ensure that she stays in remission for as long as possible, and she may need some physical therapy to help with her mobility. She may also decide to approach a fertility specialist.

With practitioners who are likely to be core to the case Pauline may also need to ask some qualifying questions on the feasibility of any treatment they prescribe. She has worked through her qualifying criteria and come up with the final part of her statement.

Pauline's end point

END POINT
remission, reduce future health risks,
eventually become drug-free

SPECIFIC GOALS
reduce inflammation (pain-free) in 3 months,
restore menses, gain weight, improve energy,
restore digestion, increase bone density

Health statement: Pauline's criteria

" Have you had experience & success in treating someone with my condition and what sort of difference do you think you can make and within what time frame? Although I am on benefit at the moment I can afford some treatment providing that it is not too expensive. My family is supportive and have offered to help. "

My Health Statement: part 3 - my criteria

	My starting point	My end point	My criteria
Why state this	You need to give a concise account of your diagnosis and treatment to date to allow the practitioner to make a judgement on whether they feel they can help you.	You need to tell the practitioner where you want to get to and then match where the practitioner can take you against your own aspirations.	You need to measure how much synergy the practitioner and their treatments share with your values, convictions and criteria.
Statement Guide	► I have been diagnosed with_____ and I have _____ (symptoms) ► I have had this condition for _____ (length of time) ► I have received medical treatment/am not on medication (indicate treatment, when you received it & length of time on treatment) ► I have been given a time frame (months/years) before my condition becomes serious. ► I have these known allergies/ inherited risks	► I would like to achieve _____ (remission/cure, improved outcome/slow progression) ► I would like to reduce my drug/ product/treatment dependency ► I would like to reduce the risk factors for my condition (name these) ► I would like to reduce my future risk/s of _____ associated with this condition ► I need help in addressing _____ (symptoms) ► I would like to see improvement in _____(within a specific time frame)	► Do you have *experience & success* in treating people with similar conditions to myself? (i.e. can you help me and with what aspect of my case?) ► Can you tell me *how long* the therapy/ treatment will last? ► What *lifestyle changes* may I need to make? ► Can you give any indication of the *costs involved?* ► Are you open to working with me if I use *a mix of conventional and alternative treatments?* ► Are you open to *collaboration or liaising with other practitioners?* ► Are you open to working with me if I *refuse any medical intervention?* ► My religion/culture *forbids specific treatments,* can you still work with me?
What the answers mean to me	► If the practitioner can help me; ► What, specifically, the practitioner may be able to help me with; ► How far they can take me & how long I can expect improvement; ► Whether I can undertake the treatment (afford it, lifestyle limitations); ► Whether I will "get on" with the practitioner.		

Share your starting point, your end point and your journey road map with every practitioner, but share the individual goals with those practitioners who have the expertise. By sharing your journey road map, each practitioner can make sure that they are not taking you further way from your end point and that they are offering measurable value.

Pauline's Health Statement

Pauline's end point

END POINT

remission, reduce future health risks, eventually become drug-free

SPECIFIC GOALS

reduce inflammation (pain-free) in 3 months, restore menses, resolve anaemia, gain weight, improve energy, restore digestion, increase bone density, get pregnant

Health statement: Pauline's starting point

" I was diagnosed with rheumatoid arthritis 5 years ago and iritis this year and have recently had an acute episode. I have had corticosteroids in the past which brought me into remission, but I have been off drugs for 3 years. My rheumatologist has said that if the inflammation doesn't reduce within 3 months I will need to take medications. "

Health statement: Pauline's end point

" I am looking to improve my condition and to try and get into remission, without using drugs, if possible. I need to reduce the pain and inflammation and I can use this as a marker for progress. "

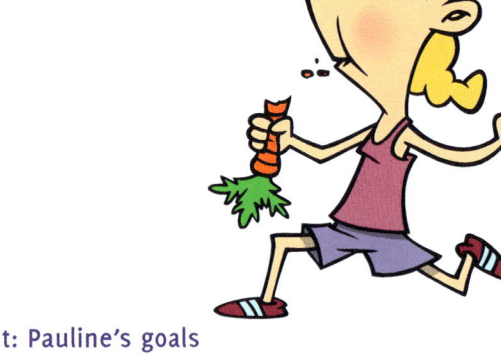

Health statement: Pauline's goals

" I am looking to improve........&/or I need help in addressing............in order to achieve .... , without using drugs, if possible. "

Pauline will present specific goals to practitioners that are within their field of expertise.

Health statement: Pauline's criteria

" Have you had experience & success in treating someone with my condition and what sort of difference do you think you can make and within what time frame? Although I am on benefit at the moment I can afford some treatment providing that it is not too expensive. My family is supportive and have offered to help. "

Why do I need to rate each practitioner?

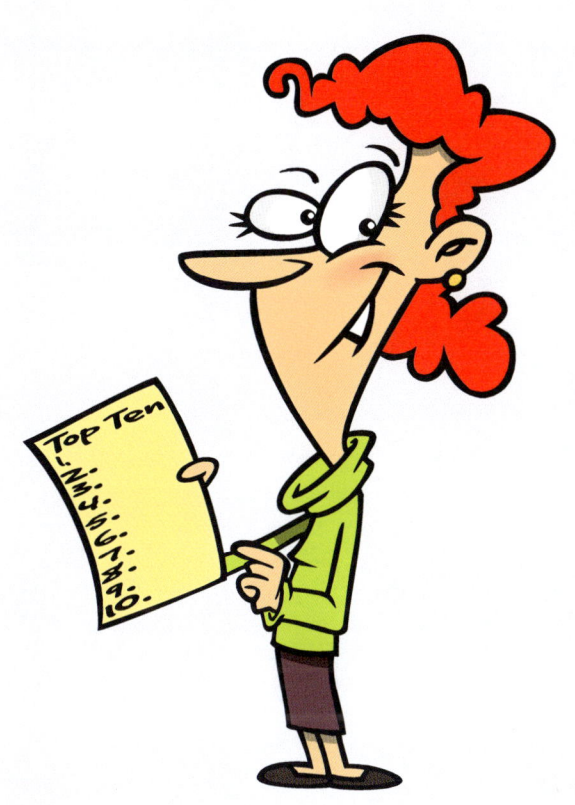

Because you have to know which leg of your journey they can help you with and how far this will take you.

3 Rate the value of each practitioner to your end point

Once you have decided which practitioners may be able to help, you will need to set up the various appointments. The aim of the first appointment is not simply to get treatment but to find out how far each practitioner can take you. So you need to come away with a fair idea of the practitioner's end point and how closely it is aligned with your own. If you look at the diagram below you will see how this is depicted on the Journey Road Map. If the practitioner's end point matches yours, entirely, then the lines will be very closely aligned, but if the practitioner can only partially match your end point, or only be able to help you reach one of your goals then they will not be closely aligned to the end point, but more aligned to a goal. This will not undermine their value to you so long as they are taking you in the right direction. They may simply be important for one leg of the journey.

The objective of the initial consultation is to:

▸ identify your practitioner's end point; ⬜1

▸ see how far it aligns with your end point; ⬜2

▸ identify which goals they can help you with; and ⬜3

▸ if possible, to plot a line that predicts where they think they can take you ⬜4

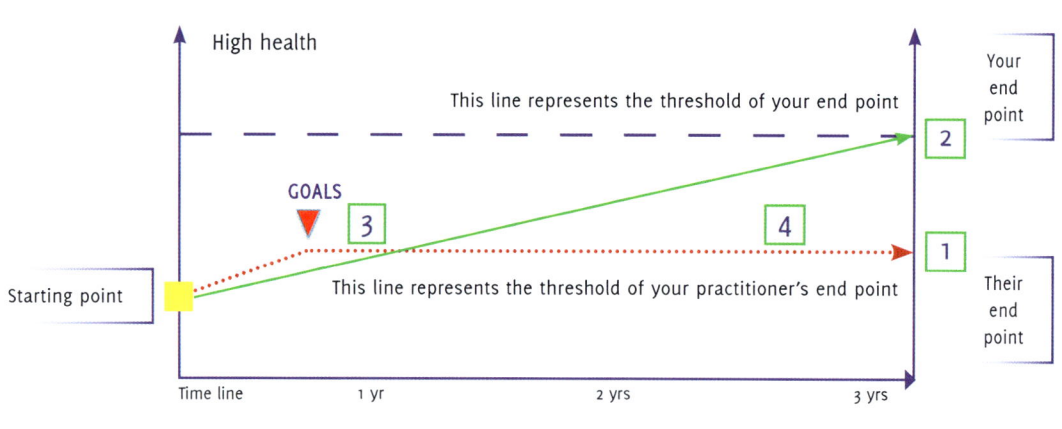

This line represents where your practitioner thinks they can take you

The initial consultation

Before you attend your appointment use *A Conversational approach: how far can they take me (p95)* to prepare your questions. Invariably there may be limited opportunity to ask all the questions you may have as much of the appointment may be spent on making a case assessment and then formulating a strategy and treatment plan. So make sure you go armed with questions that will give you an idea of their end point *What is the aim of your therapy and what will this achieve for me?* This will enable you to determine what goals they can help you with and how far they are aligned to your end point. For example, if you want to reduce your symptoms of excess stomach acidity (goal) and improve your health (end point) you would need to ensure that the practitioner's recommendations in helping you meet your goal are also going to improve your overall health. You would not want to reduce the stomach acidity at the expense of increasing future health risks as you could find yourself further away from your end point down the track.

Once you have determined your practitioner's in principle end point draw a dotted line across your graph that represents their threshold. Practitioners that check all your aspirational end points will be closely aligned with your own end point.

You also need to ascertain *What improvements can I expect and within what time frame?* This information will enable you to draw a prediction line which represents where they can get you in relation to your end point and within what time frame. You may also enquire *What are the odds of the therapy working in my case and, if it doesn't work, what will we do then?* This will allow you to factor in the chances of their therapy getting you to where you wish to be and whether they can offer you additional help.

Although you may also have questions on the actual proposed treatment/s at this appointment, it is important to focus on where the practitioner is heading, or their overall strategy and direction. Remember, the strategy focuses on where they are taking you, and the products and/or treatments on how they will get you there.

The strategy is the direction; the treatment is the means of getting there.

It's important to separate these two parts, the *strategy* and the *means*, as you may end up fudging the actual pathway and instead narrow your focus to just the means. If you do this then you could end up driving blind without a compass (destination end point) and with no clear way points to monitor your progress. For example, you may decide to take a bus *(means)* for one leg of your journey, but you need to get on the right bus so that you end up in the right location. You can then check each bus stop *(way points)* making sure you are heading in the right direction, and disembark when you get there. So you need to check that your practitioner knows where they are going, what improvements they are looking for (i.e. how they will monitor and when) and also what they will do if the treatment doesn't work.

In many cases it may be difficult for a practitioner to give assurances as to how much they can help or even give a time frame, but this may not mean that they cannot offer something meaningful. Under these circumstances don't try to pin the practitioner down, as it is better to have an honest answer than be promised the earth. You can simply determine where they are likely to benefit you and then monitor yourself, and if you don't see results within a time frame you can choose to change your therapist or the treatment.

When you have established the strategy you can then ask about the treatment bearing in mind that if you don't have time to cover all your questions you can research each treatment in your own time before making any final decision.

Remember, asking a practitioner to qualify their treatment beyond what, in principle, it will do or could achieve for you is outside the general scope of an appointment where one is seeking treatment. Seeking clarification on treatment is acceptable, but requesting detailed qualification would come under the scope of self-education, and any expectation on practitioners to fulfill this service could prejudice the patient-practitioner relationship.

Andrew's weight loss program: where will it take him?

Andrew is overweight and has high blood pressure, high blood sugar and high cholesterol. He has been told he needs to reduce his weight. He goes on a high protein/low carbohydrate diet and at 3 months his blood pressure, blood cholesterol and blood sugar have reduced to within normal limits and at 4.5 months he has lost 10 kg. He thinks he is heading in the right direction but at 6 months after starting the program he ends up in hospital with kidney stones. He comes off the diet and within a year he has not only regained all the weight he lost, but packed on additional weight as well. Although while on the dietary program Andrew achieved many of his goals, the program did not take him in the right direction of improved overall health that was sustainable. He needed to embark on a lifestyle change, a diet that he could adopt for life and one that would not tax his kidneys.

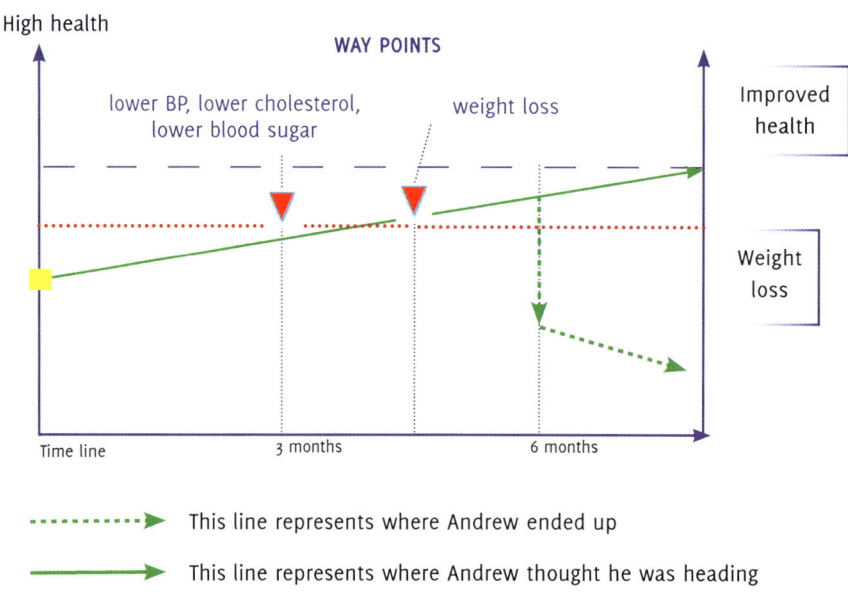

This line represents where Andrew ended up

This line represents where Andrew thought he was heading

A conversational approach: how far can you take me?

QUESTIONS	Where can you take me?
Why ask these questions?	You need to find out what stretch of your journey they can help you with.
Questionnaire guide	▸ What is the aim of your therapy?
	▸ Which aspects of my condition will it address?
	▸ What sort of improvement/s can you offer me?
	▸ What results can I expect on this program? (Worst, median, best case scenario.)
	▸ Within what time frame will I see an improvement?
	▸ Will the improvement last and how long will it last?
	▸ How long will I need to be on your program?
	▸ Could the program fail in my case (produce little or no response) or is there any chance that it could worsen my condition?
	▸ In your clinical experience how effective do you think your program will be for me? (Clinical outcome: what are the odds on your treatment working for me?)
	▸ Later on if I require additional treatments on your program when could this be? (If yes, then the same questions will apply for each program: how successful would it be and how long would the improvements last?)
	▸ What would you advise if your program doesn't work?
	▸ How will we monitor the program (and how frequently) to make sure that it is working as predicted?
How does this relate to my journey? *You need to match where they can take you against where you wish to go.*	▸ How core is the practitioner to getting me to my end point?
	▸ Which part of my journey can they help me with?
	▸ How far can the practitioner take me on my journey?
	▸ What goals can the practitioner help me with?
	▸ How fast can they take me there?
Factor in their professional criteria	▸ They can only work within their field of expertise
	▸ Their end point may be aligned to part of my journey but not to my end point
	▸ Their end point may not be aligned to my journey or my end point

Meeting your goals does not necessarily mean that you are heading in the right direction. Always check that you are on track and aligned to your end point.

Where Pauline's specialist can take her

Pauline's rheumatologist has indicated that if Pauline does not start treatment within the next three months then she will prejudice her chances of achieving remission and will risk irreversible inflammatory damage to the joints which will impair her mobility. However, if she goes on medication she will be symptom-free within a very short period of time and if she remains on the medication and has good results, they could start tapering the dose and hopefully she would be able to come off the treatment within a year and enter remission. The rheumatologist cannot say for sure how long this remission would last, but when pressed she indicated that given Pauline's case history and her inherited susceptibility she felt Pauline could stay in remission for at least three years, if not longer.

From the conversation Pauline can establish that the rheumatologist's end point is to control her condition with drugs with no guarantee of long-term remission. The alignment with Pauline's end point is to bring her into remission and come off the drugs but only for a period of time.

Pauline then asked what the treatment would be when the disease relapsed. The rheumatologist said that she would have to go back on the corticosteroids and that if she didn't go into remission, then she may remain on these indefinitely. Pauline then asked what the consequence of this would be and whether her general condition would remain stable. The specialist said not to worry about the long-term effects and that there were other drugs that could be given, if required, to offset the side-effects of say, osteoporosis. The rheumatologist could not make any recommendations as to what lifestyle factors may reduce her risks and doesn't believe that any changes Pauline makes will be of significant help.

Pauline draws her specialist's prediction line and makes some important decisions. Although she recognizes that at this late stage she may have to take the drugs she decides to try and find someone who may be able to help address her risk factors which will improve her outcome and potentially enable her to remain in remission indefinitely. She realizes that she will need to adopt a healthy lifestyle, and decides to investigate if there are any non-toxic treatments that may help her stay in remission for longer (once off the drugs) in order to take her to her end point.

You can see from this map that the overall strategy of the specialist is going in the opposite direction to where Pauline wants to be. Therefore Pauline has no option other than to seek further advice to see if any other practitioners can improve her overall outcome. Pauline is using this map as the benchmark against which to monitor overall progress. Her first goal is to resolve the inflammation and her second is come off the drugs as quickly as she can; and her third goal is to exceed the prognosis of a three year remission.

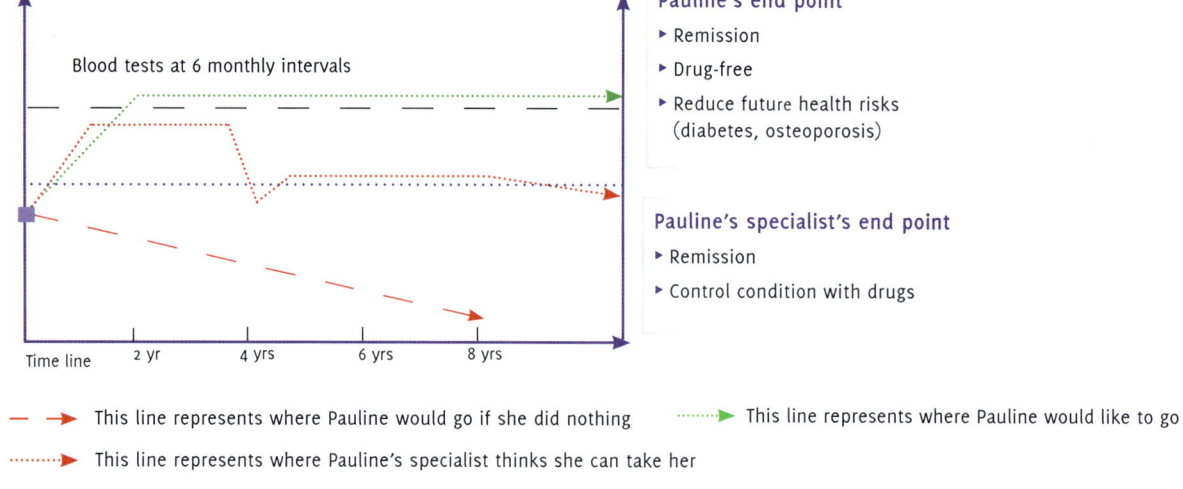

Blood tests at 6 monthly intervals

Time line   2 yr   4 yrs   6 yrs   8 yrs

Pauline's end point
- ▸ Remission
- ▸ Drug-free
- ▸ Reduce future health risks (diabetes, osteoporosis)

Pauline's specialist's end point
- ▸ Remission
- ▸ Control condition with drugs

— — ▸ This line represents where Pauline would go if she did nothing

·········▸ This line represents where Pauline would like to go

··········▸ This line represents where Pauline's specialist thinks she can take her

Where Natalie's specialist can take her

❝I am 22 years old and have been diagnosed with polycystic ovarian syndrome, haemorrhagic ovarian cysts and endometriosis. I have had one surgery two years ago for a ruptured haemorrhagic cyst. I have tried progesterone to try and control my symptoms, but this aggravated them, particularly the migraines and vomiting. I may require further surgery but currently I need help with my symptoms of painful & flooding periods, migraine, vomiting, unwanted hair growth, acne and depression as at the moment I don't have a life, I have to take a lot of time off work and I look five months pregnant for two weeks out of each month. I am looking for better control of my symptoms. **❞**

Natalie's condition is incurable. Since her first surgery at 20 years for the haemorrhagic ovarian cyst, her condition continued to deteriorate. Her GP prescribed progesterone treatment which had adverse effects and failed to stop the monthly symptoms. In addition, it managed to aggravate Natalie's acne, weight gain and nausea. She stopped the treatment and was referred to a surgeon who specialized in laparoscopic surgery for women with her condition and was considered to be one of the best around. He assured her that she could expect at least a 2 year remission from symptoms, and at best a 5 year remission, although he indicated that her chances of remaining symptom-free would be increased if she could take some form of hormonal treatment.

Natalie was very hopeful and saw that her surgeon's end point was very closely aligned with her own and therefore she opted to go with this treatment with careful monitoring.

Natalie's journey road map

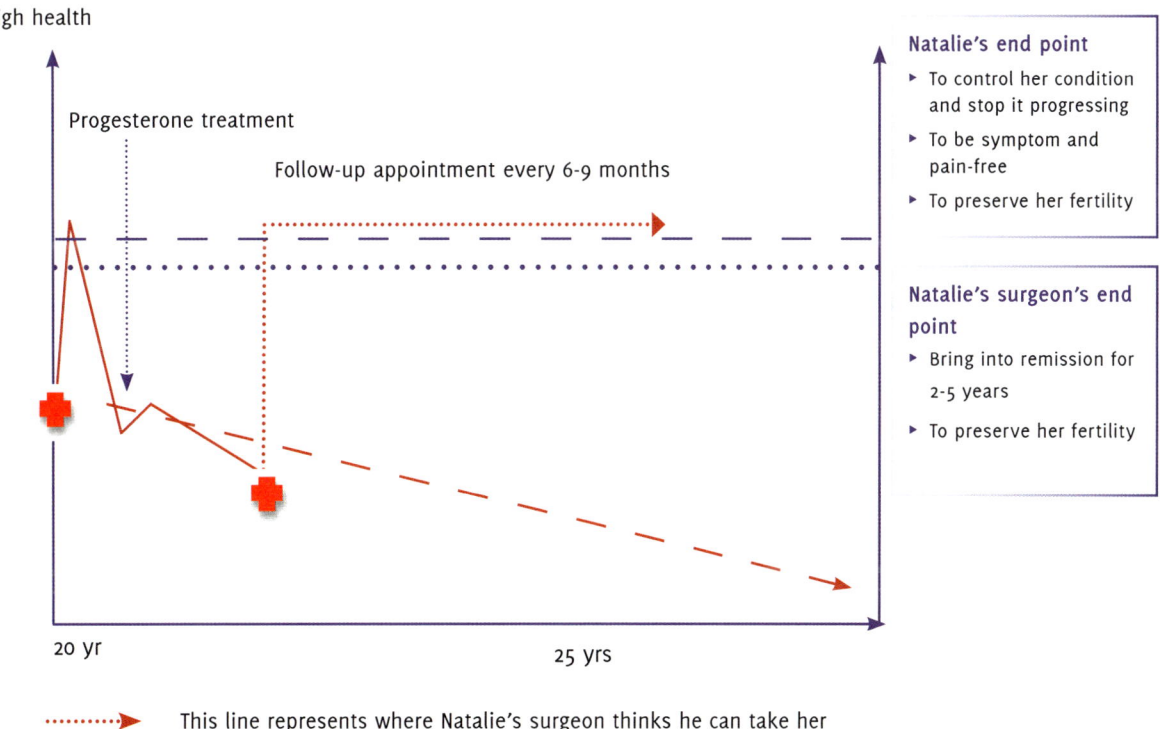

High health

Progesterone treatment

Follow-up appointment every 6-9 months

Natalie's end point
▸ To control her condition and stop it progressing
▸ To be symptom and pain-free
▸ To preserve her fertility

Natalie's surgeon's end point
▸ Bring into remission for 2-5 years
▸ To preserve her fertility

20 yr   25 yrs

······▸ This line represents where Natalie's surgeon thinks he can take her

Tips on prediction lines

▸ Make sure that any prediction lines relate to your aspirational end point and not to your goals. Goals are what you may need to achieve in order to get to your end point, and they will be prioritized. Remember, many goals make a match, but the individual goals are not the match themselves.

▸ If you have a chronic condition then draw a prediction line representing *where my doctor or medical specialist can take me* and use this as a benchmark against which you can monitor your actual progress against time.

▸ Use this line to compare your progress if you choose to reject medical treatment in favour of other treatments, or if you are going to take the recommended treatment but try to improve your outcome using adjunct treatments. It then becomes a useful tool to compare and measure the value of other treatments in getting you to your end point.

▸ I would recommend that you draw a prediction line *where will I be if I don't do your treatment?* This is useful as it will highlight your potential risks relating to your condition and you can be doubly sure of making an informed decision. If the doctor indicates specific risks if you don't take treatment, then you should plot these on your road map.

▸ Use the prediction line *if I don't take treatment* to compare your actual progress should you decide not to take conventional treatment. You can then evaluate which direction you are heading and change course should you need to. This is particularly useful if you have been given a window of opportunity to see if you can make a difference before taking conventional treatment.

▸ If other allied or alternative practitioners can make a prediction of where you will end up and within what time frame on their treatment, then you can draw these lines in also.

▸ Generally, each practitioner will concentrate on the specific aspect of your case that is within their area of expertise and therefore may be more goal-orientated. Under these circumstances you need to ensure that you match the value of their treatment against your end point (how far they can take you) and not simply against your goals.

▸ Make sure you enter way points against your time line as these will determine when you need to monitor your progress.

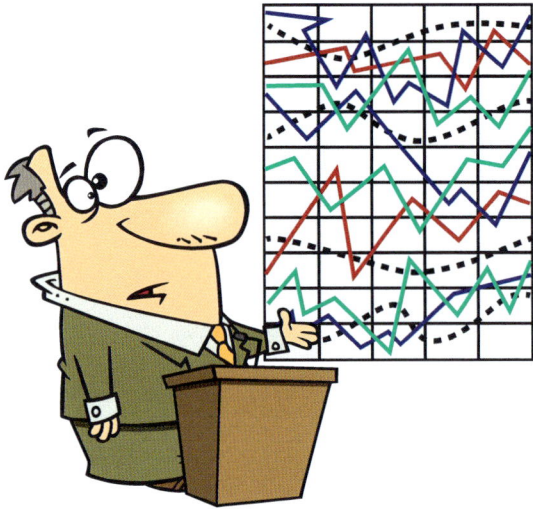

The end point is the match: many goals make a match, but are not the match themselves.

Rating each therapy

After your initial appointment with each practitioner you can fill out your *Therapy Alignment Rating Template* (below & p233). This template simply matches the therapy's end point (What is its end point?) to your end point (How does it align to my end point?) so that you can score each practitioner according to how far they can take you to your end point.

If you have taken your *Therapy Alignment Template* (pp83, 232) to your consultation you will have confirmed which goals the practitioner may be able to help you with and how they will monitor progress. You can use this template to help you fill in the Therapy Alignment Rating Template.

Next you will rate each practitioner: practitioners who address the causes, the most immediate risks, or your high/medium risk goals will score the most highly.

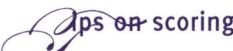

Tips on scoring

▸ therapies that address the causes will take you the furthest and will score highly;

▸ therapies that deal with your immediate risks will also score highly;

▸ therapies that can help with your high priority goals will score highly;

▸ therapies that promise no measurable benefits/results (either subjective or objective) that relate to your end point will not score well; and

▸ therapies that cannot be monitored for progress that relates to your end point will not score well.

Therapy Alignment Rating Template

Therapy	What is it	What is its end point?	How does it align to my end point?	Rating

Follow the tips for completing the *Therapy Alignment Rating Template* on the next page and look to see how Pauline has filled hers in, and then fill yours in rating each treatment.

Once you have done this go to the *Full Alignment Template (p224)* and enter the name of each therapy in the therapy column next to the goals it will address. These goals will already be aligned to an end point so it is easy to see how each therapy may support your journey.

Next enter prediction lines on *My Journey Road Map* (as Pauline and Natalie have done; see also p184) which will represent how far each practitioner can take you in terms of your end point. It is useful to add the practitioner's end point to each graph so that you are clear as to where they are heading and you can get some idea of how aligned they may be to your own end point.

Tips on completing the Therapy Alignment Rating Template

Therapy	What is it?	What is its end point?	How does it align to my end point?	Rating
List each proposed therapy	State what each therapy offers. This will be a general appraisal of the therapy and will not specifically relate to your condition. For example, imagine if someone was to ask you what acupuncture was, you wouldn't go into a lengthy explanation of your condition, you would just say what the therapy was (it is a method that....) in order to (.......[rebalance energetic disturbances])	This is the goal of treatment or the direction it can take you. It will relate to what it can achieve regarding your specific condition. Some therapies will address specific goals/symptoms that you may have. If you need clarity on where each practitioner is heading, just ask each practitioner of each therapy what their goal is in your specific case, or what they hope to achieve *(where can you take me, what symptoms will you fix?)*.	Return to your aspirational end points and match each therapy's end point against one or more of your end points *(in principle, will the therapy take me in the right direction?)*. Again, this is a general statement but it ensures that you do not lose sight of your own end point. If one of your goals is particularly significant to your progress, you may wish to enter it here also *(what will the therapy help me achieve and within what time frame?)*.	Score each therapy 1-10, Those that are most closely aligned to your end point will score the most highly. The purpose of rating each therapy is so that you can prioritize the therapies that offer you the most promise in helping you get to your end point *(how far can you take me?)*. Be cautious about therapies that can't be monitored or those that offer you no measurable value that relates to your end point or goals. These therapies operate on "trust" and without being able to monitor progress you will have no idea on which direction they are taking you - whether beneficial or counter-productive.

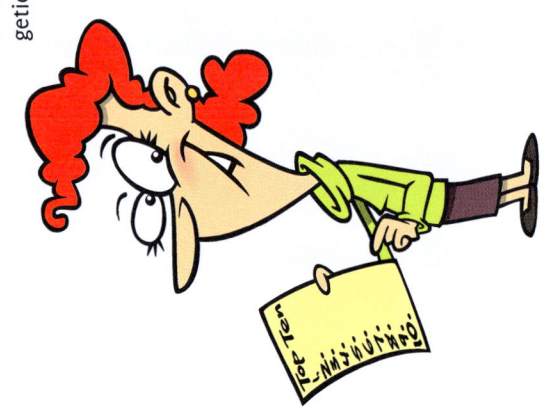

Pauline's Therapy Alignment Rating Template

Therapy	What is it?	What is its end point? *in relation to my condition*	How does this align to my end point?	Rating
Rheumatology	Addresses rheumatic conditions using pharmaceutical drugs; uses medical tests for diagnosis & monitoring.	To suppress inflammation, control disease progression and treat acute exacerbations with drugs.	Get me into remission, fast Act if I deteriorate or condition becomes acute Reduce long-term risks of inflammation Monitor, order tests	9
General Practice	Address conditions using pharmaceutical drugs; uses medical tests for diagnosis & monitoring.	Control chronic and acute symptoms with drugs.	Monitor, order tests, refer if condition becomes acute	5
Diet therapy	Promotes general health and addresses health conditions using diet.	Restore nutritional status, improve digestion, identify food allergy/intolerance that could worsen my condition; improve energy, gain weight.	Will improve general health and reduce health risks (anaemia, increase weight, osteoporosis) May help with remission	8
Traditional Chinese Medicine (herbs & acupuncture)	Uses acupuncture, herbs and dietary advice to resolve energetic imbalances which underpin disease.	To reduce inflammation, restore menses and improve digestion; reduce side effects of drugs.	May alleviate symptoms May alleviate side effects of drugs May help reduce drug dependency Support in disease management, remission	8
Physiotherapy	Uses physical methods to restore functional ability to help mobility.	To restore mobility, reduce pain and improve muscle, tendon and ligament strength, and help increase bone density.	May help reduce my pain Improve my mobility Reduce risk of osteoporosis	6

Scoring rationale:

Pauline has given the top score to the rheumatologist as she has found that no other therapy can reduce the degree of inflammation in the short period. However, she realizes that unless she takes steps to improve her general health and reduce some of her risks she may end up becoming drug-dependent. She also needs to make good any nutritional deficiencies (iron for her anaemia and vitamin D for her bones), and also increase her weight in order to increase her chances of improving her fertility. She has found a TCM practitioner who can prescribe herbs which will help reduce some of the side-effects of the corticosteroids and may also enable her to reduce the drugs and increase her chance of long-term remission. Next Pauline rates her physiotherapist who is able to design an exercise regime to improve joint mobility and increase muscle strength. At this stage of the journey her rating for her GP is marginal, however, he plays a key role in the medical system and would be Pauline's first port of call should the steps she has put in place fail or should she suffer a relapse.

By placing each therapy next to the goals they can help with (which also indicates how they align with Pauline's end point) it's easy to see where each practitioner fits and what leg of the journey they can help Pauline on. It's obvious that the rheumatologist may not have a long-term involvement in the case but may be important at the start of the journey or if Pauline relapses; the physiotherapist will be instrumental while Pauline is gaining mobility; the TCM practitioner (Traditional Chinese Medicine) may have a longer-term involvement to help with fertility and increasing Pauline's chances of long-term remission without drugs but ultimately, as Pauline would like to be product, treatment and drug independent, then her diet therapist is likely to accompany her for most of her journey ensuring that she can maintain her health with lifestyle changes and a dietary program that meets her needs and will not exacerbate her condition. (See also *Pauline's Journey Road Map* on p184.)

Prioritized list of goals (measurables)	End point alignment	Therapy
reduce inflammation	‣ remission, reduce future health risks	‣ rheumatology ‣ TCM ‣ diet therapy
restore mobility	‣ reduce future health risks (osteoporosis)	‣ physiotherapy
resolve digestive problems	‣ remission, reduce future health risks	‣ diet therapy ‣ TCM
gain weight	‣ fertility, reduce future health risks	‣ diet therapy
restore menses	‣ fertility (get pregnant)	‣ TCM ‣ diet therapy
improve bone density	‣ reduce future health risks (osteoporosis)	‣ diet therapy ‣ physiotherapy
improve energy	‣ reduce future health risks	‣ diet therapy
restore nutritional status	‣ reduce future health risks	‣ diet therapy

Pauline's condition:

‣ *Symptoms &/or diagnosis:* inflammation in the joints, skin and eyes from autoimmune conditions, amenorrhoea, fatigue, digestive problems, anaemia, underweight, osteopaenia, iron & vitamin D deficiencies

‣ *Future health risks:* immobility, impaired vision, increased risk of other autoimmune conditions, osteoporosis

‣ *Risk factors:* unremitting inflammation, poor diet, poor digestion, possible food allergy/intolerance, nutritional deficiencies, alcohol, stress, low weight, no exercise

Pauline's destination end points:

‣ remission;

‣ be drug-free; and

‣ reduce future health risks.

Pauline's Full Alignment Template

WHY	NOW		FUTURE HEALTH RISKS
Causes/Risks	**Tests**	**Diagnosis**	**Prognosis**
▲ gender (female)	Medical	▲ rheumatoid arthritis	▲ Lose mobility
▲ age	▲ blood test	▲ iritis	▲ Impaired eyesight
▲ inherited predisposition	▲ eye test	▲ osteopaenia, vit D deficiency	▲ Osteoporosis
▲ inflammatory condition can cause anaemia	▲ X-rays	▲ anaemia (iron deficiency)	▲ General deterioration of health
▲ low weight can cause anovulation	▲ bone densitometry	▲ amenorrhoea	▲ Infertility
▲ lack of exercise (osteoporosis)		▲ psoriasis	▲ Develop other autoimmune conditions
▲ stress			
▲ alcohol			
▲ dietary deficiencies			
▲ dietary intolerance/allergy			

Non-medical		
End Point		
▲ remission		
▲ become drug-free		
▲ reduce future health risks		

Symptoms &/or diagnostics	Prioritized list of goals (measurables)	End point alignment	THERAPY
▲ pain & stiffness in joints	reduce inflammation	▲ remission, reduce future health risks	▲ rheumatology, diet therapy, TCM
▲ inflammation in eyes, skin	restore mobility	▲ reduce future health risks (osteoporosis)	▲ physiotherapy
▲ no periods	resolve digestive problems	▲ remission, reduce future health risks	▲ diet therapy, TCM
▲ underweight	gain weight	▲ fertility, reduce future health risks	▲ diet therapy
▲ fatigue, anaemic	restore menses	▲ fertility (get pregnant), reduce future health risks (osteoporosis)	▲ TCM, diet therapy
▲ low bone density	improve bone density	▲ reduce future health risks (osteoporosis)	▲ diet therapy, physiotherapy
▲ mineral & vitamin deficiencies	improve energy	▲ reduce future health risks	▲ diet therapy
	restore nutritional status	▲ reduce future health risks	▲ diet therapy

My journey Road Map: where will each practitioner take me?

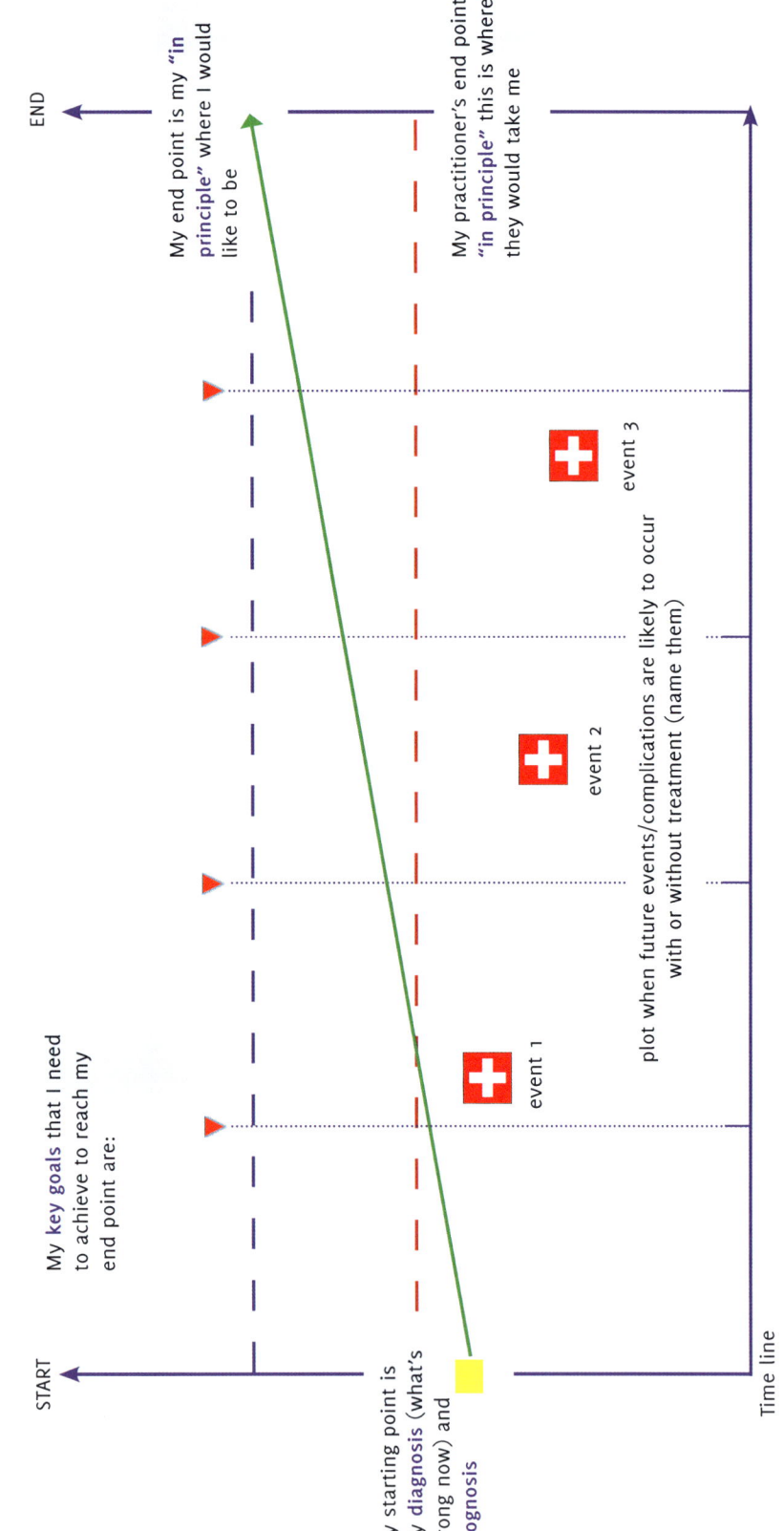

START

My key goals that I need to achieve to reach my end point are:

My starting point is my diagnosis (what's wrong now) and prognosis

event 1

event 2

event 3

plot when future events/complications are likely to occur with or without treatment (name them)

Time line

END

My end point is my "in principle" where I would like to be

My practitioner's end point "in principle" this is where they would take me

▶ Way points for monitoring progress

Fostering Collaboration

Collaboration is fundamental to getting you to where you want to go

My advice is that you choose practitioners that you can form a good working relationship with as you may need your practitioner to collaborate with others on your team, such as the sharing of records, test results or progress reports. It can all go sour when practitioners are dogmatic and unwilling to work with their patients or other practitioners, and vice versa when a patient does not respect the doctor's professional code, their medical responsibility and duty of care for the management of a case, or if they expect a practitioner to comment on and resolve issues that are outside of their field of expertise or that have been incurred by other practitioners involved on the case.

When conflict occurs patients can easily be put into the "too hard basket" and slip through the net. The best results are achieved with collaboration and in today's environment, where patients are looking to improve their outcome by using conventional treatment alongside alternative therapies, it is even more important to acknowledge these options or adjuncts as valid. Furthermore, patients who are active in trying to achieve better outcomes should be embraced by any fraternity.

However, there is an art to fostering collaboration: it can only be built on mutual trust and respect; it can only evolve when both parties are willing and the patient can demonstrate to each member of their team that they are making informed decisions that have been thoroughly investigated, and where they acknowledge and take responsibility for any of the risks involved.

Factoring in professional criteria

To cultivate respect within medical relationships you need to factor in any professional criteria of taking on and managing a patient. If you disregard this then you could run into insurmountable problems. Difficulties arise for patients when they are trying to manage their chronic condition by opting for more natural treatments that their doctor or specialist can't offer, or if they are implementing an integrative approach without informing their primary health care worker (usually their doctor) or giving sufficient information so that the doctor can understand the treatment and its potential impact on the case. Under these circumstances if the patient is asking their doctor to monitor their progress while they are on another therapy it may lead to a situation that is untenable for the doctor for reasons that are important for the patient to understand:

▸ they are professionally obliged to treat and monitor you in accordance with their own current medical guidelines;

▸ the doctor, as your primary health care worker, has a duty of care and a responsibility to fulfil this obligation. When a patient chooses not to follow conventional treatment or the recommendations of the doctor, but needs medical monitoring due to the chronic nature of their condition with its risk of acute or adverse events, then the doctor could run the risk of medical negligence if the condition deteriorates and an adverse event arises; and

▸ if the doctor does not understand the chosen treatment and what outcomes can be expected and within what time frame, they may consider the patient's request for monitoring unreasonable. They may also feel that they are being used simply to monitor, rather than for what they are professionally trained to do: to manage the patient's chronic condition with drugs.

This poses many problems for both the practitioner and the patient. A doctor, under most circumstances, would be reluctant to deny treatment or monitoring if there were sufficient medical grounds to justify making the request. The problem for the patient is that they may need their doctor's assistance for monitoring as there may be no other avenue for them to obtain the necessary requests or referrals. Monitoring is vital to the journey as patients need to know that they are travelling in the right direction so that they don't get caught on the back foot if a medical emergency arises.

So you need to remember these key points when working with your health professionals:

Each professional will:

- ▸ work within their field of expertise;
- ▸ prescribe treatment procedures/pathways endorsed by their medical body & based within their field of expertise;
- ▸ recommend treatment based on medical risk/ benefit criteria which has been endorsed by their medical body; and
- ▸ follow procedures for monitoring their own treatments endorsed by their medical body.

Your role

As you will be in the driving seat it falls on you to determine the value of each pathway offered in terms of what the therapy addresses and where it will take you, along with time frames for monitoring progress and the risks involved. If a pathway promises measurable outcomes then you need to provide these details to other health professionals along with an explanation of why you have opted for that therapy. From here you can work out a clear strategy for monitoring.

What may not go down too well is if you ask a practitioner to comment on, or help you decide on a range of treatments, particularly if these are outside their field of expertise and you have little or no supporting evidence to offer. In other words, it pays to do the research and seek clarification from a practitioner who has sufficient expertise on that treatment. You can then be discriminative about the merits of each treatment and how they would fit into your strategy and simply seek confirmation from other practitioners on your case that the treatment wouldn't conflict with their treatments that may be core to the case.

In the current climate of escalating chronic disease and with conventional treatment being unable to offer cure but only greater drug-dependency, medical professionals need to understand that it is not so much that patients rule out conventional strategies, as we all may have requirement for them at some stage in our lives, but simply that we are looking for an optimal outcome where we may need input from several practitioners. An integrative approach is valuable when each modality can offer something that the other cannot.

Avoid getting caught-in-the-web scenario

This situation occurs when you get conflicting advice from different practitioners on your case, who may either be from the same discipline or from different medical disciplines. The problem for the patient is how to determine who is correct, or which therapy/practitioner offers the most appropriate pathway for their individual case.

Stress for the patient

Problems arise when practitioners do not fully explain where they are taking the patient in terms of what outcome they can expect and within what time frame, or how much benefit the treatment will have for the patient after factoring in the full risks. The most that the patient can do under these circumstances is to seek enough clarification to satisfy their own criteria. However, it is not without considerable stress for the patient, particularly if they run the risk of getting a medical practitioner off-side, and especially one who is core to their case, experienced in their field and to whom they may need to return in the future.

Stress for the practitioner

Practitioners may also feel the stress when the patient appears to be on board with the strategy, where they are in agreement with the diagnosis and they feel that the practitioner can get them to their end point, but there are aspects of the strategy that they may wish to tweak. For example, they may have read from various sources a slightly different application of the therapy. The patient may want the practitioner to either comment on this, or to justify their stance. If the practitioner feels that the changes or "tweaking" could be counter-productive, send the patient in the opposite direction or slow their progress they may indicate this, or if the changes are marginal they may embrace these and see how the patient fares.

However, it is rarely that simple as what the patient may really require is a detailed explanation on a medical or scientific topic in order to be able to understand the ramifications within the context of their own case, which falls outside the practitioner's role or scope of diagnosis, interpretation and treatment recommendations. The practitioner may begin to feel like a car salesman who has already recommended what they feel is the best form of transport, but is suddenly asked to open the bonnet, go through all the mechanical details, and then make adjustments to main parts of the engine which they know, through experience, will reduce the performance of the vehicle.

Once you go down this track there may be no easy meeting ground and at the end of the day decisions on moving forward (by both parties) are determined by the level of respect and trust that is fostered by both sides. However, patients need to be mindful that a health professional has the right to refuse a case when their recommendations are either rejected or if they believe that the chosen pathway/changes are detrimental to the overall case.

Practitioner bias

Situations also arise when a practitioner is biased against another modality that a patient wants to incorporate into their strategy. This may have far-reaching implications on the practitioner-patient relationship, particularly if the practitioner is basing their recommendations on hearsay, prejudice or rational ignorance (sounds good but not based on fact) rather than clinical experience or a working knowledge of the therapy they are commenting on.

Under these circumstances the patient will have to weigh up the advice accordingly, do further research around the validity of the statements made and then rate the value of that advice.

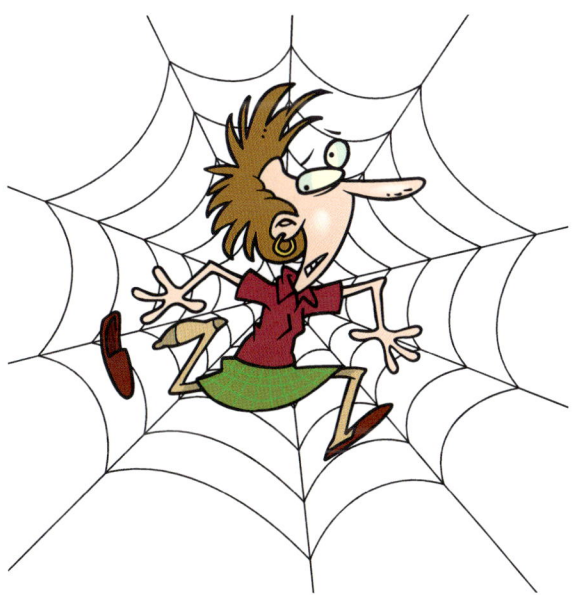

End note

In collaboration you need to remember there is a big difference between seeking *clarification* and *qualification*.

Clarification is simply making sure of key details which may cover:

- that you have grasped the recommendations correctly;
- that the treatment can be monitored (when and how);
- which aspect of the case the therapy or treatment/s align with (goals, end point, reducing risks);
- the time frame within which you may see improvements, and what these may be; and
- any known risks of treatment for the individual case.

Qualification implies a requirement for proof or justification which is another kettle of fish and needs to be undertaken diplomatically. On the one hand it is legitimate to seek qualification that the recommended therapy or treatment works, either from a statistical or clinical evidence position but, as you have seen, it is easy to breach the professional line where you are questioning the expertise of the health professional and asking them to justify their stance. So you need to be mindful of this and try to keep your main questions on seeking clarification.

When you are going through the therapy alignment module, remember that you are choosing from a range of therapies that may each have inherent value in your case and you will be rating them according to how important (core) they are in getting you to your end point. Try not to become waylaid in the ins and outs of the finer details of treatment at this stage, but wait until you have done the fundamental mapping or the "in principle" where will the therapy take me?

The principles of collaboration & negotiation

It's unlikely that you will find a practitioner who can tick all your boxes. For example, a practitioner may be kind, gentle and easy to talk to, but they may offer no overall value in helping you get to your end point. Alternatively, another practitioner may be curt and to the point, lack any bedside manner but what they can offer may be critical to your case.

In a paternalistic medical environment patients often forfeit the opportunity to be a key decision-maker in choosing treatment options, but in the new, evolving environment patients are seeking relationships of shared responsibility. Responsibility is the key word here and in order to take responsibility you need to make informed decisions against an understanding of your case.

It is how you, the patient, negotiate with your health specialists that will make or break relationships and increase or decrease the capacity for collaboration. So understanding your case and its risks, where you are trying to get to and the value of each treatment to your case, should form the basis of all your negotiations.

Collaboration and negotiation are two sides of the same coin: getting a meaningful outcome.

The flow chart below shows the relationships and key principles for collaboration and negotiation. Always bear these principles in mind when trying to establish working relationships for generating meaningful outcomes.

COLLABORATION

All parties must be:

Honest

Transparent

Outcome orientated

NEGOTIATION

Any negotiation must focus on achieving meaningful value:

to the end point; and/or

to a goal

MEANINGFUL OUTCOME

You need to understand and rate the value of each input and share your findings with others

"The doctor of the future will give no medicine, but will educate his patients in the care of the human frame, in diet, and in the cause and prevention of disease."

Thomas Edison 1847-1931

"There are three kinds of lies: lies, damned lies, and statistics."

Mark Twain 1835-1910

What treatments will offer me the most value?

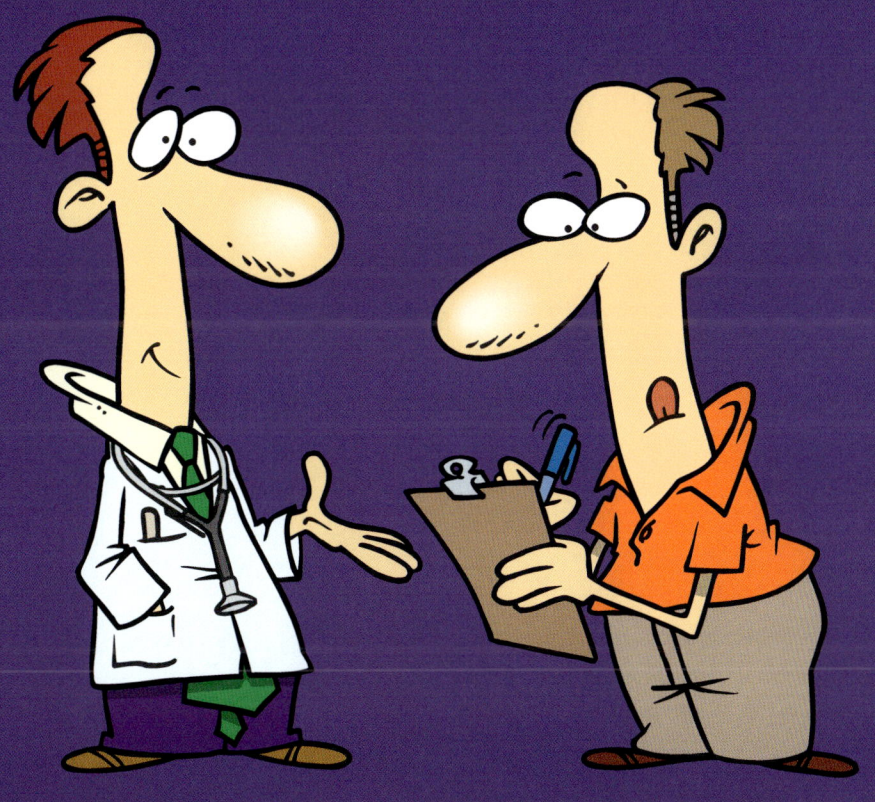

To do

1 Research treatments offered

Select a range of questions from *A conversational approach: what treatments can help me?*

Short list and prioritize those treatments that are core to getting you to your end point.

2 My benefit/risk assessment

Revisit *My Value Template* & select your measuring criteria.

Use the *SWOT analysis* and the *Quadrant chart* to help evaluate treatments.

3 Rate the value of each treatment to your end point

Complete the *Treatment Alignment Rating Template* to compare the value of each treatment.

Why do I need to make sense of the treatments?

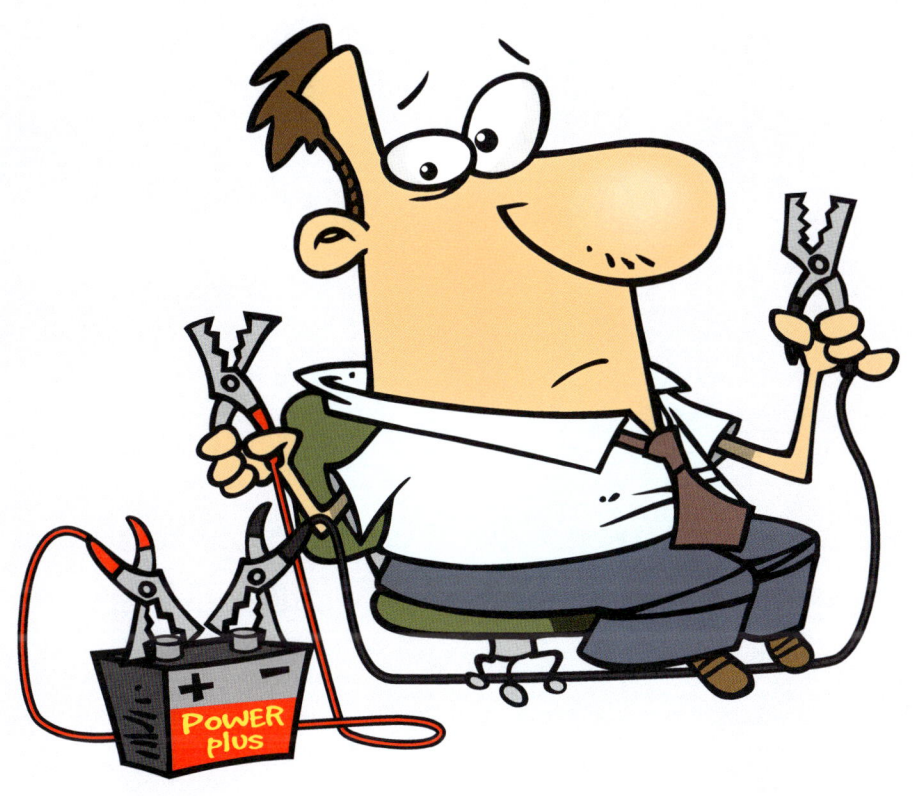

Because if you don't know how it works or what it treats,
you won't know how far it will take you.

"

I saw a naturopath about this time last year and had the live blood analysis test done which worked in conjunction with a supplement program. I decided to do it because I am hypoglycemic, always tired etc.

I wondered if I had a hormone imbalance. However, I didn't find the program that helpful really in that *it was very tailored to the program rather than the person*. In actual fact I felt worse than I did in the beginning.

Eventually I gave up before we got to the "liver and kidney part". It was also getting expensive.

"

1 Research treatments offered

*H*aving chosen a therapy or a range of therapies that are most aligned to your end point, you may now be in the unenviable position of being presented with a wide range of treatments or products that are recommended by the practitioner. You may feel that you need to ask about each treatment or product in order to determine what its specific value is to you, particularly if treatment is going to prove expensive and appears to offer only marginal or questionable value.

This is often where the nightmare begins, and without a framework to evaluate treatments for the individual case many people will come unstuck and may waste valuable time, energy and money on treatments that will take them nowhere (or worse still further away) and, by default, miss out on treatments that could be of more help.

If possible try to obtain an accurate diagnosis as this will indicate the cause. Treating the cause will take you the furthest. If you don't have a diagnosis you will either end up treating what you think the cause is or just the symptoms which can result in a hit and miss approach. If you don't know the cause, then you won't know what needs treating, what the treatment should be, or whether the treatments recommended are core to your case.

There are 3 key aspects to bear in mind when starting your evaluation process:

‣ A treatment needs to deliver *measurable* improvements within a given time frame. *What improvements can I expect and how soon?* Treatment may become a risk if it cannot deliver measurable benefits within a given time frame.

‣ A treatment needs to be *meaningful* in that it must align with and take you nearer to your end point. The most meaningful treatments are those which are *core* to your case; and

‣ You must be able to *factor in any risks* for the treatment particularly to your individual case: what you gain on the one hand you do not want to lose on the other.

Core treatments: are those that treat the cause, the greatest health risks, the risks and/or exacerbating factors - in that order. These treatments will take you the furthest toward your end point. Core treatments may also need to deliver results within a given time frame.

Adjunct treatments: treat secondary issues that are not core to the case, treat the side-effects of treatments or may be palliative. These treatments have inherent value but will NOT get you to your end point.

The framework for researching treatments

What will it do?
How does the treatment work?
What will the treatment achieve for me?

Is it high or low priority?
What aspect of my case will it treat?
(*core or adjunct*)

How long will it take?
When can I expect results?
How long will I be on treatment?

Benefit/Risk
Are there any risks of treatment?
Will the benefits outweigh the risks?

Where does my treatment fit?

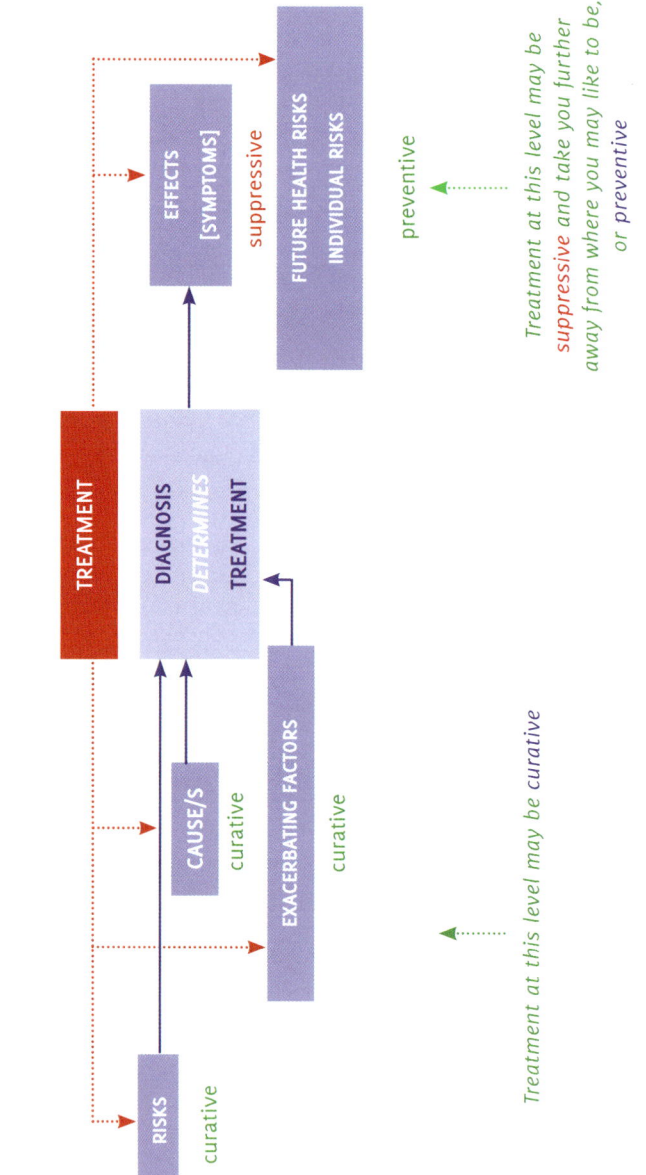

TREATMENT

RISKS
curative

CAUSE/S
curative

EXACERBATING FACTORS
curative

DIAGNOSIS
DETERMINES
TREATMENT

EFFECTS
[SYMPTOMS]
suppressive

FUTURE HEALTH RISKS
INDIVIDUAL RISKS
preventive

Treatment at this level may be curative

Treatment at this level may be suppressive and take you further away from where you may like to be, or preventive

If you don't know what your treatment does then you won't be able to monitor whether it's working.

Treating the symptoms: the band-aid approach

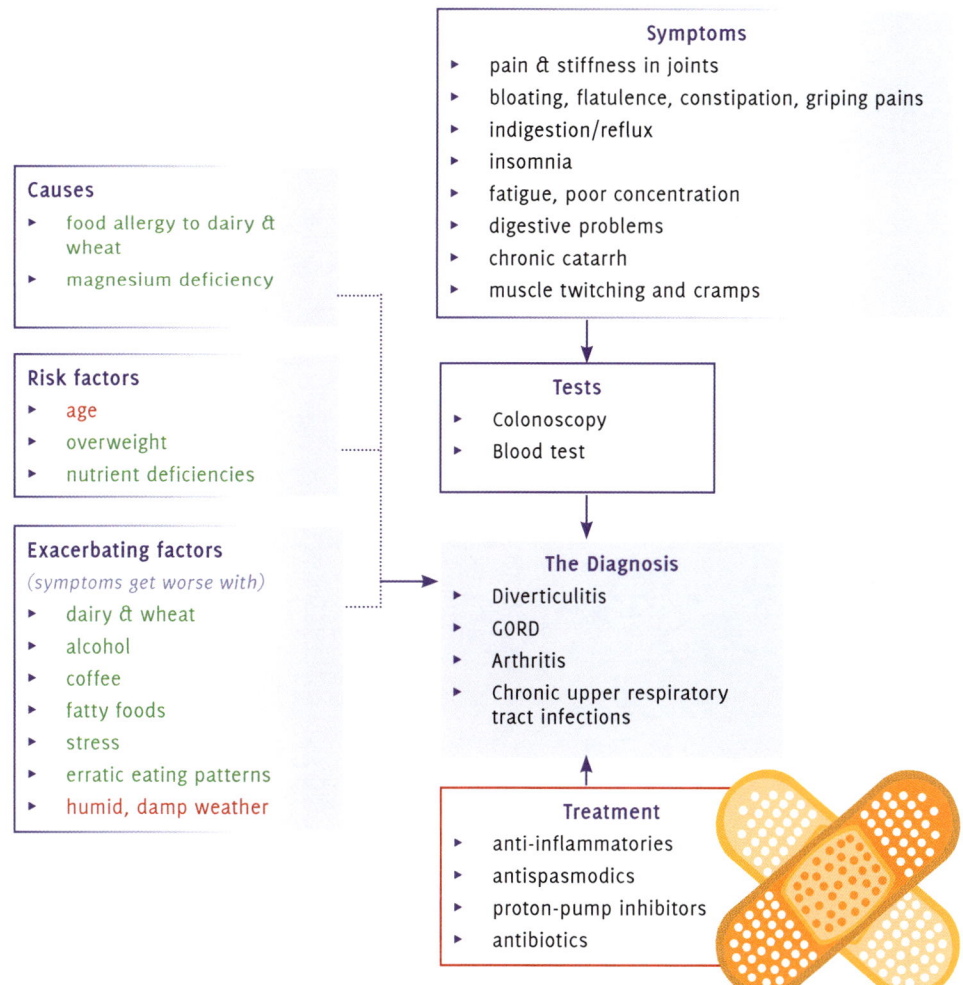

Symptoms
- pain & stiffness in joints
- bloating, flatulence, constipation, griping pains
- indigestion/reflux
- insomnia
- fatigue, poor concentration
- digestive problems
- chronic catarrh
- muscle twitching and cramps

Causes
- food allergy to dairy & wheat
- magnesium deficiency

Risk factors
- age
- overweight
- nutrient deficiencies

Exacerbating factors
(symptoms get worse with)
- dairy & wheat
- alcohol
- coffee
- fatty foods
- stress
- erratic eating patterns
- humid, damp weather

Tests
- Colonoscopy
- Blood test

The Diagnosis
- Diverticulitis
- GORD
- Arthritis
- Chronic upper respiratory tract infections

Treatment
- anti-inflammatories
- antispasmodics
- proton-pump inhibitors
- antibiotics

Graham was 51 yrs old. Three years previously he had been diagnosed with GORD (gastric oesophageal reflux disease), diverticulitis and arthritis. He was taking anti-inflammatory drugs for his arthritis, but these made the digestive problems worse, so he was prescribed a proton-pump inhibitor to reduce the amount of acidity his stomach produced. Since his teens he had been plagued with chronic sinus infections that had been treated with antibiotics, and at 39 years he had surgery on his septum (septoplasty) to try and resolve the problem. However, he was still suffering sinus problems and was prone to chest infections. Graham's current symptoms were reflux, indigestion, bloating, flatulence and constipation, heavy catarrh in the upper respiratory tract (lungs and sinuses), joint pain and insomnia. He was suffering from extremely low energy and poor concentration.

Graham's medical treatment focused on the symptoms. This is a band-aid approach. If he was to resolve his problems then he would need to address the causes, risk factors and exacerbating factors. In Graham's case it was fairly easy to determine the root of most of his problems: food intolerance, namely dairy and wheat. This had led to the chronic catarrh since childhood, the diverticulitis and digestive problems, and also his arthritis. Graham was surprised that his arthritis was so closely connected with the inflammation in his gut, but delighted to be drug-free, even though it meant a considerable lifestyle change in order to achieve this.

Flow Chart for Evaluating & Validating treatments -
steps 1 & 2

Step 1

Core or adjunct

Determine what the treatment does

▸ how does it work; and

▸ what aspects of my case does it treat.

Match the claims of treatment against your end point & goals to prioritize and determine the value of treatment.

Step 2

Measurable & meaningful

Determine how you will *measure* progress

▸ objective (tests, scans etc.)

▸ subjective (resolution of symptoms)

and how *meaningful* this will be to the overall case:

▸ which leg of my journey will it help with?

▸ how far will it get me to my end point?

If you can't monitor progress then there is no way of knowing the value of treatment.

Steps 1 & 2: To formulate your questions use *A Conversational Approach: what treatments can help me*; to formulate your criteria use *My Value Template* column 4 *Any practitioner/product/service must demonstrate a value in helping me with my journey* and *My Criteria for Evaluating Advice*. Complete your *Treatment Alignment Template*.

Step 5

Treatment alignment rating

Use *My Treatment Alignment Rating Template* and select the various treatments which may help, indicate how they may work/what they will do and what benefit they offer in helping you get to your end point. Make sure that the treatment can be monitored. Next rate each treatment and make your decision on which treatments will offer you the most value.

Step 3

Benefit/Risk assessment

Complete the *SWOT analysis* and the *Quadrant chart* when you need to factor in:

- ▸   the risks of treatment in your individual case;
- ▸   the risks of not doing treatment; or
- ▸   when the benefits of treatment are unknown.

These charts will facilitate decision-making when there is an absence of scientific proof or clinical data for a treatment, or when you need to make a decision based on a range of criteria which include how your condition and the potential treatment could affect your life. These charts are invaluable as they will provide a basis for collaboration and help clarify your position to all parties.

These charts can be completed with simple information provided at an appointment and require no medical expertise. They do not require reference to scientific data. The quadrant chart can be used as a visual platform to match the relative value of many therapies and/or treatments to the patient's end point.

Step 4

Scientific & Clinical Validation

Use *My value template* (column 4) to select your own criteria for validating treatments. Then use the simple steps from the *Evaluating scientific evidence* chart to determine how appropriate the treatment is to your case and its potential value in getting you to your end point.

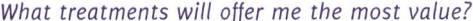

A conversational approach:
what treatments can help me?

QUESTIONS	What value are your treatments to me?	Research: Is the treatment suitable for me?
Why ask these questions?	You need to know how effective the treatment will be in your case or how far it will get you to your end point.	You need to know the risks of the treatment and if there are any additional individual risks for you.
Questionnaire Guide	<ul><li>How does the treatment work? (scientific basis)</li><li>What aspect of my case will it treat? (cause, risk factors, symptoms)</li><li>In your clinical experience how effective do you think this treatment will be for me? (clinical outcome/what are my odds?)</li><li>Within what time frame will I see an improvement?</li><li>Will the improvement last and how long will it last?</li><li>How long will I need to be on this treatment?</li><li>Will you be able to monitor my progress and, if so, how will you do this and how frequently?</li></ul>	<ul><li>Is the treatment recommended appropriate for my condition/symptoms?</li><li>Does the treatment match my profile?</li><li>Are there any specific contraindications for the treatment that would apply to me?</li><li>Are there any health risks for the treatment, both in the short and long-term and, if so, what are they and how great are those risks?</li><li>Are there any side-effects/adverse reactions and, if so, what would these be and how would we monitor for them?</li><li>Could this treatment fail in my case (produce little or no response) or is there any chance that it could worsen my condition?</li></ul>

Professional criteria

- to only prescribe treatment procedures endorsed by their medical body and based within their field of expertise;
- to recommend treatment based on medical risk/benefit criteria which may not factor in long-term or individual risks, or a range of variables that have not been scientifically proven;
- to follow procedures for monitoring treatment, the results of which may not have a bearing on the patient's overall clinical condition; and
- to prescribe only the products from their own retail range.

If you use the questions provided to give yourself a head start, then from here you can use the internet to further your research on treatments, their benefits and risks and any individual risk that the treatment may carry for you. There are many good websites and a wealth of health forums for you to find out what has worked for others with your condition.

You need to be mindful that each professional will be working within their own field of expertise and may be required to follow treatment procedures as laid out by their governing body. From a medical perspective frustration may arise on both sides due to a medical stance that may rely heavily on statistical evidence from clinical trials rather than the clinical outcome for the individual patient. On the other hand, the doctor may show concern if there is a lack of scientific evidence to support other options which the patient may favour. However, if you, as the patient, do due diligence using this framework for all treatments then you can show your road map and demonstrate to each practitioner that you are making informed decisions.

As you will be receiving advice from each practitioner, not only on your case but also for the treatments they prescribe, it is best if you can determine at the outset your own criteria for evaluating their general advice and the value of each treatment. In order to help you, you may choose your criteria from column 4 Any practitioner/product/service must demonstrate a value in helping me with my journey of *My Value Template (pp122, 226-227)* and from *My Criteria for Evaluating Advice (p123)*.

If a practitioner is offering you a range of treatments for a single condition, then it is important to clarify what aspect of the condition each treatment is addressing. For example, you may be offered two treatments that deal with two different symptoms relating to the same condition. For each treatment offered you need to do a separate evaluation as each may come with its own inherent risks.

From this interview you should be able to gain sufficient information to understand how the treatment works, what aspects of your case it will help and how far it will take you. You can also find out the potential risks of the treatment both in the long and short-term. If possible, plot a line on your journey road map that predicts where each treatment could take you and within what time frame.

My Value Template

will help me filter out all the things that will not work for me so I can look more closely at what might work best for me

Any choice of treatment must work for me

Any choices must fit my life-style

Any choices must fit with my own values & convictions

Any practitioner/product/service must demonstrate a value in helping me with my journey

Prerequisites

Clinical outcome

Time frame

Cost

Capacity to embrace lifestyle changes

My stance on medicinal treatments

Religion &/or culture

Level of expertise in treating my condition

Proof that it works/how far it will take me

Be able to monitor treatment

Criteria for measuring value

Clinical outcome / Time frame

Cure
Reversal of condition
Remission/slow the disease process
Longer survival
Improved health/recovery potential
Maintain my health
Give me better quality of life
Reduce exacerbating factors (list these)
Reduce risks associated with my condition & prognosis (list these)
Reduce future health risks associated with my condition (list these)
Reduce drug/product dependency
Be symptom-free (name these)
Improved symptom-management/symptom relief (name these)
Specific goals: eg. to increase my fertility, reduce weight etc.

Must work within my time frame

Cost / Capacity to embrace lifestyle changes

Cost (within my specified budget)
I need to be able to do at home
It must fit with my family
I can travel for treatment
I must be able to carry on working/education
I can take time off work
I have no physical impairments
I have physical impairments
I require a specific diet
I can change my diet
I can make lifestyle changes (name these)

My stance on medicinal treatments / Religion &/or culture

natural/nontoxic only
conventional treatment only
integrative (both conventional & alternative)

my religion &/or culture forbids specific treatments (name these)

Level of expertise / Proof / Be able to monitor treatment

Must be experienced in my condition
Must have success in treating my condition
Must be able to collaborate with other practitioners

clinical proof
scientific proof
anecdotal
faith-based
makes sense that it could help
indicate how far it will it take me
be core to my case
the benefits must outweigh the risks

Must be able to monitor results objectively (what my tests say)
Must be able to monitor results subjectively (how I feel)

My Criteria for Evaluating Advice

Here is a range of criteria for measuring advice or opinions on treatment. Choose from this list your own criteria for measuring the validity of any advice. This will help you rapidly filter through any advice or opinion at the outset.

▸ Any advice must be based on the person's/practitioner's clinical *experience*

▸ Any person/practitioner offering advice must have sufficient *working knowledge* of the treatment/topic that they are commenting on

▸ I will accept advice based on *trust*

▸ I will accept advice that *"something is better than nothing"*

▸ I will accept an opinion *"to be on the safe side"* by a medical professional

▸ I will accept advice on the basis *"it makes sense to me"*

▸ I will accept *"try this and see"* as feasible advice or recommendation

It can be very difficult for a patient to see the wood from the trees when the advice given is emphatic. However, decisions rarely have to be made on the spot and there is usually always time to deliberate and do your own research. However, you can short circuit your research if you can find out what's behind the advice, or what it's based on. For example, a patient may receive advice to try a treatment and find that the person giving the advice is not qualified to do so, or if they are qualified they may be recommending it because they *don't know what else to suggest*, or on the basis that *something is better than nothing*. Further investigation of what the treatment is for/how it works and what you can expect can easily validate the advice, or not!

On the other hand, a practitioner may forbid a specific treatment that you want to try as an adjunct. You may have investigated the treatment and found that it has merit and that you are not willing to forfeit the treatment

without understanding why. Upon questioning you may find that the opinion is based on *professional prejudice*, or that there is scientific or even clinical evidence which indicates that the treatment is either of no use or incompatible with your core treatment. Equally, the practitioner may be concerned that the treatment could *conflict with their treatment*, but they have no proof of this, but want *to be on the safe side*. You will then need to make up your own mind. Invariably, medical practitioners may be opposed to natural treatments when they need to be on the safe side or if they feel that the patient is placing too much emphasis on the claims or capability of the treatment.

All in all, if a treatment is known to address the cause or a main risk or exacerbating factor, and improvements can be measured, then it should not be discarded on the basis of prejudice or ignorance.

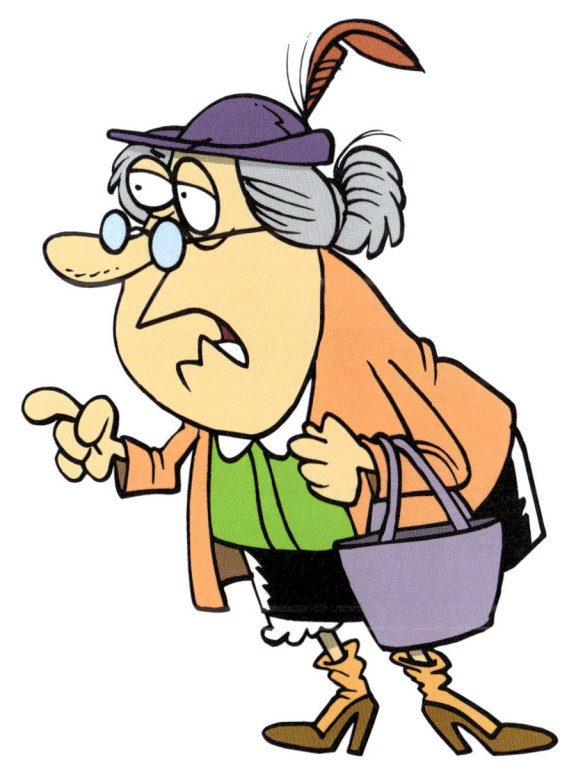

Case study: conflicting advice

Geraldine was 42 years old when she was hospitalized with acute cholecystitis. An ultrasound revealed that her gallbladder was distended and inflamed and contained multiple small stones (<3mm) and lots of biliary sludge.

Geraldine tailored her already good organic diet and took some natural treatments. A follow-up ultrasound six weeks later revealed that although there was still some inflammation in the gallbladder, there were no stones or sludge. The medical advice was that her gallbladder should be removed as she would continue to get acute crises and her condition would worsen. Geraldine was hoping to continue with her dietary and herbal treatment to see if she could continue to improve her situation as she wanted to avoid surgery, if possible. We prepared the following questions:

1. In your expert opinion how soon do you think I could have another gallbladder attack given my recent history and my reports?

2. What are my risks if I leave surgery for now? Could I:

▸   narrow my chances of being offered just this surgery if I have another flare-up/attack;

▸   risk having to have more extensive surgery; or

▸   risk a life-threatening or more chronic situation?

"The surgeon was very negative about my situation, and got quite cross with me for asking questions. He did not want to discuss it at all and only had one response, surgery and the sooner the better. He was going to schedule me in for one month's time, but I've put it off.

My doctor, when I saw her, thankfully was the complete opposite. She recommended not to have my gallbladder removed for a number of reasons including that my long term digestion may never be the same and she also didn't think it was urgent or life-threatening. She suggested that I work on my diet and see how I go - she was very supportive of my program and wants to monitor me every month to see how I'm going, including blood tests and an ultrasound of the gallbladder.

She wrote me a certificate so I now have time off to concentrate on my wellness regime! She also wanted to check that things were progressing well, so that if I have to have surgery I can have it while I'm on leave in a couple of months. I'm working really hard to improve my health situation."

Update: "I had 6 months of absolutely no pain and feeling great, and suddenly I had gone to the other extreme and couldn't even eat anything or do anything without pain. I had so many terrible attacks that I decided I had no option but to get my gallbladder out. The attacks were acute and came on within five minutes, usually from eating anything - it didn't have to be fatty. I couldn't even exercise I was so unwell. By the time I made my decision to have the removal, I was at peace with it. I felt that I had given it the best shot I could and knew that it was time to accept the removal of it and move forward. I met with my surgeon and explained how concerned I was about getting it out, and how worried I was about suffering from digestion issues etc. He was wonderful and explained in great detail how he would do the procedure so that he could ensure he didn't cut anything he shouldn't etc., and he was so nice and reassuring I felt I was in good hands. The best part was that he told me (without me asking anything) about how my gallbladder issue may have come about, and said that excess oestrogen or oestrogen dominance was assumed to be a contributing factor! (Apart from my doctor, everyone else had said this was ridiculous.)

I ran into the opposite when I made the decision to have it out. Most of the people who had originally wanted me to have it out were all for it and thought that it was about time, and the "alternative" people were full of more ideas of how I could save it and trying to convince me not to do it. I felt pressure in the opposite way! However, I knew it was right for me and that I had tried harder than most to avoid the operation.

I had the procedure and I'm pleased to say that it went fine. At first I looked in the jar they gave me and there were just a couple of tiny, sticky looking lumps (my "stones"). I felt that perhaps I shouldn't have had the operation, as I was still convinced that I could rid myself of all stones and sludge over time. However, the surgeon told me that my gallbladder was in a very bad way, it was the wrong colour and was extremely scarred. He said the duct was so mushed up and scarred that the bile wasn't getting through anymore, and despite trying for a long time he couldn't get his scope down it to check. I felt a little better in a way, and knew that even though I had fought hard to save my gallbladder, it had been too late to reverse the severe damage that had already occurred.

The good news is that I had spent 6 months working on myself and had lost nearly 18 kgs, my shape had changed and I felt fantastic once it was removed."

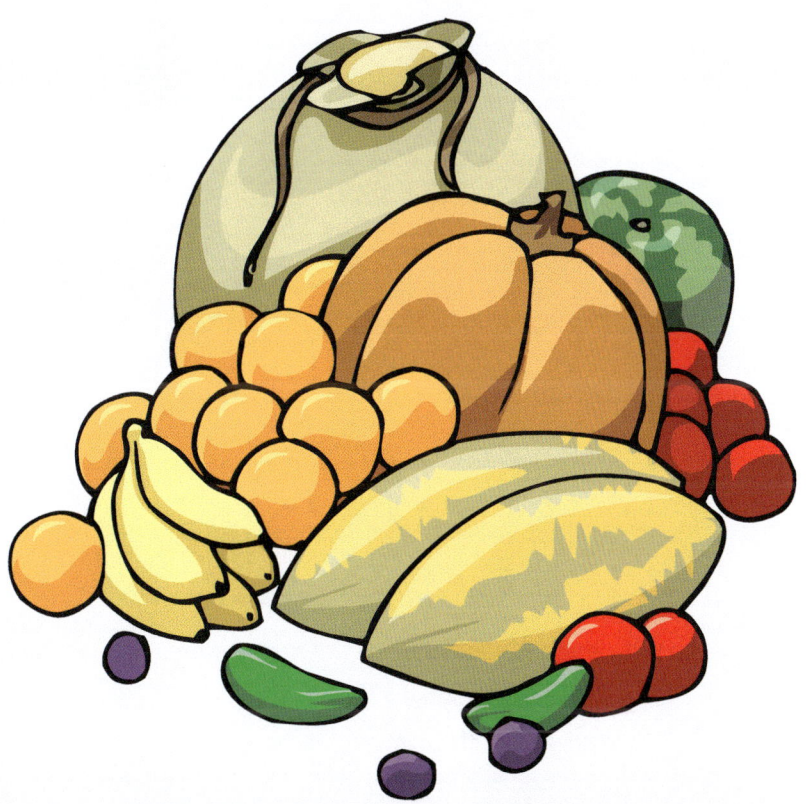

Treatment Alignment Template

TREATMENT	DRUGS (name of)	HERBS (name of)	SUPPLEMENTS (name of)	HOMOEOPATHIC (name of)	SURGERY
My aspirational end point					
List of prioritized goals					
Tests for monitoring					

This template enables you to do a quick cross check where you can try and match each treatment's claim against your end point and prioritized goals. By asking the right questions at your consultation you should be able to fill in the template fairly easily. Otherwise, you can research each of the recommended treatments and then seek further clarification from your practitioner. By doing this exercise you will discover which treatments will take you the furthest, or what leg of your journey they will help you on.

Add your aspirational end point criteria and your list of prioritized goals in the fields provided. Then place each treatment that has been recommended in the top row, one at the head of each column.

At your appointment don't forget to ask each practitioner how they will monitor progress to make sure that the treatment is working.

Pauline's treatment alignment template

TREATMENTS		Corticosteroids	Vitamin D / Iron	Diet therapy	TCM herbs	Physiotherapy
Pauline's end point	remission	✓		?	?	
	become drug-free			?	?	
	reduce future health risks		✓	✓	?	✓
List of prioritized goals	reduce inflammation	✓		✓	✓	
	restore mobility	✓			✓	✓
	resolve digestive problems			✓	✓	
	gain weight			✓		
	restore menses			✓	✓	
	improve bone density		✓ (D)	✓		✓
	improve energy		✓ (Iron)	✓		
	restore nutritional status		✓ (D, Iron)	✓		
Tests for monitoring	blood tests	✓	✓	✓		
	bone densitometry			✓		✓
	Pulse and tongue diagnosis				✓	

Pauline has done her research and confirmed what each treatment can do and how it works. She makes provisional ticks against her aspirational end points and sees that the corticosteroids offer the best hope of bringing her into remission quickly. She has been told that anti-inflammatory TCM herbs may be prescribed during the period when she is reducing the corticosteroids and they may offer her a longer remission period, but she may still be dependent on herbs if the cause of the condition is not addressed. Diet therapy addresses most of her goals and it will most certainly reduce her future health risks. Nutritional supplements will be good for addressing her iron and vitamin D deficiencies which will improve her anaemia (and hence her energy) and increase calcium uptake for bone density, respectively. Pauline has yet to factor in the risks of long-term corticosteroids.

Troubleshooting treatments

Your end point	▸ Assess whether the treatment is aligned with the direction you are heading (your "in principle" end point)
	▸ Work out what that alignment is
Your goals	▸ Find out which goal/s the treatment will address
	▸ Match its claims of what it can achieve and within what time frame
Your symptoms	▸ Find out how the treatment works and how it will address your symptoms
	▸ Find out whether it could create any new symptoms (side-effects)
Prioritized list	▸ Determine whether the treatment is core or adjunct. Treatments that address the cause or reduce your risks/exacerbating factors will take you the furthest
Benefit/Risk	▸ Make sure that the treatment does not conflict with other treatments, particularly core treatments
	▸ Make sure that any benefits outweigh the risks

Tips

▸ Make sure you are in agreement with the diagnosis and its causes (*what has caused the problem, what aggravates the problem*) as this will determine the treatment and your potential outcome.

▸ If you don't know the cause of your condition then identify a possible range of causes and select treatments based on these and monitor carefully.

▸ Research how a treatment works and what aspects of your case it claims to address (*core or adjunct*). For example, hormone treatment may claim to fix lethargy, but if the lethargy is not caused by an hormonal imbalance then it may not help or, worse still, could have inherent risks for your case.

▸ If a practitioner has not done a full case study then they may not be able to give an interpretation or factor in any inherent risks of treatment.

▸ Treatments that cannot deliver a measurable clinical improvement (what health improvements can I expect) or cannot be monitored should be discarded. Many treatments rely more on the science than clinical outcome.

▸ Treatments that assist with symptoms may be important, but may not get you to your end point.

▸ Testing and diagnostics are aligned to treatment if they can identify the cause or monitor the efficacy of treatment. Understand what each test is for, what it will show and how it can be interpreted in relation to your treatment (see p207).

Focus on the journey rather than the individual treatments
by aligning each treatment to your end point.

Why do I need to work out the risks of treatments?

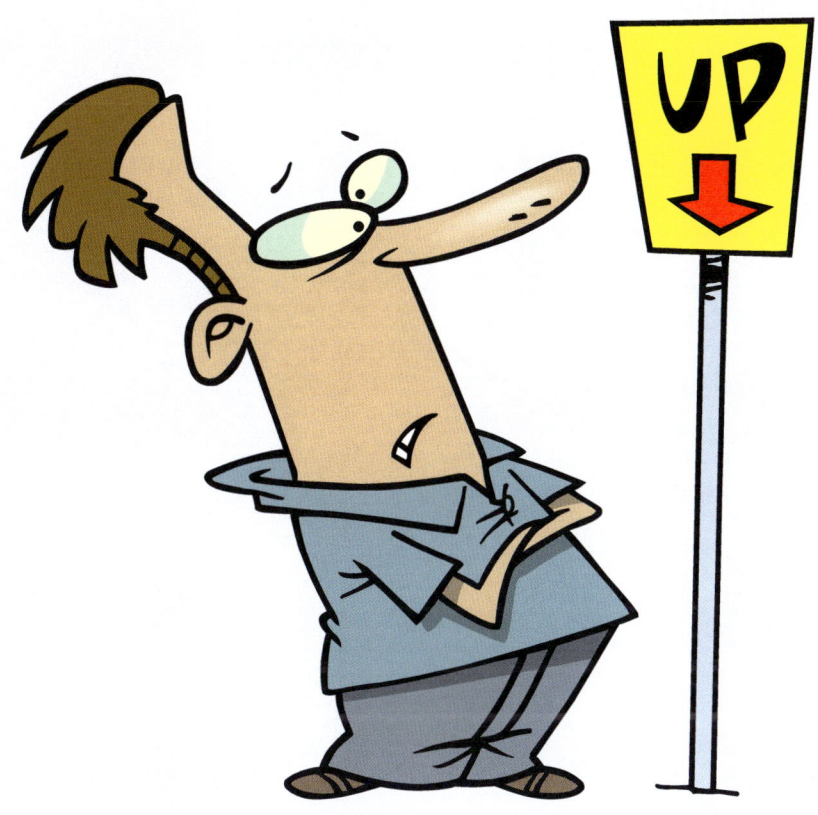

Because you have to make sure that what others
advise will take you to where you want to go.

Flow Chart for Evaluating & Validating treatments: step 3

Step 1

Core or adjunct

Determine what the treatment does

- how does it work; and
- what aspects of my case does it treat.

Match the claims of treatment against your end point & goals to prioritize and determine the value of treatment.

Step 2

Measurable & meaningful

Determine how you will *measure* progress

- objective (tests, scans etc)
- subjective (resolution of symptoms)

and how *meaningful* this will be to the overall case:

- which leg of my journey will it help with?
- how far will it get me to my end point?

If you can't monitor progress then there is no way of knowing the value of treatment.

Step 5

Treatment alignment rating

Use *My Treatment Alignment Rating Template* and select the various treatments which may help, indicate how they may work/what they will do and what benefit they offer in helping you get to your end point. Make sure that the treatment can be monitored. Next rate each treatment and make your decision on which treatments will offer you the most value.

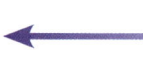

Step 3

Benefit/Risk assessment

Complete the *SWOT analysis* and the *Quadrant chart* when you need to factor in:

▸ the risks of treatment in your individual case;

▸ the risks of not doing treatment; or

▸ when the benefits of treatment are unknown.

These charts will facilitate decision-making when there is an absence of scientific proof or clinical data for a treatment, or when you need to make a decision based on a range of criteria which include how your condition and the potential treatment could affect your life. These charts are invaluable as they will provide a basis for collaboration and help clarify your position to all parties.

These charts can be completed with simple information provided at an appointment and require no medical expertise. They do not require reference to scientific data. The quadrant chart can be used as a visual platform to match the relative value of many therapies and/or treatments to the patient's end point.

Step 4

Scientific & Clinical Validation

Use *My value template* (column 4) to select your own criteria for validating treatments. Then use the simple steps from the *Evaluating scientific evidence* chart to determine how appropriate the treatment is to your case and its potential value in getting you to your end point.

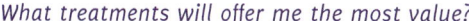

2 My Benefit/Risk Assessment:
the SWOT analysis & Quadrant Chart

The problem for most patients is that they don't automatically want to go where their medical practitioner wants to take them: they may not share the same criteria, they definitely do not see themselves as a statistic and, most importantly, they may not like their odds. However, when you're diagnosed with a serious health condition you can get trapped in a world of fear where it becomes impossible to make informed decisions particularly when the only choice that's put before you is the very one you don't want to have to face.

Patients can rarely comment on the statistics that are presented and may have no answer to a medical rationale that is too complex to grasp. However, no-one disputes that it is your body and that it is you that has to carry all the risks. So it pays to have a framework where you can make an informed decision without being a medical expert. The *SWOT analysis* and the *Quadrant Chart* are two frameworks which will help you in your decision-making and should also provide a platform for you to collaborate with any medical professional. Both of these charts will help you weigh up the risks of treatment versus the risks of the disease, as it is on this basis (or the risk of doing nothing) that decisions are often made.

The SWOT analysis

The SWOT analysis provides an opportunity for the patient to separate the two worlds: the objective medical perspective and their subjective world, or how their condition affects them on a day to day basis. Often choices are presented to patients using just medical criteria, such as statistical or scientific evidence, without taking into account any other criteria that the patient may hold. Patients with a chronic condition often find it difficult to make decisions purely on statistical evidence particularly if that treatment cannot offer cure but only long-term drug-dependency and all the inherent risks that this brings.

SWOT stands for **S**trengths, **W**eaknesses, **O**pportunities & **T**hreats.

The *strengths & weaknesses* columns will refer to the medical benefit/risk analysis for the specific treatment recommended, according to medical criteria. You may also need to factor in any individual risks based on your case. Risks are either due to any potential side-effects of the treatment (which could cause related or new conditions that you may be predisposed to) or because you have another condition which is a contraindication for the treatment.

The *opportunities & threats* columns will determine how the treatment measures up to your personal aspirations and how much it may negatively impact or positively improve your quality of life. This is where you reference any individual risks for treatment which may not be reflected in the purely objective statistical approach. This approach also helps patients when they are trying to make a decision between different treatment options. By completing a SWOT analysis for each treatment patients can judge according to the opportunities and threats that each option delivers. Generally patients decide on the merits of treatment and whether the opportunities outweigh the threats according to their own criteria of what is important.

So the SWOT analysis provides a way for the two worlds to meet: the specialist's world of benefit/risk assessment dominated by science and statistics, and the patient's world dominated by symptoms and suffering. While a specialist may feel that the benefits of treatment far outweigh any potential risks from a medical stand point, they should be mindful that these criteria may not carry the same weight for the patient and it is this area where discussion and collaboration often needs to occur.

The SWOT analysis allows you gain a broader perspective of your total situation so that you can discuss your condition, your fears and your aspirations intelligently. It allows you to factor in the medical criteria, but at the same time takes into account your own criteria and what outcomes you need to achieve in order to fulfil your aspirations. The SWOT analysis then becomes a platform for collaboration: the practitioner will have made their case

Your specialist's side of the fence		Your side of the fence	
Strengths	**Weaknesses**	**Opportunities**	**Threats**
Science & Statistics		*Symptoms & Suffering*	
Benefits or strengths of treatment according to my specialist	Risks or weaknesses of treatment according to my specialist &/or my research	If it works for me I will be able to:	The possible consequences for me are:

for how they wish to treat you, and you will be able to make your case along the lines of what the treatment will mean to you in your day to day life. Sometimes when the patient feels that the negative effects of treatment outweigh all the perceived benefits they are then faced with a difficult decision, and one that may not gain the empathetic support of their attending specialist or doctor.

By doing the SWOT analysis you will be surprised at how much clarity you gain in your decision-making. It has the capacity to shed a different light on your situation and focus you on the total impact of your condition on your life. It will help you voice your concerns within the context of your case, which may not necessarily be within the medical context. When decisions are very difficult, such as "if I do I'm damned, and if I don't I'm damned" it will steer you towards looking at your future and what opportunities a treatment may give you, or the opportunities a treatment may rob you of. You can then weigh up the positives against the negatives and make your decision based on quality of life.

If you follow Pauline's case on the following page, where she was faced with the decision of accepting corticosteroid treatment, you will see how she completed her SWOT analysis and came to her final decision.

Why do I need to identify all my individual risk factors?

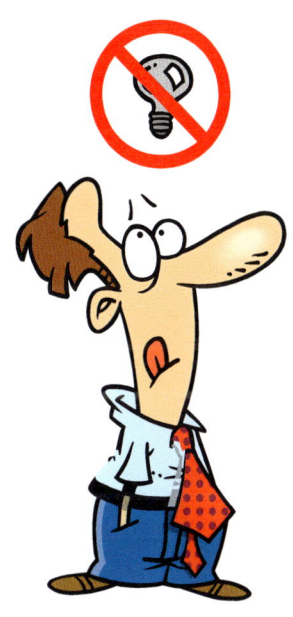

Because you can't assume that each practitioner will cross reference any contraindications of the treatment they prescribe against all your risk factors. This becomes essential when you are being treated by multiple parties.

Pauline's SWOT analysis

STRENGTHS	WEAKNESSES	OPPORTUNITIES	THREATS
Benefits or strengths of treatment according to my specialist:	Risks or weaknesses of treatment according to my specialist/my research:	*If it works for me I will be able to:*	*The possible consequences for me:*
▶ it will stop my disease progressing while I am on the treatment;	▶ remission may only last a year;	▶ continue in my day to day life without pain;	▶ I would be worried about getting pregnant on the drug;
▶ it may bring me into remission where I don't need to take the drugs; and	▶ it will worsen my osteopaenia;	▶ stay on at work, have less days off work; and	▶ it may add to my depression about my future if the remission period is short;
▶ it will manage the symptoms of my condition and stop the pain.	▶ it will make me retain fluid;	▶ feel better in myself in that some areas of my life will have more quality for a period of time.	▶ it will add to my anxiety about osteoporosis and lowered immunity;
	▶ it will lower my immunity;		▶ my self-esteem is going to go down as I will likely gain a lot of weight;
	▶ it will break down my body protein (muscle, liver, skin, bones); and		▶ I am worried about diabetes as I have this in my family; and
	▶ it can lead to diabetes.		▶ it may increase my drug-dependency and future health risks.

Pauline has an acute disease crisis which needs to be controlled. The only treatment that can offer sufficient value is corticosteroid treatment. As Pauline's end point is to be drug-free and reduce her future health risks, then corticosteroid treatment could take her in the opposite direction as it will increase her risks for osteoporosis & diabetes and she could become dependent on drugs for the continued control of her condition. Pauline needs to do her own benefit/risk assessment based on the fact that if she does nothing, or if she chooses a treatment that is ineffective, then her risks increase. Bearing in mind that Pauline has plotted out her main goals against a time line, which she believes are realistic, she is going to have to put in place a longer-term strategy for treatment options if she wishes to get to her end point.

There may be no easy meeting ground between Pauline and her rheumatologist. On the one hand Pauline cannot expect her rheumatologist to monitor her on her chosen treatment, but on the other hand it is Pauline who has to live with both the risks of treatment and the risks of the disease. So she needs to make an informed decision based on a range of criteria that will include those of her specialist and also factor in how her condition affects her life. There are two sides of the fence, and providing that Pauline does not cross the line into her specialist's territory (the objective benefit/risk evaluation of the treatment) then she should not run into any problems. Pauline was able to present her case and she did decide to take the corticosteroids, but her rheumatologist was sympathetic and sensitive to her concerns and more than willing to continue to monitor her during her remission even though by that time Pauline had elected to go with a number of alternative and complementary therapies.

Productive conversations are more likely to occur if the patient can present their case from how their condition affects them, the subjective evaluation (symptoms and suffering). This will provide a meeting ground where the ultimate criteria that both parties should share are patient autonomy and quality of life decisions.

Pauline's Journey Road Map

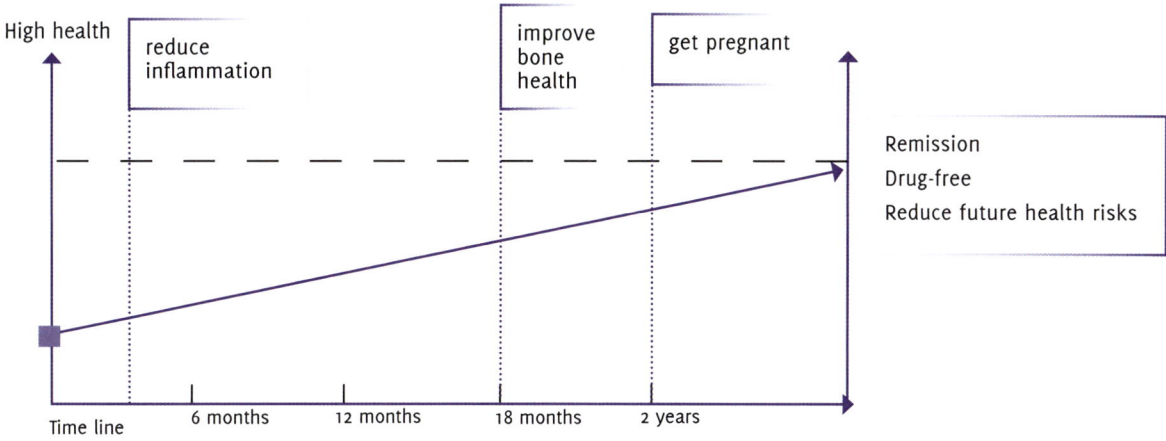

Pauline's Health Flow Chart

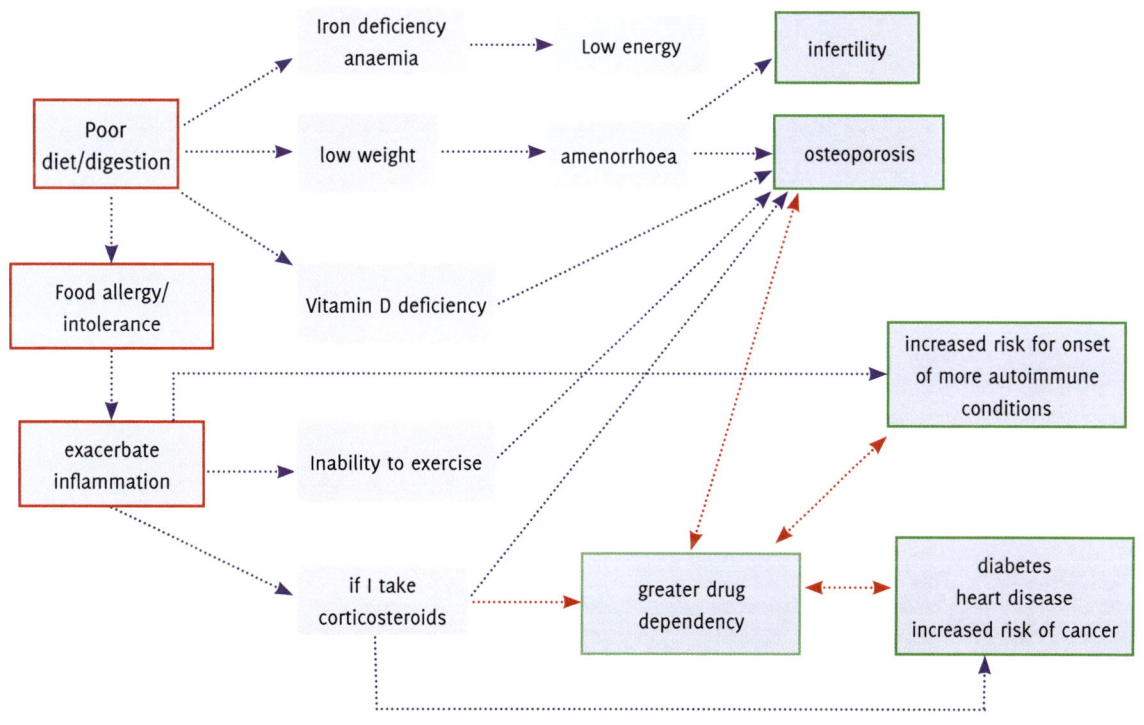

My Benefit/Risk Assessment: the Quadrant Chart

The quadrant chart is used to aid you in determining how far a treatment is likely to help you get to your end point. The beauty of this chart is that you do not need to have researched treatments in depth in order to complete it, but you simply need to know the following:

▸ what are my risks if I do not take treatment *(where could I end up)*;

▸ what are my risks if I do take treatment *(which direction will it take me in)*; and

▸ what is the value of treatment as it relates to my end point *(how far will it take me)*?

This chart orientates you to your end point. It is like a ready reckoner where you will be making subjective assessments of where, in principle, you could end up on a given treatment. Importantly, it encourages you to assess your risks both with and without treatment, which may be an over-riding consideration if time is not on your side.

The chart is divided into 4 sections, A, B, C and D. The arrow going up on the left hand side measures the benefit or value of treatment, or how far it aligns to your end point, and the arrow along the bottom measures the risks, or how far a treatment may set you back. The arrows move from low to high benefit or risk, respectively.

The diagonal line represents the benefit/risk threshold - so anything that is placed on that line will indicate that the benefits and risks are equal. Treatments that have low risk but also low benefit would be placed on the diagonal line in quadrant D, while treatments that have high benefit but also carry a high risk would be on the diagonal line in quadrant B. All treatments where the benefits outweigh the risks would be placed above the diagonal line, and treatments where the risks outweigh the benefits would go below the diagonal line.

Obviously, to determine benefit the treatment needs to be measurable. So if a practitioner can't indicate what a treatment can do for you, but you still feel it's worth pursuing as it may be of value and the treatment carries no inherent risks, then you may place this treatment in quadrant D above the diagonal line. In other words it may not get you to your end point, but it is of low risk. But if your health risks are high and you take a low-risk treatment that can't make a measurable difference within a specific time frame, then this treatment of undetermined benefit may end up in quadrant C by virtue of the fact that ineffective treatment, by default, may take you further away from your end point by allowing the disease to progress.

Treatments that fit into quadrant A are the ones that will take you the furthest towards your end point.

So quadrant A represents your destination end point, and any treatments that match or are aligned to these aspirations may be placed in this field.

The quadrant chart can also be used when you need to compare a range of possible treatment options against each other. It's a very easy chart to complete and it highlights the true risks of any decision that you may make. For example, we often get fixated on the risk of treatment rather than on the risk of not taking a treatment. With any condition that carries high risks one needs to weigh up the consequences, particularly if the condition deteriorates, as you may narrow your future treatment options leading to a poorer outcome.

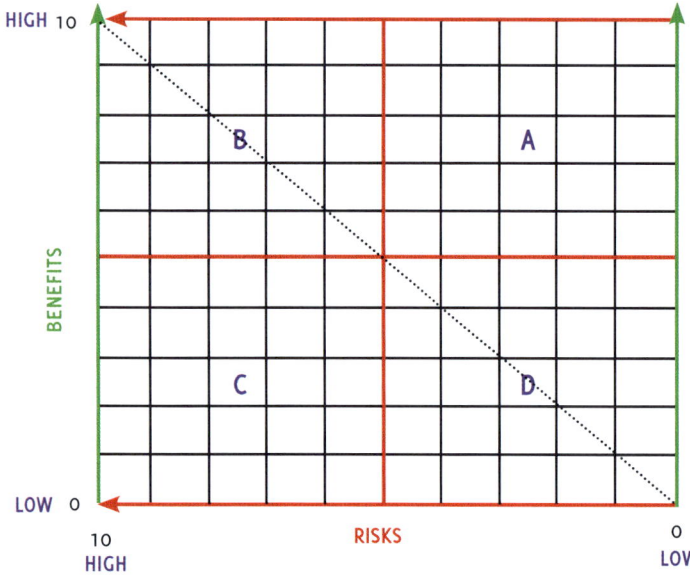

Pauline's quadrant chart

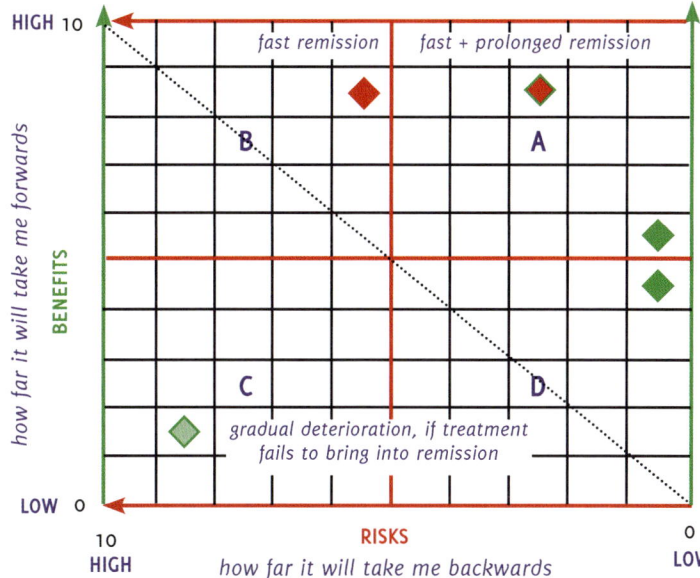

Quadrant A represents Pauline's end point: *long-term remission; reducing future health risks*

TCM: may bring into remission, but not within time frame; no additional health risks/side effects

Diet therapy: no fast remission; will address other health risks and may reduce inflammation

et's take Pauline's case. Quadrant A represents long-term remission and reducing her future health risks, such as osteoporosis.

♦ If Pauline decides to go with corticosteroids as a stand-alone treatment, then we would place the symbol in quadrant B, where the benefits at this stage will outweigh the risks of doing nothing as Pauline needs to reduce the inflammation fast. However, long-term treatment could carry a heavy health debt and could eventually end up in quadrant C.

♦ Pauline researches diet therapy and quickly realizes that as a standalone treatment it may not bring her into remission quickly, but long-term application will help her reduce her future health risks. If she finds that diet plays a major role in controlling inflammation, then this symbol may well be elevated to quadrant A. Next Pauline researches TCM herbal treatment (Traditional Chinese Medi-

cine) and finds that this treatment could bring her into remission without any of the side-effects, but the practitioner cannot make any guarantees on an early remission. Pauline places the symbol in quadrant A, above the diet therapy.

♦ If Pauline decided to rely on a combination of two or more alternative approaches, although they may be of low risk if they can't reduce the core threat of uncontrolled inflammation then they carry a high risk for not getting her anywhere quickly and therefore could be placed in quadrant C.

♦ Pauline can now start to appreciate the value of an integrative approach. If the corticosteroid treatment was part of an integrated program which could address other risk factors and enable her to reduce her medication faster and stay in remission for longer, then the symbol could appear in quadrant A. There would still be some risks regarding getting into remission quickly, as without meeting this criterion she could go backwards.

Troubleshooting your options

When treatment determines diagnosis

Harry has presented with acid reflux and his GP gives him a drug which is a proton pump inhibitor to resolve the symptoms. Harry's end point is simply to feel comfortable and be rid of the symptoms. As far as he is concerned the treatment fits into quadrant A (high benefit/low risk) as he is assured there are no risks or contraindications for the drug.

However, the diagnosis is wrong. The symptoms are reduced but the real problem is undiagnosed stomach cancer. The condition is allowed to progress and by the time the diagnosis is made it is too late for surgery and very little may be offered. So in actual fact the treatment should be placed in quadrant C: low benefit and very high risk for a poor clinical outcome.

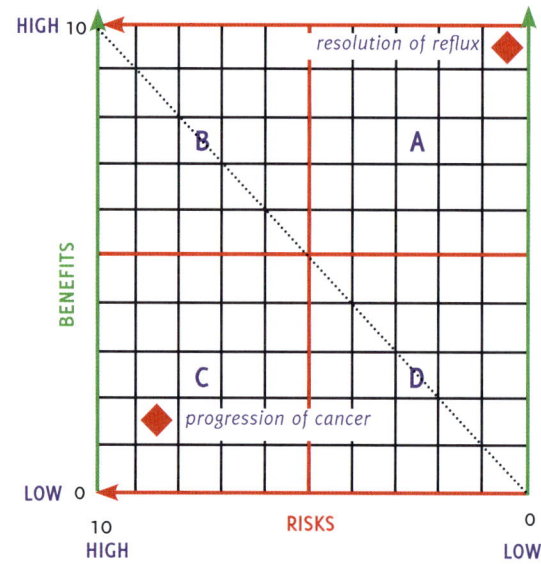

When time is on your side

Brenda has recently had surgery for rectal cancer, stage 2. She has elected not to have chemotherapy as she only has one kidney and felt that the risks may be too great. She has been told that without chemotherapy she only has a 58% chance of surviving 5 years. Her destination end point is to remain in remission for as long as possible and to eradicate any remaining cancer cells. She needs to find a treatment that could offer this. She chooses radiowave therapy which is of low risk, but is unable to offer any statistics or research material pertinent to her case that can confirm exactly what value the treatment could be to her, or how far it could take her toward her end point. Brenda feels that she has nothing to lose and possibly a lot to gain. The treatment is placed in quadrant D as there is no imminent risk from her disease, the cancer has been removed by surgery and her latest scan is clear so there is no critical time frame or present danger. Quadrant D is where a lot of alternative treatments fall – they may be chosen for their low risk, but may not be able

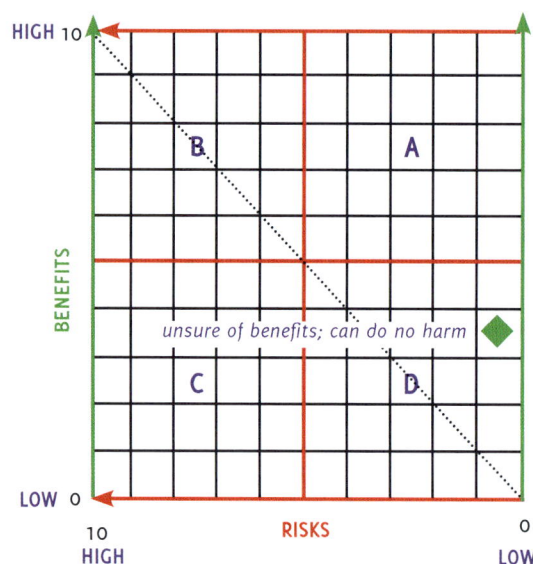

to offer much measurable benefit, which may not be a problem for a patient who is not facing any imminent health risks.

When time is not on your side or when treatment is ineffective

Karen has been diagnosed with cervical cancer which has spread to the neighbouring tissues. She has been told that she will need chemotherapy prior to surgery in order to give her the best outcome. Karen refuses the chemotherapy, but would like the surgery, however this is not an option. Karen decides that she will go the natural route as the cancer is a low grade (slow growing). She finds a practitioner who advises on diet, herbs and supplements, but does not ask whether the treatment will work and how she should monitor. Karen goes on trust and feels that the treatment should have benefit as it is "good" for her. She places this treatment in quadrant A - low risk/high benefit.

Over the next few years Karen feels well until one day she has some bleeding. It is discovered that the tumour has grown and that her options on treatment have now narrowed. She is told that she must have chemotherapy, and possibly some radiotherapy prior to surgery. However, the surgeon indicates that she now requires extensive surgery (pelvic exenteration to remove her uterus, rectum, anus, pelvic floor, labia, tailbone and part of her sacrum followed by reconstruction of the area from the abdomen) and that he will not treat her unless she accepts the entire procedure. The natural treatment Karen has been following is now placed in quadrant C.

The surgeon indicates that his treatment (combined with chemotherapy and radiotherapy) has a 60/40 chance of arresting the disease process and slowing the progression of the cancer. As the potential benefits outweigh the risks of following the current pathway, but the odds on success (ar-

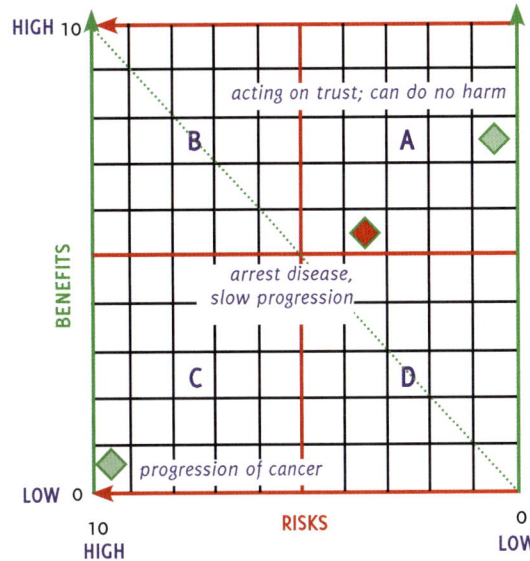

resting the disease) are marginal, Karen decides to combine this treatment with a complementary diet therapy that has a proven track record with cancer, and so places this combined treatment in quadrant D, just above the diagonal line. The treatment will leave her with disabilities, but Karen is hoping for an increased survival time and increased quality of life. Karen recovered well and went on to exceed her whole medical team's expectations.

If Karen had asked her surgeon at the outset what would happen and within what time frame if she refused his treatment, she could have used this time frame to monitor her condition and make a decision before it was too late. By leaving things she not only had narrowed her options, but was now much further away from her end point.

Quick Reference

Quadrant A: good clinical outcome

Quadrant B: good clinical outcome, but treatment carries inherent health risks

Quadrant C: high risk for poor clinical outcome (when time is not on your side, misdiagnosis, or failing to monitor for any individual risks for the treatment itself)

Quadrant D: little or unknown value, but little risk of setting you back (a feasible option only if time is on your side and there are no imminent health risks).

Weighing up the odds

◆ David has a life-threatening heart condition which requires immediate surgery. If the surgery is successful then he will have his life back, but there is a 50/50 risk of death. Any treatments that offer 50/50 will fall directly onto the diagonal line where the benefits are equal to the risks. As the risk of death is the ultimate risk one would pay, then David places the surgery at the highest risk rating of 10 in quadrant B. David decides to seek a second opinion from another heart specialist to see if he can increase his chances for a better outcome.

This specialist uses a different technique and has a higher success rate. He indicates that although there is always a risk of death, he can confidently say that the risk would be around 20%, and that David would see an 80% improvement in his current condition. David places this treatment in
◆ quadrant A but also decides to improve his overall health by addressing some of his risks, such as his weight.

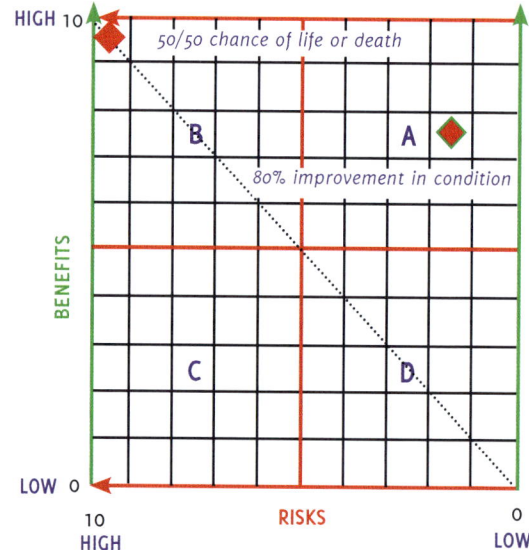

Treating the blood results

◆ Paul has a high cholesterol level. His end point is to reduce his cholesterol and reduce his future health risks with drugs. He opts for medication which will guarantee a reduction in cholesterol. His test results indicate that the treatment is successful in accomplishing this. The treatment goes into quadrant A. Although the treatment carries some health risks, his GP says that the benefits outweigh the small, unimportant risks and a follow-up is not requested to check for contraindications.

◆ Unfortunately Paul does have some side-effects which go undiagnosed. This puts the treatment in quadrant C, where the risks outweigh the benefits and may take Paul further away from his end point, particularly if he wants to reduce all his future health risks.

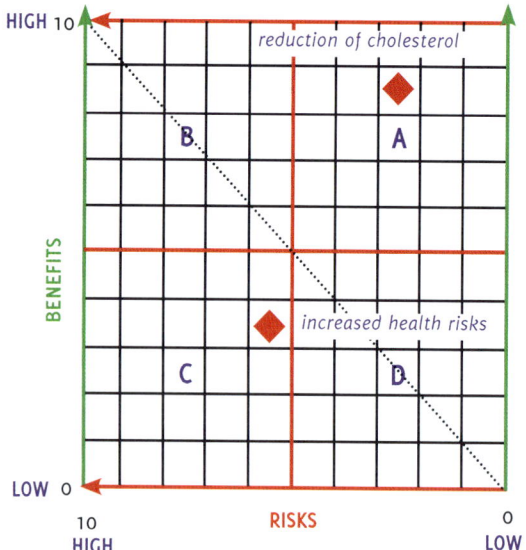

Why do I need to understand statistics?

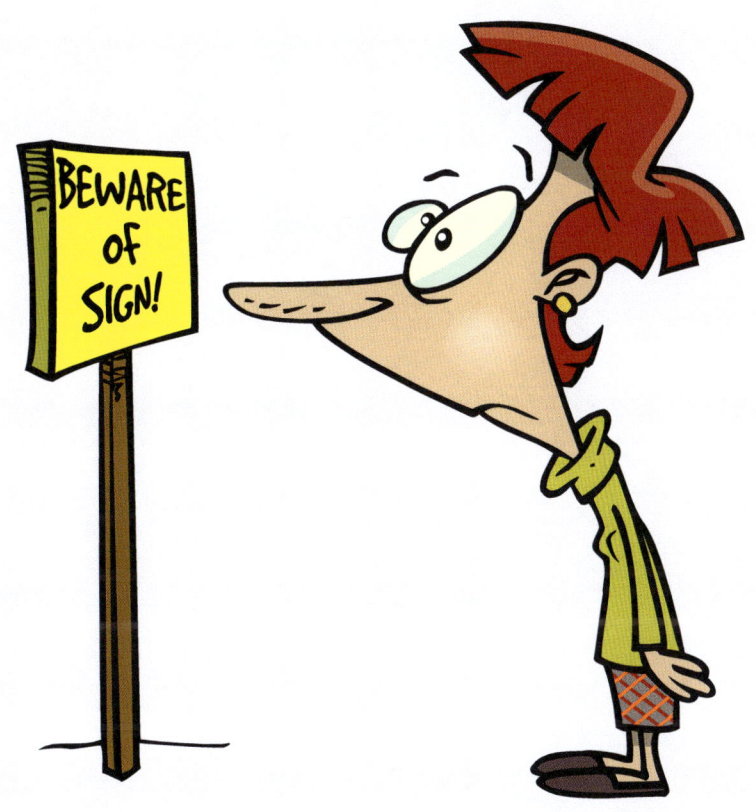

Because you have to know what your REAL odds are.

Flow Chart for Evaluating & Validating treatments: step 4

Step 1

Core or adjunct

Determine what the treatment does

- how does it work; and
- what aspects of my case does it treat.

Match the claims of treatment against your end point & goals to prioritize and determine the value of treatment.

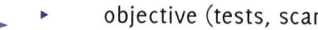

Step 2

Measurable & meaningful

Determine how you will *measure* progress

- objective (tests, scans etc)
- subjective (resolution of symptoms)

and how *meaningful* this will be to the overall case:

- which leg of my journey will it help with?
- how far will it get me to my end point?

If you can't monitor progress then there is no way of knowing the value of treatment.

Step 5

Treatment alignment rating

Use *My Treatment Alignment Rating Template* and select the various treatments which may help, indicate how they may work/what they will do and what benefit they offer in helping you get to your end point. Make sure that the treatment can be monitored. Next rate each treatment and make your decision on which treatments will offer you the most value.

Step 3

Benefit/Risk assessment

Complete the *SWOT analysis* and the *Quadrant chart* when you need to factor in:

▸ the risks of treatment in your individual case;

▸ the risks of not doing treatment; or

▸ when the benefits of treatment are unknown.

These charts will facilitate decision-making when there is an absence of scientific proof or clinical data for a treatment, or when you need to make a decision based on a range of criteria which include how your condition and the potential treatment could affect your life. These charts are invaluable as they will provide a basis for collaboration and help clarify your position to all parties.

These charts can be completed with simple information provided at an appointment and require no medical expertise. They do not require reference to scientific data. The quadrant chart can be used as a visual platform to match the relative value of many therapies and/or treatments to the patient's end point.

Step 4

Scientific & Clinical Validation

Use *My value template* (column 4) to select your own criteria for validating treatments. Then use the simple steps from the *Evaluating scientific evidence* chart to determine how appropriate the treatment is to your case and its potential value in getting you to your end point.

....A University of NSW professor of clinical pharmacology, Ric Day, said there was no doubt a lot of Australians had been prescribed statins when their total risk of heart disease was not high. "It's a bit of a pity because you are taking a drug that doesn't contribute much to your protection at all," he said....

....Statins have long been touted as a miracle drug, with some doctors and researchers pushing for their use in all older people. But Professor Le Couteur said that was unwise. "Unfortunately the history of medicine is chequered with hopes that have turned out to be dashed and even caused harm," he said....

....The chief executive of the service, Lynn Weekes, said Australia's high use of statins compared to the OECD indicated it was likely low-risk people were being treated. "If they are at low risk of heart disease you shouldn't be putting them at risk for something else," she said....

....But the director of the Baker IDI Heart and Diabetes Institute, Garry Jennings, said people should not stop taking statins.

"I hope that pretty much everyone who is on a statin in Australia is on it for a very good reason, although there might be a few lower-risk people on the fringe," he said. "Statins work and there have been tens of thousands of people in trials … the overall benefit is clear.

About 500 people would need to take statins for one new case of diabetes to develop, while a major cardiac event would be prevented for every 150 people taking them....."

http://www.smh.com.au/national/health/miracle-drugs-put-thousands-at-risk-20120229-1u3ia.
html#ixzz1nosnBn60

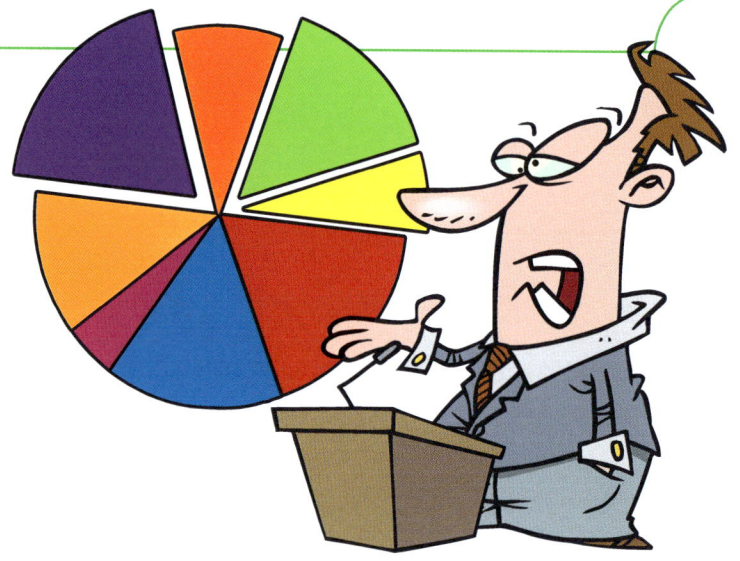

My Benefit/Risk Assessment: Understanding statistics

Statistics are simply a method of measuring your odds. There are various ways you can present statistics and depending on what you need to convey, then statistics will usually oblige. It's fairly easy to talk up the benefits of a drug using statistics to give the impression that it promises more than it does, so if your end point is not to be drug-dependent and yet you have been told that you should take medication to reduce your risks, it's a good idea to determine your odds and discover just how much the treatment offered is likely to reduce your risks.

When you are offered a drug you need to seek *qualification* as to why you are being offered it (what is the research and what does it show) and then you may need help in interpreting the clinical trial data. This may be difficult as statistics are hard to explain, and if you go for a second opinion you are likely to get another take both on your diagnosis and treatment.

So it pays to do your own checks and balances and find out what the results mean and whether they apply to you. This does not only apply to conventional medicine but also alternative and complementary medicines. If your condition does require treatment then you may need to ascertain how well your chosen option is going to work for you.

Guidelines for Evaluating Scientific Evidence

When evaluating scientific evidence you need to make sure that the product that has been tested is the one that's being offered to you, and that the people on the trial have the same condition as you. For example, if a heart drug was tested on people who were over 65 years of age, had high cholesterol and already had suffered a heart attack, but you were only 45 years old and had never had a heart attack - then the trial data would not apply to you.

Similarly, if a product has only been tested on animals, or in a test tube (in vitro) then any clinical results obtained may not apply to a human. Complementary or alternative treatments often fall into this category where "promising data" is cherry picked and forms the basis of marketing propaganda.

Working through the statistics is a hurdle in itself, but with a bit of practice you can become proficient enough to make an informed decision. The point to remember is that relative statistics are meaningless - you need the absolute statistics or the real numbers, not simply the difference between those that got sick in both arms of the trial presented as a ratio.

It's also important to take into account the absolute statistics of those in the control arm (without treatment) who did not get sick. If, for example, 80 percent of people with high cholesterol in the control arm did not go on to have a heart attack then your odds on the likelihood of suffering an acute event may be small (5:1) and you may decide against a treatment, particularly if it carries additional inherent risks.

Use the table *Evaluating Scientific Evidence* on the next page as a reference to validate the information you need to acquire before making an informed decision as to how far a product or treatment will help you get to your end point.

Don't forget to factor in any risks of treatment and see if these would apply to you. If you feel that the risks of treatment in your individual case are high and the benefits not worth it, then by having done this exercise you will not only be confident in your decision on treatment, but also when discussing options with your specialist.

Use this table as a check list and read through the following case studies to make sure you understand the mechanics of evaluating trial abstracts and interpreting statistics. There are many examples given in this chapter to help you understand how to work out the value of treatment from scientific data.

Guidelines for Evaluating Scientific Evidence

PRODUCTS/TREATMENT	CLINICAL TRIALS	STATISTICS
▲ What is it that has been tested? *(Product name, active ingredient.)* ▲ How has it been tested? *(In a test tube [in vitro], on an animal or on a human [in vivo].)* ▲ What has it been tested for? *(The condition that the product was tested for.)* ▲ What is the therapeutic dosage? *(The amounts used to achieve the specific end point.)*	▲ Does the selection criteria fit my profile? *(People who have the same condition as me.)* ▲ Is the drug/product tested the same as the one offered to me? ▲ Are the research outcomes relevant to me? *(Does the primary end point match what I want to achieve?)* ▲ Was the length of the trial long enough to give meaningful results? *(Short trials will not indicate long-term or meaningful results.)* ▲ Were enough people enrolled on the trial? ▲ Are there any conflicting trial results? ▲ Were any adverse events reported and, if so, what were these and could these risks apply to me?	What do the statistics measure: ▲ people *(the % of the group)* ▲ time *(duration of time of improvement)* ▲ response rate *(reduction in frequency of medical events, shrinkage of tumour)* Are the statistics: ▲ absolute *(give the actual percentage of people in each arm, the actual time, and/or the actual response)* ▲ relative *(compare the reduction/ increase in risk between each arm. These are often irrelevant and meaningless to the patient)*

Note: if more than 60% of people in the control arm (or untreated group) of a trial remain well then the odds of risk for the condition will be in your favour. However, some people, due to their higher risk factors, could fall into the higher risk bracket. By identifying these risks and taking other steps to address and reduce them then your odds of remaining well could increase.

Statistics: what do they measure?

Statistics either refer to the percentage of a group that reach a specific end point on a given treatment, or compare the difference in outcome between groups to determine how much a treatment reduces or increases the risk. Absolute statistics represent the actual percentage, whereas relative statistics represent the difference between the numbers of people who get sick on all arms of a trial as a ratio. Relative statistics are often used by clinicians as these tend to give a more favourable impression than the absolute statistics of what the treatment can achieve.

In this example we have two groups: group A is the control group (untreated group) and group B, the treated group. In group A 12 percent got sick but in the treated group B only 8 percent got sick. The absolute statistics for group A would be 88 percent remained well and 12 percent got sick, and for group B, 92 percent remained well and 8 percent got sick. You can see there is a difference of 4 percent between the two groups and it is this 4 percent that indicates the reduction of risk for the treated group.

You can see from the diagrams how this 4 percent is converted to a relative statistic. The 4 percent represents

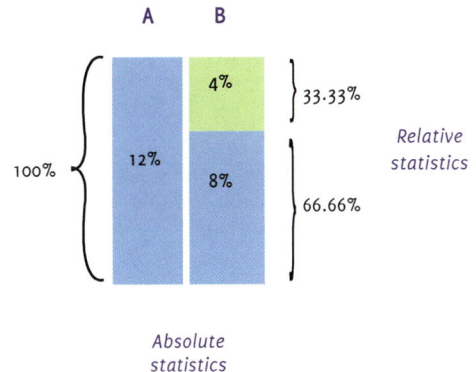

the absolute reduction of risk (if you take the treatment then 4 people out of every hundred that would normally get sick won't) but when expressed as a ratio of the 12 percent translates as a 33.33% *reduction in risk* on the treatment. You can begin to appreciate why relative statistics can give an exaggerated impression of the actual benefit of treatment. Furthermore, if the side-effects or risks of treatment were high then this could influence decision-making on treatment particularly if the absolute benefits were low.

Absolute statistics: the number of people expressed as a percentage of the whole group.

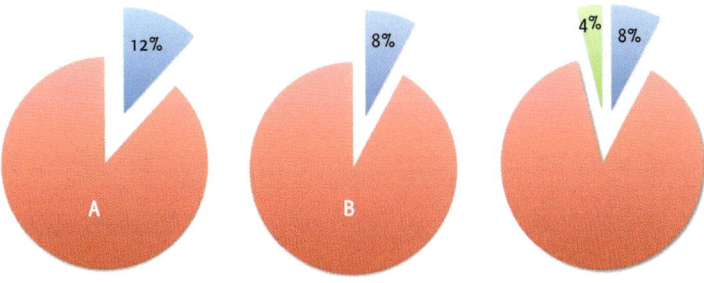

Relative statistics: a comparison between the absolute percentage of people who got sick in two or more groups expressed as a ratio. They are used to indicate which treatment may work best at reducing risk, rather than the actual numbers of people that may benefit. It is better to ask for the absolute statistics than rely on the relative, as the absolute statistics are more meaningful.

Working out the math

Relative Reduction of Risk

How much is my risk of getting sick reduced by going on the treatment?

Before you even do any math you can see that one third less people got sick in group B than in group A (8 as opposed to 12). So you would be told that your risk would be reduced by 33.33% if you take the treatment. There is still a 66.66% risk of getting sick, so the treatment doesn't reduce your risk completely.

The math is worked out like this:

$$8 \div 12 = 0.6666$$

or 66.66% chance of getting sick on the treatment

$$1 - 0.6666 = 0.3333$$

or 33.33% chance of not getting sick on the treatment

Relative Increase in Risk

How much is my risk of getting sick increased by not going on the treatment?

Again, without doing any math you can see that half-again the number of people get sick without treatment (12) than those on treatment (8), which means that your risk would be increased by 50% if you don't take the treatment.

The math is worked out like this:

$$12 \div 8 = 1.5$$

where a ratio of 1 means no difference, 2 means double the risk and 1.5 means that the risk is increased by 50%

Always ask for the absolute statistics.
If statistics indicate
"we can reduce your risk by .... %" or
"there is a reduction of risk of.... %"
then you will know that these are relative, not absolute.

Working out the odds

What does this mean to me?

What are the odds of the treatment helping me?

Statistics, whether absolute or relative, may still mean absolutely nothing in terms of how meaningful a treatment could be to you. Most statistics do not even convey the numbers of people on trials who remain disease or event-free, which is true particularly when relative statistics are presented. To see how meaningful the results are you have to be able to work out what your odds are of the treatment helping you. This treatment, which is taken over 5 years, helps 4 percent of patients. So the odds are 100:4 or 25:1. This means that for every 25 people treated over 5 years only 1 person will benefit.

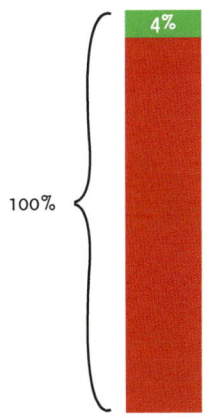

Working out the odds

To work out the odds you simply take the absolute "difference" between those who got sick on the treatment and those who got sick in the control arm (not doing any treatment). In this case the absolute difference is 4 in every 100. 100:4 expressed as a ratio is 25:1. So the odds on the treatment helping any individual would be one in twenty-five. The odds are often presented as numbers needed to treat (NNT) which, in this instance, would be "we would need to treat 25 people in order to benefit 1 person" where the "benefit" would be determined by the end point criterion, such as reduction of adverse events, overall survival or remission.

Don't be put off – it may seem difficult but working out the odds is as easy as figuring out how to plug in a cable!

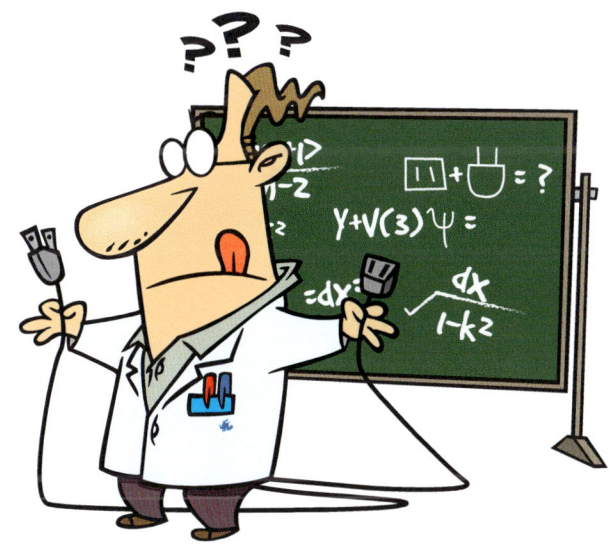

Working out absolute & relative statistics

Brian is a 56 year old man who has recently suffered a heart attack. He has average cholesterol levels but his specialist says that if he goes on Pravastatin (a cholesterol-lowering drug) then he can reduce his risk of heart attack by 23%. Brian is concerned as he has had some other health issues in the past and is keen to improve his outcome using more natural methods. He asks for further information on the research. The specialist refers him to the CARE 5 year study (below). All Brian has to do is look at the abstract and then put the relevant information into context. He finds the study and begins his assessment. He looks for the absolute statistics and makes a note of these. He finds that there is, in fact, only a 3 percent absolute reduction of risk for him on the drug. Brain has been presented with the relative statistics which seem impressive but are irrelevant. He needs to work out exactly how meaningful the treatment would be for him.

The effect of Pravastatin on coronary events after myocardial infarction in patients with average cholesterol levels.

Cholesterol and Recurrent Events Trial investigators

http://www.ncbi.nlm.nih.gov/pubmed/8801446

Study group: average cholesterol and LDL levels who had already suffered myocardial infarction

Drug: Pravastatin 40mg

Length of time: 5 years

Number of people: 4,159

Primary end point: to measure the incidence of fatal coronary event or a non-fatal myocardial infarction (i.e. to see if it reduced the rate of heart attack).

Findings:

Reduction in risk: 23% relative reduction in risk of heart attack (the absolute frequency was 10.2% in the Pravastatin group and 13.2% in the placebo group, or a 3% absolute reduction of risk).

Increase in risk: no significant differences in overall mortality from non-cardiovascular causes.

Abstract

BACKGROUND: In patients with high cholesterol levels, lowering the cholesterol level reduces the risk of coronary events, but the effect of lowering cholesterol levels in the majority of patients with coronary disease, who have average levels, is less clear.

METHODS: In a double-blind trial lasting five years we administered either 40 mg of Pravastatin per day or placebo to 4159 patients (3583 men and 576 women) with myocardial infarction who had plasma total cholesterol levels below 240 mg per deciliter (mean, 209) and low-density lipoprotein (LDL) cholesterol levels of 115 to 174mg per deciliter (mean, 139). The primary end point was a fatal coronary event or a nonfatal myocardial infarction.

RESULTS: The frequency of the primary end point was 10.2 percent in the pravastatin group and 13.2 percent in the placebo group, an absolute difference of 3 percentage points and a 24 percent reduction in risk (95 percent confidence interval, 9 to 36 percent; P = 0.003). Coronary bypass surgery was needed in 7.5 percent of the patients in the Pravastatin group and 10 percent of those in the placebo group, a 26 percent reduction (P=0.005), and coronary angioplasty was needed in 8.3 percent of the Pravastatin group and 10.5 percent of the placebo group, a 23 percent reduction (P=0.01). The frequency of stroke was reduced by 31 percent (P=0.03). There were no significant differences in overall mortality or mortality from non-cardiovascular causes. Pravastatin lowered the rate of coronary events more among women than among men. The reduction in coronary events was also greater in patients with higher pretreatment levels of LDL cholesterol.

CONCLUSIONS: These results demonstrate that the benefit of cholesterol-lowering therapy extends to the majority of patients with coronary disease who have average cholesterol levels.

http://www.ncbi.nlm.nih.gov/pubmed/8801446

Measuring the rate of adverse events

Brian needs to work out the benefit of taking the drug in his individual case. In the diagram below Brian has placed the incidence of heart attack in the untreated group (A) against the incidence in the treated group (B). As you can see there is an absolute reduction of risk of 3% in group B.

Calculating the Absolute Reduction in Risk (ARR):

Untreated group: 13.2% had a cardiac event in 5 years

Treated group: 10.2% had a cardiac event in 5 years

ARR: 13.2 - 10.2 = 3% of people

As we can see the absolute benefit appears small (3%) but by changing the absolute into relative statistics the benefits can appear much larger.

Relative statistics are simply a comparison of two results expressed as a ratio. You divide the highest risk by the lowest risk to get the relative increase in risk, or the lowest risk by the highest risk to get the relative reduction in risk.

The highest risk divided by the lowest risk will give you a ratio greater than 1 (which means that the risk is increased) and the lowest risk divided by the highest risk will give you a ratio less than 1 (which means that the risk is reduced).

Calculating the Relative Reduction in Risk (RRR):

10.2 ÷ 13.2 = 0.77 or a 77% relative risk of cardiac event which means a 23% relative reduction of risk (1 - 0.77 = 0.23 or 23%).

Calculating the Relative Increase in risk:

13.2 ÷ 10.2 = 1.29. This means that if Brian decides not to take the drug then he is increasing his risk of a cardiac event by 29%.

If all this is double dutch, then simply look at the diagram below and you can see that the space representing the 3% is roughly 25% of 13.2%. So the relative reduction in risk is 23%.

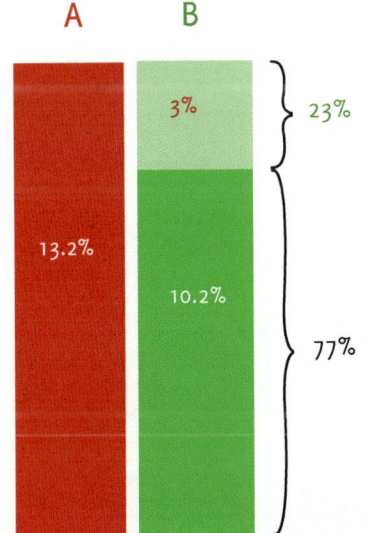

A   B

13.2%

10.2%

3% } 23%

} 77%

absolute risk reduction 3% (ARR)

relative risk reduction 23% (RRR)

What are Brian's odds?

These figures are still meaningless to Brian who has to make a considered decision being that he has had a serious liver complaint in the past and this is one of the contraindications for the drug. To work out his odds he needs to take the absolute advantage (3%) and make this a ratio of 100

100:3 or 33:1

Translated, this means that 33 people would need to be treated for 5 years to prevent one heart attack.

Brian decides that as he is in the low risk group (lower pretreatment levels of LDL cholesterol) then the risks could outweigh any benefits in his individual case.

To recap

In five years the frequency of heart attack was 10.2% in the treated group and 13.2% in the untreated group, which gives an absolute reduction of risk of 3% (ARR). To ascertain the relative reduction of risk you simply divide the lowest risk by the highest risk to get a ratio: 0.77 [10.2 ÷ 13.2 = 0.77] or a 77% relative chance of relapse which means a 23% relative reduction of risk (RRR) [1 - 0.77 = 0.23 or 23%].

To calculate the increase of risk of not taking the drug you simply divide the highest risk by the lowest risk 13.2 ÷ 10.2 = 1.29. This means that there is a relative increase in risk of 29% for those not taking the drug.

- ▸ A ratio of 1 means that there is no difference in outcome on treatment
- ▸ A ratio ‹1 means that the risk is reduced
- ▸ A ratio of 0.5 means that the risk is halved
- ▸ A ratio ›1 means that the risk is increased
- ▸ A ratio of 2 means that the risk is doubled

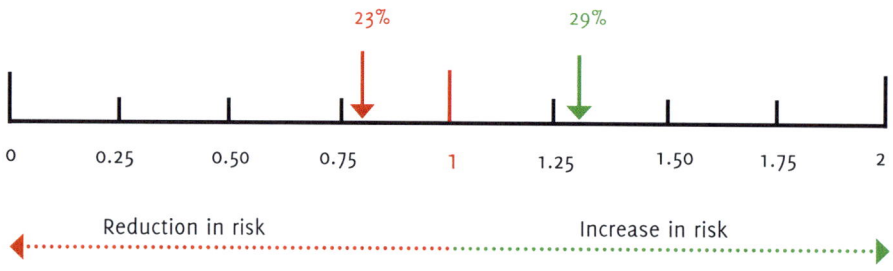

To calculate the odds simply take the absolute number of those who benefited (3 percent or 100:3) and convert it to a ratio (33.3:1). Working out the odds is the easiest method of determining just how valuable a treatment may be to you.

Measuring the rate of adverse events: cont'd

*C*armel was 56 years old. She had gone through menopause and a recent bone density scan revealed that she was slightly osteopaenic in her hip (T-score: -1.9) and osteoporotic in her lumbar spine (T-score: -2.7). Her GP recommended that she start taking a biphosphonate which he said would increase her bone density and significantly reduce her risk of fracture. Carmel's dentist had warned her against this class of drug, so she decided to do some research.

Effect of Alendronate on Risk of Fracture in Women With Low Bone Density but Without Vertebral Fractures

Fracture Intervention Trial

http://jama.jamanetwork.com/article.aspx?articleid=188299

Study group: Women aged 54 to 81 years with a femoral neck BMD of 0.68 g/cm^2 or less but no vertebral fracture.

Treatment: 5 mg/d of alendronate sodium for 2 years followed by 10 mg/d for the remainder of the trial. All participants reporting calcium intakes of 1000 mg/d or less received a supplement containing 500 mg of calcium and 250 IU of cholecalciferol (D3).

Length of time: 4.2 years

Number of people: 4432 were randomized to alendronate or placebo. (4272 completed the trial, or an average of 2136 in each group.)

Primary end point: To test the hypothesis that 4 years of alendronate would decrease the risk of clinical and vertebral fractures in women who have low bone mineral density (BMD) but no vertebral fractures.

Findings:

Average findings: in the control group (A) 312 suffered fractures (312/2136 x 100 = 14.6%); while in the treated group (B) 272 suffered fractures (12.7%). (The absolute reduction of number of fractures is 40 but the percentage difference [absolute reduction of risk] between the two groups is 1.9% (14.6% - 12.7% = 1.9%). The odds are 100:1.9 (or 50:1) which means that the NNT (number needed to treat) to prevent one fracture is 50 (i.e. you would need to treat 50 women for 4 years to prevent one fracture). However, in women with baseline osteoporosis at the femoral neck the relative reduction of risk was more than tripled (100:6.5 or 15:1) or the NNT to prevent one fracture is 15. Alendronate decreased the absolute risk of radiographic vertebral fractures by 1.7% (treatment control difference) which means that the NNT to prevent one vertebral fracture is 60.

CONCLUSIONS: In women with low BMD but without vertebral fractures, 4 years of alendronate safely increased BMD and decreased the risk of first vertebral deformity. Alendronate significantly reduced the risk of clinical fractures among women with osteoporosis but not among women with higher BMD. The results indicated that there was no significant reduction of risk amongst those in the osteopaenic range.

My comment: although Alendronate increased BMD at all sites, the study was to identify whether, and by how much, increasing bone density prevented fracture. The drug was only effective (15:1) in those with existing osteoporosis. It can be misleading to the consumer when presenting a reduction of risk as a ratio between the total number of fractures sustained by each group, rather than as a percentage of the group that benefited, particularly when that percentage is so small, as in this case, 1.9%. For example, a fracture rate of 312 in 2,136 women simply means that 14.6% of the group sustained a fracture, and a fracture rate in the treated group of 272 per 2,136 means 12.7% of the group sustained a fracture. The absolute reduction of risk (1.9%) may appear insignificant; the relative reduction of risk of 13% (12.7 ÷14.6 = 0.87 or 13% relative reduction of risk) will appear less so, but when the odds on reducing risk (50:1) are worked out, then these figures offer a more meaningful assessment of the drug's true capability to the health consumer.

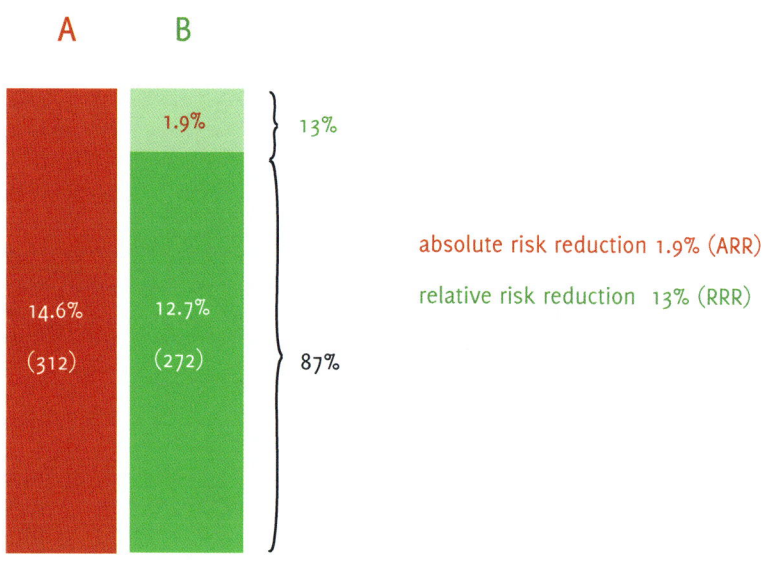

What are Carmel's odds?

100:1.9 = 50:1

but as Carmel was already osteoporotic (in her lumbar spine) then her odds may be:

100: 6.5 = 15:1

Carmel decided to do some further research as no long-term studies using this drug had been concluded and she was nervous about what may happen to her bones when she came off the drug. As she had a sedentary lifestyle, she knew that lack of exercise would have a negative impact on her bones. After some researching she came across this study (opposite) and concluded that just with exercise alone she could not only stop her bones becoming weaker, but also improve their density. She decided to embark upon a healthy lifestyle and exercise regime which she knew would stand her in good stead for years to come.

Benefits of 2 years of intense exercise on bone density, physical fitness, and blood lipids in early postmenopausal osteopaenic women

Erlangen Fitness Osteoporosis Prevention Study

http://www.ncbi.nlm.nih.gov/pubmed/15159265

Study group: early post-menopausal women with no medication or illness affecting bone metabolism

Treatment: 50 women undertook 2 group training sessions per week and 2 home training sessions per week (EG); 33 women in control group (CG). Both groups were individually supplemented with calcium and cholecalciferol.

Length of time: 26 months

Number of people: 83

Primary end point: To determine whether exercise improves bone mineral density and bone formation, lipid levels, and other menopausal symptoms including pain.

Findings:

BMD percentage changes over base line for lumbar spine and total hip in the CG were -2.3% and -1.7% respectively, and in the EG +0.7% and -0.3% respectively. Serum lipid changes over base line for cholesterol and triglycerides in the CG were +4.1% and +23.2%, respectively and in the EG -5.0% and -14.2% respectively.

CONCLUSIONS:

Exercise maintains bone mass, with marginal increase in the lumbar spine, and significantly improves blood lipids. General purpose exercise programs with special emphasis on bone density can significantly improve strength and endurance and reduce bone loss, back pain, and lipid levels in osteopaenic women in their critical early postmenopausal years.

My comment: *exercise training programs have been found to prevent or reverse almost 1% of bone loss per year in the lumbar spine or femoral neck in both pre and post-menopausal women.*

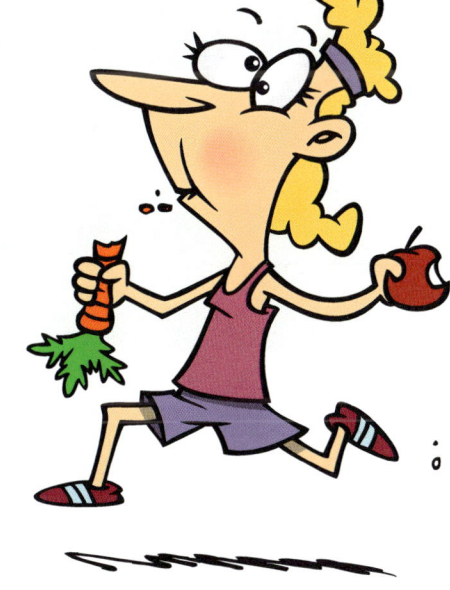

Measuring time & rate of relapse

*B*arbara has been recommended long-term medication to reduce the risk of relapse of her ulcerative proctitis. She is already in remission following treatment but in the past she has experienced relapses within 6 months of entering remission so she is keen to check out the drug mesalamine that is being recommended to her by her specialist. She finds a study which looks very promising.

Long-term use of mesalamine (Rowasa) suppositories in remission maintenance of ulcerative proctitis

http://www.ncbi.nlm.nih.gov/pubmed?term=10925979

Study group: patients with ulcerative proctitis in clinical and endoscopic remission

Drug: Mesalamine 500mg at night

Length of time: 2 years

Number of people: 65

Primary end point: to evaluate the efficacy and safety of mesalamine as a maintenance therapy for patients with ulcerative colitis

Findings:

Median duration of response: Mesalamine increased the median duration of response 2.87 fold (the time to relapse was 2.87 times longer)

Rate of relapse: Mesalamine reduced the risk of relapse at 12 months by 63%

Measuring duration (time): the average length of time for both groups (treated and untreated) that patients stayed in remission before relapse.

Median duration: for each arm you add up the total number of months until relapse and then divide by the number of people in that arm of the trial to get the average number of months. This means that some people would experience a much longer duration of response, while others a much shorter duration of response.

Untreated group: median duration of remission of 5.64 months

Treated group: median duration of remission or 16.2 months

16.2 ÷ 5.64 = 2.87 which nearly triples the duration of response in the treated group.

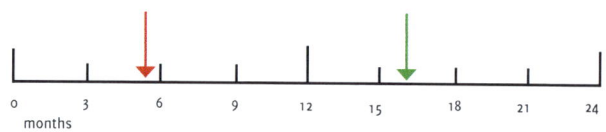

Measuring rate of relapse (people):

Untreated group (A): 86% relapsed at 12 months

Treated group (B): 32% relapsed at 12 months

ARR: 86 - 32 = 54% benefit for the treated group

Relative Reduction in risk:

32 ÷ 86 = 0.37 (37% relative risk of relapse on the drug). This translates as a 63% relative reduction in risk (1.0 - 0.37 = 0.63 or 63%).

RRR: 32 ÷ 86 = 0.37 or 63% relative reduction of risk of relapse

Relative increase in risk for the untreated group:

86 ÷ 32 = 2.68 fold (268% or nearly 3 times more likely to have a relapse if untreated).

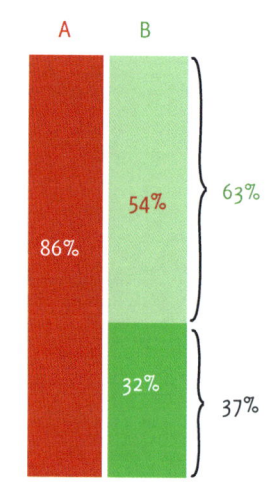

absolute risk reduction 54% (ARR)
relative risk reduction 63% (RRR)

Measuring response rates: reduction in exacerbation rates

Sally is considering taking a drug to reduce the number of multiple sclerosis exacerbations. On average she is currently having one attack a year. Her specialist wants her to take Interferon. She finds a study which indicates that she could reduce her current annual exacerbation rate from 1 to 0.84, where nearly 30% of this group were free from exacerbations. She doesn't like the look of the potential side effects, but the bonus of reducing MS activity in the body was a plus for Sally. She was concerned that the trial was short and there was no long-term follow-up to see if the adverse effects of the drug would ultimately outweigh these initial benefits. Having viewed all the evidence Sally decided to take the drug and see how she felt on it over the next 6 months, but if she had any side-effects she would review her position.

Interferon beta-1b is effective in relapsing-remitting multiple sclerosis

The IFNB Multiple Sclerosis study group

http://www.ncbi.nlm.nih.gov/pubmed?term=8469318

Study group: ambulatory patients with relapsing-remitting multiple sclerosis (MS) with entry criteria including an Expanded Disability Status Scale (EDSS) score of 0 - 5.5 and at least two exacerbations in the previous 2 years.

Drug: One-third of the patients received placebo, one-third 1.6 million international units (MIU) of IFNB, and one-third 8 MIU of IFNB, self-administered by subcutaneous injections every other day.

Length of time: 2 years

Number of people: 372

Primary end point: differences in exacerbation rates and proportion of patients remaining exacerbation-free.

Findings:

- 34% relative reduction in risk of exacerbation in the high dose group over the control group

- 29% of this group remained exacerbation free which is double those taking 1.6 MIU of IFNB

- A significant change in disability could not be discerned in this trial

- In serial MRIs, MS activity was significantly less in the high-dose group

What are we measuring: The difference between the average annual exacerbation rate in patients in the treated groups (1.6MIU and 8.0 MIU interferon-beta 1b) and the untreated or control group.

Control group: average exacerbation rate per annum 1.27

1.6 MIU INFB: average exacerbation rate per annum 1.15

8.0 MIU INFB: average exacerbation rate per annum 0.84

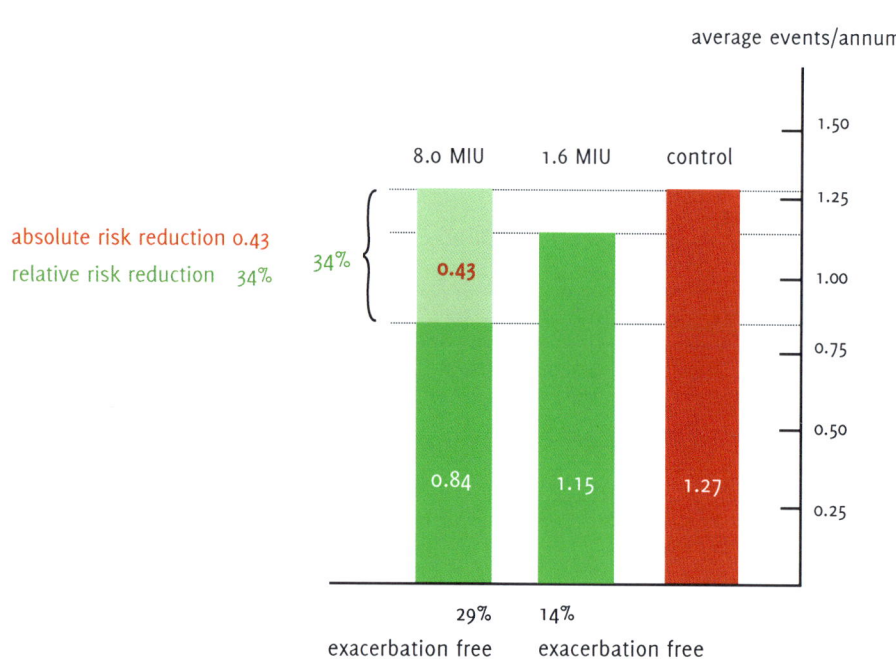

absolute risk reduction 0.43
relative risk reduction 34%

Absolute reduction in exacerbation is *0.43* (1.27 - 0.84 = 0.43)

This means that you have to treat 232 patients for 2 years to prevent 1 exacerbation per year. (100:0.43 = 232:1)

Relative reduction in exacerbation between the high dose group and the untreated group:

0.84 ÷ 1.27 = 0.66 or a 66% chance of exacerbation which means a *34% relative reduction in exacerbation* (1.0 - 0.66 = 0.34 or 34%).

However, as almost double the number of people remained exacerbation-free on the high dose compared to the lower dose (no figures given for the control group), then this would suggest that some people responded much more favourably than others to the treatment.

Understanding statistics in cancer

When interpreting statistics in cancer you need to determine what the statistics are measuring and the criteria used for measuring value. I would recommend that you take the lead and ask the questions rather than wait for the specialist to offer statistics which support their recommendations. As you will have seen statistics can be offered as absolute (more relevant to the patient) or as relative.

Statistics offered will be measuring either people, time or response.

▸ People: what percentage of people respond to treatment, survive for a specific period of time, or survive, disease-free, for a specific period of time

▸ Time: how long a group of patients survive on one treatment relative to a similar group on another treatment. These statistics are generally relative. So if group A survives 6 months and group B survives a year, then group B doubles the survival time of group A; or if group A survives 6 months and group B, 9 months, then the relative survival time is increased by 50% for group B.

▸ Response: degree of shrinkage. Complete response (CR) indicates that no tumour can be seen; partial response (PR) indicates the degree of shrinkage that is likely to be expected measured as a percentage.

So, for example, if a specialist indicates that a recommended treatment will give 75% chance of success, what does this mean? Does it mean that 75% of patients have an overall survival of 5 years; does it mean that it will increase survival time by 75% (and 75% of what); does it mean that the tumour should shrink by 75%; does it mean that 75% of people will see tumour shrinkage; does it mean that there is a 75% relative reduction in risk of death?

Relative versus absolute statistics

It will be much easier for you to work with absolute statistics as these are more meaningful. Absolute statistics will measure absolute benefit or absolute reduction in risk, whereas relative statistics are often used when comparing the risk of one treatment over another where the difference is expressed as a percentage. For example,

on treatment A there may be an 80% overall survival (OS), compared with 70% OS on treatment B. In absolute terms this represents a 10% benefit for treatment A. However, 10 as a percentage of 30 (number of those who died on treatment B) is 33% ([80-70]/30 x 100). This is the relative statistic which translates as a 33 percent relative reduction in risk of death on treatment A.

Treatment options: a statistical analysis

Combinations of treatments are often offered for cancer patients, including local (surgery, radiation), systemic (chemotherapy) and targeted treatment (specific drugs that target a risk factor for the cancer). It's useful to understand the difference in value between the various treatment combination options, and particularly the value of second line treatments (targeted treatment) as these can improve the outcome significantly.

Unfortunately, rarely are studies conducted against a base line that doesn't include chemotherapy, so it may be impossible for a patient to do a risk/benefit analysis comparing a treatment with or without chemotherapy. This can be a particularly difficult situation for patients that present with cancer at an early stage, where it can be surgically removed and where there are good second-line targeted treatments (such as tamoxifen, herceptin or other monoclonal antibodies) which have a proven track record for reducing recurrence and offering survival advantage. These patients fall into two groups: those that wish to have chemotherapy as they believe it to be of benefit; and those that do not wish to take chemotherapy as there may be insufficient trial data or lack of compelling evidence to make a decision particularly when the long-term risks of chemotherapy may outweigh any perceived advantages. Under these circumstances, these patients may be refused a second line targeted treatment as a first option if they refuse the chemotherapy.

When weighing up treatments it is useful to fill in a chart, such as the examples on pp160, 162. Find out what treatment options are available and add these in the header columns. If combination therapies are recommended then you need to state the exact combination. Then add the advantage that each treatment or combina-

Weighing up treatments from a statistical perspective

DIAGNOSIS
adenocarcinoma of oesophagus
stage 4 (metastases to lymph nodes and liver)
poorly differentiated (aggressive)
size of main tumour; 5cm

PROGNOSIS
9-12 months survival with treatment recommended

TREATMENT OPTIONS

		surgery	radiotherapy	chemotherapy
Survival	Years/months	symptom-relief only	symptom-relief only	9-12 months
	% of group			?
Remission (disease-free survival)	Years/months			nil
	% of group			
Response (shrinkage)	Stabilization (Years/months)			?
	% of shrinkage			30%-50%
	% of group			85%-90%
Practitioner's clinical experience/opinion of cases like mine	Years/months (best/worst/median)			?
	% of their treated group			0.5% survived 5 yr 50% managed OK 50% stopped chemo

This example illustrates how the clinician's input radically changed the prognosis for the patient. Statistics for this condition indicate that 85-90% of patients respond to treatment with an expected 30-50% shrinkage of the tumour. Upon clarification this patient found that at most (but not necessarily) he could expect his tumour to shrink by 30-50%; but that in his clinician's experience 50% of patients had to drop out of treatment, and that of the 50% remaining, 85-90% could expect some tumour reduction. In reality, this means that in her clinical experience only 43%-45% of patients responded. She also said that she had seen only 1 person out of 200 with a similar condition survive 5 years.

tion of treatments will offer. Make sure to check that you are given the absolute statistics rather than the relative statistics.

Help in formulating the questions

Overall Survival: *(survival simply means still being alive. It does not indicate if the patients are well and disease-free)*

There are 2 parts to this where you need to determine for each of the treatments offered:

▸ the time line in years and/or months; and

▸ how many, in terms of the percentage of the group, survived?

In other words, what percentage of the group survived and for how long?

Disease-free survival: *(the length of time the patient is in remission or disease-free)*

There are 2 parts to this where you need to determine for each of the treatments offered:

▸ time line in years and/or months of remission before the cancer returned; and

▸ how many, in terms of the percentage of the group, achieved remission for this period of time?

You may also ask what further treatments would be offered were the disease to relapse.

Response: *(degree of shrinkage of tumour)*

When the treatment proposed produces a remission then a complete response (CR) is achieved (i.e. no sign of the cancer). A partial response (PR) indicates the degree of shrinkage that is likely to be expected measured as a percentage of overall shrinkage.

There are 4 parts to this section: the patient needs to determine for each treatment offered:

▸ tumour shrinkage: by how much/what percentage are the tumours expected to shrink (best and worst case);

▸ how many, in terms of the percentage of the group, responded;

▸ for how many (in terms of the percentage of the group) did the treatment worsen the condition; and

▸ time line: how long are the beneficial results likely to last before the tumour/s regrow?

Progression-free survival: *(The length of time the patient's condition remains stable. These statistics apply when treatment can only halt the progression but not offer any degree of remission.)*

There are 2 parts to this where you need to determine for each of the treatments offered:

▸ time line (usually months) of stabilization before the cancer progresses; and

▸ how many, in terms of the percentage of the group, achieved stabilization for this period of time?

You may also ask what further treatments would be offered when the disease progresses.

Practitioner's clinical opinion

The information you will receive is drawn from the results of clinical trials, so it is always worth asking the specialist how others in a similar condition fared in their experience. Although statistics are used as a guide, the specialist may have greater insight into which bracket you are likely to fall, given your individual case and risk factors.

It is also important to ask whether you are risk from *late effects* of treatment, what these would be, how and when you would monitor and who would monitor.

If you follow the chart on the following page, this patient was diagnosed with aggressive breast cancer, stage 2, and told that treatment option A (ACT chemotherapy + herceptin) would give her a 12.5% survival advantage and a 17.6% disease-free survival advantage over treatment option B (TC chemotherapy + herceptin). The ACT chemotherapy was more aggressive and a much longer treatment with long-term risks for secondary leukaemia. When the patient looked at the absolute statistics she saw that the absolute benefit for treatment A was a 1% survival advantage and a 3% disease-free survival advantage. This patient felt that the marginal benefit was worth it, and she opted for treatment A.

It is helpful if you can also draw a graph as these can depict comparisons with greater clarity, particularly if you are measuring more than one treatment outcome. The graph on page 163 illustrates the advantage that herceptin delivers as a targeted therapy when added as a second-line treatment to chemotherapy. Conversely, you can see how a biphosphonate offers only marginal advantage (p165).

Weighing up treatments from a statistical perspective

> ### DIAGNOSIS
> Breast cancer (IDC); triple positive
> Grade 3; score 8/9
> stage 2 (metastases to axillary lymph nodes)
> size of main tumour, 3cm

> ### PROGNOSIS
> 4 year, 86% DFS with recommended treatment (surgery, radiation, ACT chemotherapy, tamoxifen & herceptin)

TREATMENT OPTIONS

		Chemotherapy A (ACT+H)	Chemotherapy B (TC+H)	
OS (overall survival)	Time	4 years	4 years	
	% of group	93%	92%	1% absolute benefit *12.5% relative benefit*
DFS (disease-free survival)	Time	4 years	4 years	
	% of group	86%	83%	3% absolute benefit *17.6% relative benefit*
Response (shrinkage)	Time stabilization	N/A	N/A	
	% of shrinkage	N/A	N/A	
	% of group	N/A	N/A	
Practitioner's clinical experience/opinion of cases like mine	Time (best/worst/median)			
	% of their treated group	All her patients on this protocol have had no recurrence in 7 years	Comment: ACT+H is a longer program than TC+H, can cause cardiotoxicity and a 1.6% risk of secondary leukaemia.	

This patient failed to qualify whether the clinician's experience applied to her specific population (stage 2, grade 8/9, triple positive) or whether it was an "in general" observation. The clinician did not rate the risk of leukaemia as being significant, as the risk of breast cancer was foremost and that the leukaemia, if it did occur, would be 10 years down the track.

Comparison of treatments recommended for HER2+ breast cancer

A 4 year study comparing a nonanthracycline regimen (Doxotaxel + carboplatin) + herceptin (TCH) against an anthracycline regimen + herceptin (ACTH) showed a 3% absolute benefit for DFS and a 1% absolute benefit for OS in the ACTH group. If one factors in the risks for the ACTH group, which include the greatly extended length of time for treatment, cardiotoxicity and secondary leukaemia [1.6%], then these surivival advantages may not look so attractive. However, you can appreciate the huge benefit that herceptin delivers when added to any chemotherapy regime for HER2+ breast cancer. (There were no results for the TC only regimen.)

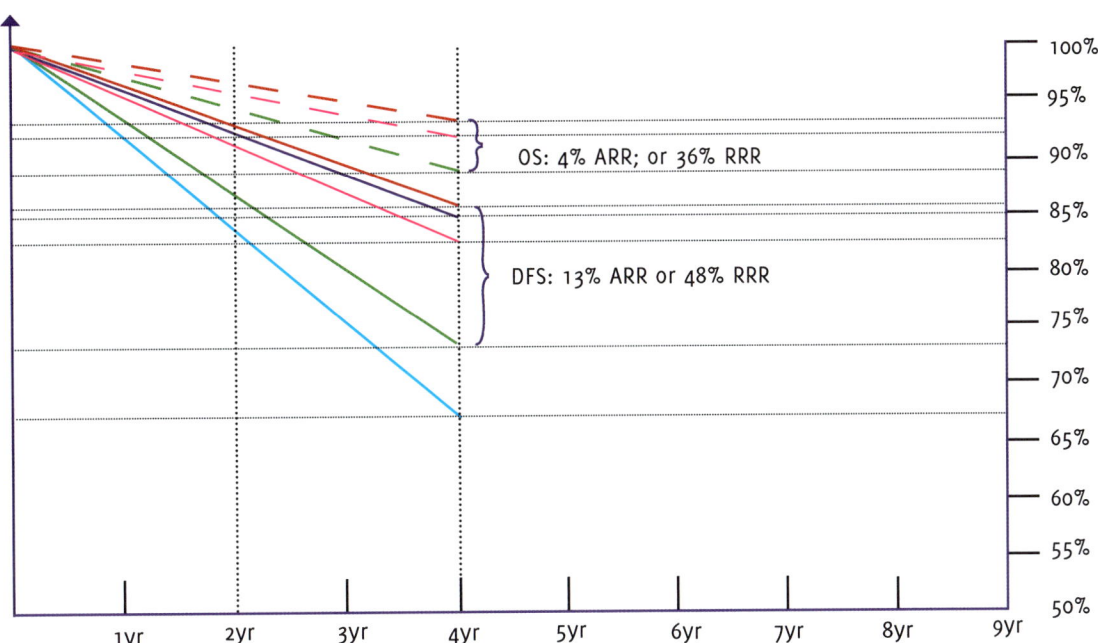

ACT+ H (anthracycline, cyclophosphamide, paclitaxel + herceptin)

— — Overall survival (93%)

———— Disease-free survival (86%)

ACT (anthracycline [doxorubicin], cyclophosphamide, paclitaxel)

— — Overall survival   (89%)

———— Disease-free survival (73%)

CMF + H (cyclophosphamide, methotrexate, fluorouracil + herceptin)

———— Disease-free survival (85.3%)

CMF (cyclophosphamide, methotrexate, fluorouracil)

———— Disease-free survival (67.1%)

TC + H (Doxotaxel, carboplatin + herceptin)

— — Overall survival (92%)

———— Disease-free survival (83%)

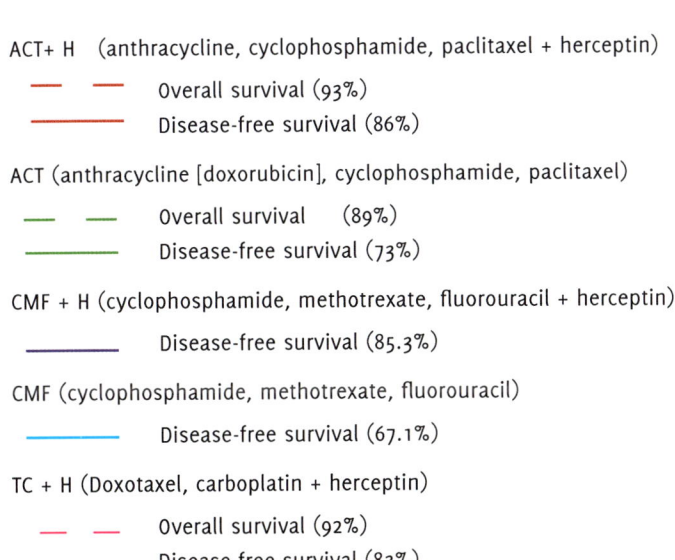

Measuring relative reduction of risk for ACTH/ ACT

OS: Relative Reduction in Risk

ACTH: OS 93% (7% died)

ACT: OS 89% (11% died)

RRR: 7 ÷ 11 = 0.636 or 36%
(1.0 - 0.64 = 0.36 or 36%)

DFS: Relative Reduction in Risk

ACTH: DFS 86% (14% recurrence)

ACT: DFS 73% (27% recurrence)

RRR: 14 ÷ 27 = 0.52 or 48%
(1.0 - 0.52 = 0.48 or 48%)

Comparison of adjunct treatments in cancer

*P*at is 36 years old and has been diagnosed with stage 1, oestrogen positive breast cancer and has been offered a biphosphonate drug to reduce the risk for relapse with bone metastases. She is unsure as she has read some negative results with this drug. But her specialist says that he can reduce her risk of relapse by 36% on the drug. So Pat does some research. She finds that over 90% of patients on the trial survived disease-free, regardless of their group placement, so the very tiny advantage would have to be weighed against the risks.

The addition of zoledronic acid (biphosphonate) to adjuvant endocrine therapy improves disease-free survival in premenopausal patients with estrogen-responsive early breast cancer

http://www.ncbi.nlm.nih.gov/pubmed/19213681

Study group: premenopausal women with endocrine-responsive early breast cancer.

Drug: 1803 patients randomized to receive goserelin (3.6 mg given subcutaneously every 28 days) plus tamoxifen (20 mg per day given orally) or anastrozole (1 mg per day given orally) with or without zoledronic acid (4mg given intravenously every 6 months) for 3 years.

Length of time: 3 years

Number of people: 1803

Primary end point: disease-free survival; recurrence-free survival and overall survival were secondary end points.

Findings:

Disease-free survival rates of:

▸ 92.8% in the goserelin + tamoxifen group;

▸ 92.0% in the goserelin + anastrozole group;

▸ 90.8% in the group that received endocrine therapy alone (tamoxifen or anastrazole only); and

▸ 94.0% in the group that received endocrine therapy (goserelin + tamoxifen) with zoledronic acid.

There was no significant difference in disease-free survival between the goserelin + anastrozole or goserelin + tamoxifen groups. The addition of zoledronic acid to endocrine therapy, as compared with endocrine therapy without zoledronic acid, resulted in an absolute reduction of 3.2 percentage and a relative reduction of 36% in the risk of relapse; the addition of zoledronic acid did not significantly reduce the risk of death.

Relative reduction of risk of relapse with bone metastases in the zoledronic acid group:

6 ÷ 9.2 = 0.65 or or a 65% chance of relapse or 35% reduction in risk of relapse (1.0 - 0.65 = 0.35)

▸ endocrine therapy + zoledronic acid: 6% suffered relapse

▸ endocrine therapy alone: 9.2% suffered relapse

4 year disease-free survival rates for premenopausal women with oestrogen responsive early breast cancer, with and without zoledronic acid

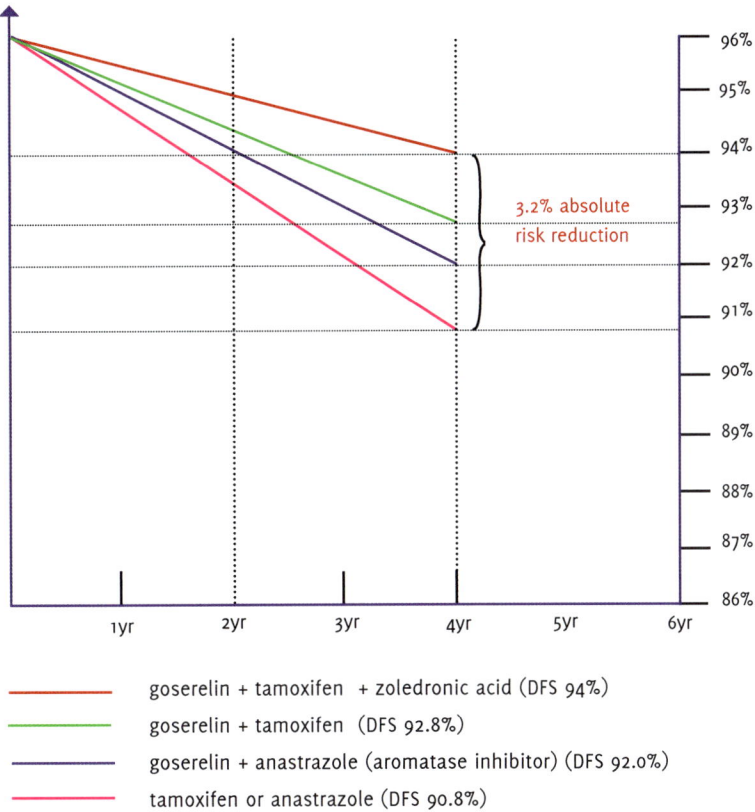

——————— goserelin + tamoxifen + zoledronic acid (DFS 94%)

——————— goserelin + tamoxifen (DFS 92.8%)

——————— goserelin + anastrazole (aromatase inhibitor) (DFS 92.0%)

——————— tamoxifen or anastrazole (DFS 90.8%)

▶ *tamoxifen* blocks the oestrogen receptors in breast tissue inhibiting oestrogen's stimulant effect on the breast cancer, but stimulates ovarian oestrogen production

▶ *goserelin* suppresses ovarian production of oestrogen, so lowers the oestrogenic burden

▶ *anastrozole* reduces the conversion of endogenous oestrogen to its active form (suppresses the aromatase enzyme) and decreases the oestrogenic stimulus, but is not strong enough to oppose ovarian production of oestrogen hence it is generally given to post-menopausal women

▶ *zoledronic acid* (biphosphonate - Zometa) slows bone turnover, and prevents calcium from being removed from the bone

*C*heryl had been diagnosed with stage 2, grade 2 invasive ductal breast carcinoma. The tumour was 3.4cm and there were 6 out of 45 lymph nodes infected. Cheryl had been offered mastectomy followed by radio-therapy and was told that she could reduce her risk of the cancer returning within 5 years by 54% if she opted for the adjunct radiotherapy. Cheryl did her research and found the study (opposite).

Measuring rate of relapse:

Untreated group (A): 23% had relapsed at 5 yrs
Treated group (B): 6% had relapsed at 5 yrs
ARR: 23 - 6 = 17%

Relative Reduction in risk:
RRR: 6 ÷ 23 = 0.26 (26% relative risk of relapse) or 74% relative reduction of risk of relapse in the treated group (1.0 - 0.26 = 0.74 or 74%).

Relative increase in risk for the untreated group:
23 ÷ 6 = 4.37 fold (437% or over 4 times more likely to relapse if untreated).

Measuring the odds:

100:17 = 5.88 (or 6:1) *(NNT = 6 people to treat to prevent 1 relapse)*

The odds are 1 in 6 (6:1) of staying disease free at 5 years with mastectomy + radiotherapy. It's always worthwhile to work out your odds as these can give a truer or more meaningful picture of what a treatment can do for you. Relative statistics can be quite misleading to the average patient. For an explanation of working out your relative risks and odds please see pp147-149.

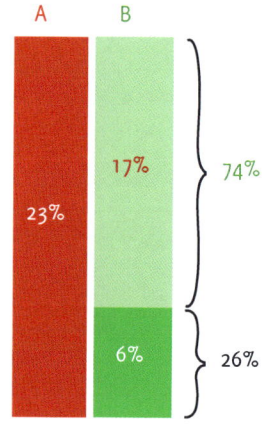

5 year rate of relapse

absolute risk reduction 17% (ARR)
relative risk reduction   74% (RRR)

Cheryl refined the information as she belonged to the sub-group who had 4 or more infected nodes.

Untreated group (A): 26% had relapsed at 5 yrs
Treated group (B): 12% had relapsed at 5 yrs
ARR: 26 - 12 = 14%

RRR: 12 ÷ 26 = 0.46 (46% risk of relapse) or 54% relative reduction of risk of relapse in the treated group

Relative increase in risk for the untreated group:
26 ÷ 12 = 2.17 (more than double the risk of relapse in the untreated group).

Measuring the odds:

100:14 (or 7:1) *(NNT = 7 people to treat to prevent 1 relapse)*

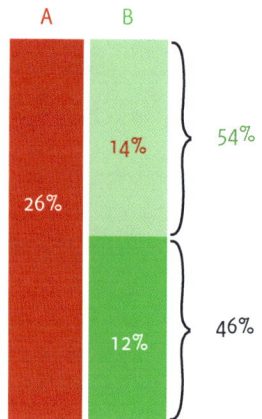

5 year rate of relapse
(4+ infected nodes)

absolute risk reduction 14% (ARR)
relative risk reduction   54% (RRR)

http://www.cancernetwork.com/cancer-management/stage-ii-breast/article/10165/1802575

The EBCTCG meta-analysis included 8,500 women who had primarily node-positive disease and were treated with mastectomy and axillary clearance. Patients were randomized to receive post-mastectomy radiation versus no post-mastectomy radiation. The 5 year risk of local relapse was significantly lower in the radiation group **B** (6%) than among those randomized to no radiation group **A** (23%). Radiotherapy produced similar proportional reductions in local recurrence, regardless of patient age or tumor characteristics. The 15 year breast cancer mortality risk (OS) was also markedly lower for the radiation patients (54.7%), compared with those receiving no radiation (61.2%). The 5-year risk of local recurrence in patients with one to three positive nodes who received radiation therapy was 4%, compared with 16% in controls. In patients with four or more nodes, the 5 year risk of local recurrence was 12% in the radiation group and 26% in the control group.

Measuring 15 year overall survival:

Untreated group (A) : 61.2% had died at 15 yrs (OS =38.8%)

Treated group (B) + radiation: 54.7% had died at 15 yrs (OS = 45.3%)

ARR: 61.2 - 54.7 = 6.5%

Relative reduction in risk:
RRR: 54.7 ÷ 61.2 = 0.89 (89% relative risk of death) or 11% relative reduction of risk of death for the treated group (1.0 - 0.89 = 0.11 or 11%).

Relative increase in risk of death for the untreated group:
61.2 ÷ 54.7 = 1.11 (11% more likely to die or a 1.1 fold increase in risk of death.)

Measuring the odds:

The odds: 100:6.5 = 15.38 (NNT = 15 people to treat to prevent 1 death)

The odds are 1 in 15 (15:1) of being alive at 15 years with radiotherapy.

The margins for 15 year overall survival were quite narrow, offering a 6.5% absolute survival advantage which translates as an 11% relative reduction in mortality risk for the treated group.

15 year overall survival (OS)

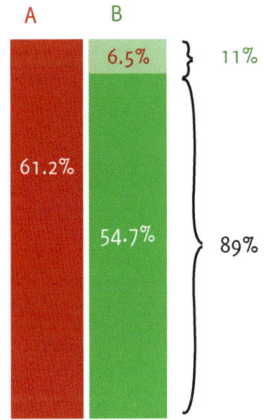

absolute risk reduction 6.5% (ARR)
relative risk reduction   11% (RRR)

Researching natural treatments

Clinical studies which demonstrate efficacy of natural products within a clinical setting can help a patient determine whether a product will help or not. When a product is recommended it is wise to research the product to see whether any studies have been undertaken on humans with a similar condition to yourself.

Josephine has ulcerative colitis and she wonders whether she can improve her remission if she adds a product recommended by her naturopath, curcumin. She can't find any trials with curcumin for her specific condition but she does find a trial which compares patients with ulcerative colitis taking mesalamine plus curcumin with a good outcome. Although the study is short and small, Josephine decided there were no risks involved, and after factoring in other research with curcumin in bowel cancer, she felt it could be of benefit to her.

Curcumin Maintenance Therapy for Ulcerative Colitis

Randomized, Multicenter, Double-Blind, Placebo-Controlled Trial

http://www.ncbi.nlm.nih.gov/pubmed/17101300

Study group: patients with quiescent ulcerative colitis (UC)

Drug: 45 patients received curcumin, 1g after breakfast and 1g after the evening meal, plus sulfasalazine (SZ) or mesalamine, and 44 patients received placebo plus SZ or mesalamine for 6 months.

Length of time: 6 months

Number of people: 89 (82 completed study)

Primary end point: assess the efficacy of curcumin as maintenance therapy in patients with quiescent ulcerative colitis (UC)

Findings:

In the control group (A) 20.51% relapsed (absolute number 8 out of 39 patients) while in the treated group (B) 4.65% relapsed (absolute number 2 out of 43 patients). Furthermore, curcumin improved both CAI (P = .038) and EI (P = .0001), thus suppressing the morbidity associated with UC.

CONCLUSIONS:

Curcumin seems to be a promising and safe medication for maintaining remission in patients with quiescent UC. Further studies on curcumin should strengthen our findings.

Relative Reduction in risk of relapse:

4.65 ÷ 20.51 = 0.23 (23% chance of having a relapse with curcumin). This translates as a 77% relative reduction in risk (1.0 - 0.23 = 0.77 or 77%).

From the diagram to the right you can see the difference in relapse between the treated group and the untreated group over a 6 month period.

Group A (drug treatment only): 20.51% suffered a re-lapse within 6 months

Treated group B (drug + curcumin): 4.65% suffered a relapse within 6 months

ARR: 20.51 - 4.65 = 15.86% The absolute reduction of risk of relapse is 15.86%.

Relative reduction in risk with curcumin:
RRR: 4.65 ÷ 20.51 = 0.23 or a 23% relative risk of relapse on curcumin. This translates as a 77% relative reduction of risk relapse on curcumin (1 - 0.23 = 0.77 or 77%).

Relative increase in risk of relapse without curcumin:
20.51 ÷ 4.65 = 4.41 (4.4 fold increase in risk of relapse)

Measuring the odds:

100:15.86 = 6.3 (or 6:1) *(NNT = 6 people to treat to prevent 1 relapse)*

You would need to treat 6 patients for 6 months with curcumin to prevent 1 relapse.

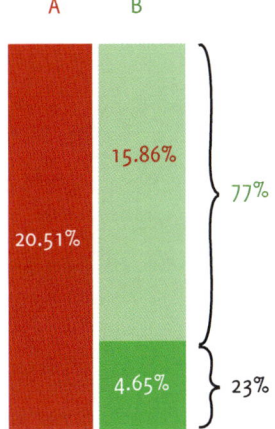

A   B

15.86%

77%

20.51%

4.65%   23%

absolute risk reduction 15.86% (ARR)
relative risk reduction   77% (RRR)

The odds are 100:15.86 or 6:1
(NNT = 6 people to prevent 1 relapse)

Weighing up the benefit of Vitamin D in breast cancer

The following is an example of marketing propaganda. When reading the latest research on vitamin D and breast cancer the consumer may be led to think that vitamin D is a miracle vitamin and therefore should be a core treatment.

"Vitamin D can reduce the risks of breast cancer by 43%. The high vitamin D group had a breast cancer risk 32% to 43% lower compared with those with the lowest vitamin intake."

"Women deficient in the "sunshine vitamin" when they were diagnosed with breast cancer were 82 percent more likely to have their cancer spread and were 73 percent more likely to die than women with adequate vitamin D levels."

However, the studies were evaluating vitamin D status at diagnosis as a prognostic marker (risk factor) for disease progression, and not as a treatment. Meaningful interpretation of these statistics, which relate to both reduction of risk (first quote) and increase of risk (second quote), requires some absolute statistics. Additionally, these quotes may mislead the consumer to believe that there is a reduced risk of getting breast cancer if you are vitamin D sufficient. The study simply compared the overall and disease-free survival in both the vitamin D sufficient and vitamin D deficient groups at diagnosis. See if you can make sense of the statistics.

Chustecka, Z; Vitamin D deficiency linked to poorer outcome in breast cancer
Medscape Medical News

Study group: women with a mean age of 50 with newly diagnosed and treated breast cancer tested for vitamin D sufficiency at diagnosis

Length of time: median 12 years

Number of people: 512

Primary end point: comparison of overall survival and disease-free survival between the vitamin D deficient and vitamin D sufficient groups

Findings:

Overall survival rates:

- 85% in the vitamin D sufficient group (15% died)
- 74% in the vitamin D deficient group (26% died)
- Absolute reduction of risk 11% (26 - 15 = 11)
- Relative reduction of risk for the D sufficient group = 42% (15 ÷ 26 = 0.58 = 58% relative risk of dying or 42% relative reduction of risk of death/less likely to die)
- Relative increase of risk for the D deficient group = 73% (26 ÷ 15 = 1.73 or 73% more likely to die)

Disease-free survival rates:

- 83% in the vitamin D sufficient group (17% had relapsed)
- 69% in the vitamin D deficient group (31% had relapsed)
- Absolute reduction of risk 14% (31 - 17 = 14)
- Relative reduction of risk for the D sufficient group = 46% (17 ÷ 31 = 0.54 = 54% relative risk for relapse or 46% relative reduction of risk for relapse)
- Relative increase of risk for the D deficient group = 82% (31 ÷ 17 = 1.82 or 82% more likely to relapse)

Overall survival rates

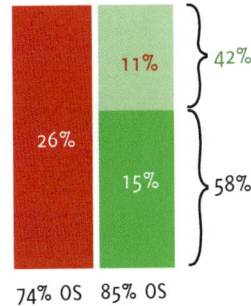

74% OS   85% OS

absolute risk reduction 11% (ARR)
relative risk reduction   42% (RRR)

Relative reduction of risk for mortality within a 12 year survival period for women pretreated for breast cancer with vitamin D sufficiency at diagnosis:

15 ÷ 26 = 0.58 (58% relative chance of dying within 12 years or 42% relative reduction of risk of dying within this period). This translates as a 42% relative reduction in risk (1.0 - 0.58 = 0.42).

Relative increase in risk of death with vitamin D deficiency:

26 ÷ 15 = 1.73 (73% more likely to die within 12 years with vitamin D deficiency)

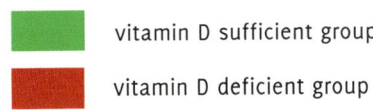

vitamin D sufficient group

vitamin D deficient group

Disease-free survival rates

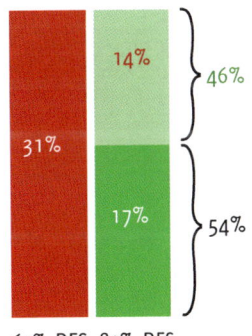

69% DFS   83% DFS

absolute risk reduction 14% (ARR)
relative risk reduction   46% (RRR)

Relative reduction of risk for disease relapse within a 12 year period for women pretreated for breast cancer with vitamin D sufficiency at diagnosis:

17 ÷ 31 = 0.54 (54% relative chance of disease relapse within 12 years or 46% relative reduction of risk of disease progression within this period).

Relative increase in risk for disease relapse with vitamin D deficiency:

31 ÷ 17 = 1.82 (82% more likely to relapse which represents nearly a 2 fold relative increase in risk of disease relapse within 12 years with vitamin D deficiency)

Cherry picking the data

Early studies show lymphoma responds to fucoidan

http://www.canceractive.com/

" Fucoidan is a natural compound found in various forms of seaweed like kombu, limu, wakame and mozuku plus animals like the sea cucumber. Researchers from the Hashemite University in Jordan at the AACR Dead Sea International Conference on Advances in Cancer Research working on previous studies said that the extract from common brown seaweed causes cancer cell death (apoptosis) and shrinks tumours, have found that fucoidan suppressed cancer cell growth and caused a significant increase in apoptosis, or cellular death, in lymphoma cancer cells while leaving healthy cells intact.

Previous research studies in 2002 and 2005 have labeled Fucoidan as an exciting new ingredient with potential for cancer treatment.

Seaweeds containing fucoidan have been found to have anti-tumor activity in mice and Japanese researchers at the Biomedical Research Laboratories have found that Fucoidan caused leukaemia, lymphoma, colorectal and stomach cancer cells to self-destruct. It has also been found to have significant immune boosting effects, and can even reduce blood cholesterol levels and is effective in cases of meningitis. Fucoidan is found in two forms: F-fucoidan, a complex sulphated polysaccharide containing the sulphuric ester L-fucose; and U-fucoidan containing the trace elements galactose, xylose, and about 20 per cent glucuronic acid. About 4 per cent of the dry weight of seaweed is fucoidan.

Lymphoma is divided into two classes, Hodgkin's and non-Hodgkin's which are, in turn, further classified into B-cell and T-cell groups.

'Some forms of B-cell lymphoma are especially resistant to standard treatment and thus new therapies are needed', said Professor Mohammad Irhimeh adding, 'in this study, we looked at a new treatment strategy using novel active compounds derived from a natural source – seaweed.' "

Let's take a look at the study.

The objective was to measure the effectiveness of fucoidan on the mobilization of hemopoietic progenitor stem cells (HPC) into the peripheral blood (PB). This could provide an alternative treatment to transplantation of surgically-harvested bone marrow in patients who are resistant to standard treatment particularly if they have been pretreated with chemotherapy.

Fucoidan ingestion increases the expression of CXCR4 on human CD34+ cells

Mohammad R. Irhimeha,J. Helen Fittona,and Raymond M. Lowenthala; Experimental Hematology 35 (2007) 989–994

Objective: To measure the increase of HPCs in peripheral blood of healthy, non-smoking volunteers following oral ingestion of either 3g of 10% Fucoidan or 3g of 75% Fucoidan taken three times daily for 12 days against a control group.

Study group: healthy, non-smoking volunteers

Drug: oral ingestion of either 3g of 10% Fucoidan or 3g of 75% Fucoidan taken three times daily for 12 days against a control group.

Length of time: 12 days

Number of people: 37

Primary end point: to determine the effects of ingested Undaria-derived fucoidan on peripheral blood

Findings:

Oral administration of fucoidan significantly amplified the CXCR4 HPC from 45% to 90% after 12 days; SDF1 and INF also increased

The ability to mobilize HPCs with high levels of CXCR4 expression could be clinically valuable. No side effects and no toxicity

You can see how you can whip up marketing propaganda for a product by cherry picking the available data on a naturally-derived compound. However, the study did not measure clinical outcome in a population with lymphoma, it merely measured how much the product could stimulate the release of hemopoietic progenitor stem cells from the bone marrow for potential collection from the peripheral blood. Whilst this is excellent research and could offer new and safer options for treatment in the future, it would be difficult to determine how it would influence the outcome of a patient with lymphoma, or even help them get to their end point. The danger lies when there is heavy reliance or expectation by consumers on these products to produce results that these products have never achieved. Although patients may choose a product on the basis that it *can do no harm,* problems arise when patients are presented with twenty or more products (that may also do no harm) as to how to determine which one/s are able to deliver measurable value or give a better outcome in their individual case.

"People don't die from the old
diseases any more.
They die from new ones,
but that's Progress, isn't it? "

Harlan Ellison, 1934 -

Why do I need to rate the value of each treatment?

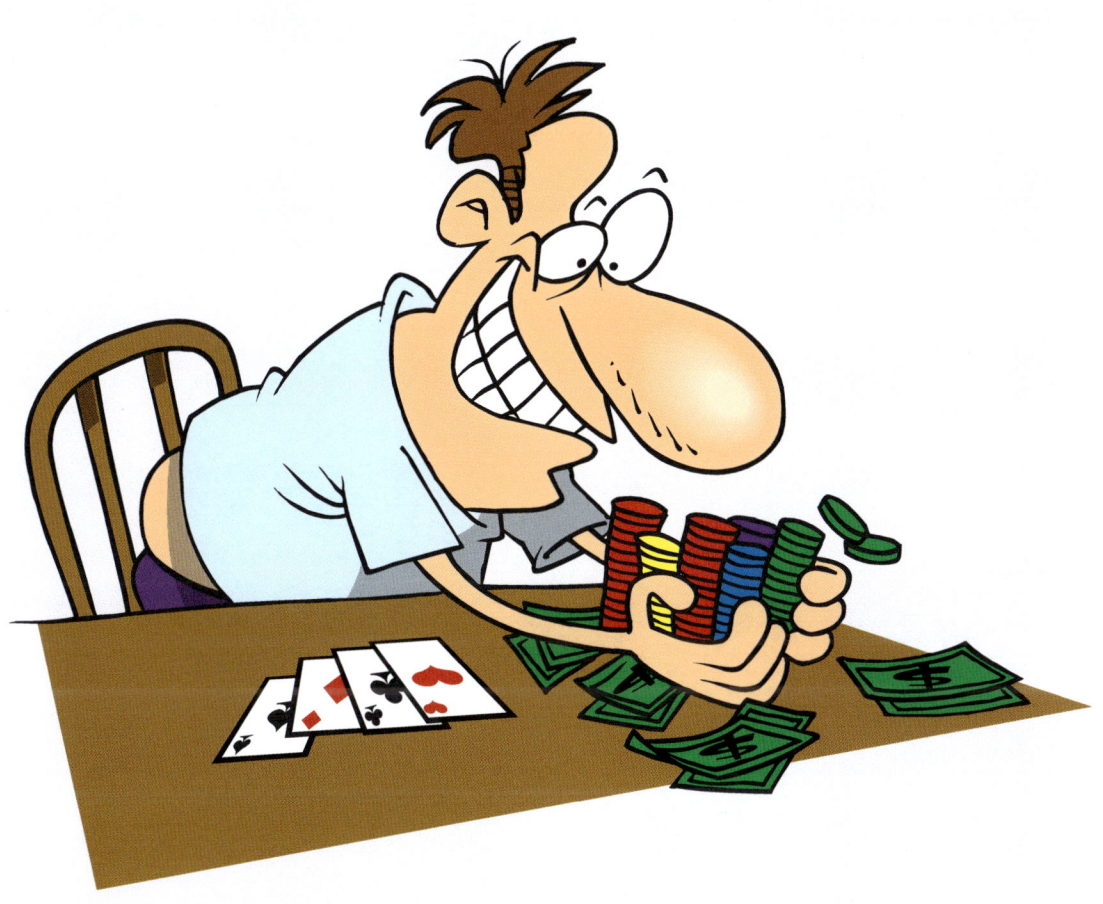

Because you have to know which option will give you the best odds!

Flow Chart for Evaluating & Validating treatments: step 5

Step 1

Core or adjunct

Determine what the treatment does

- how does it work; and
- what aspects of my case does it treat.

Match the claims of treatment against your end point & goals to prioritize and determine the value of treatment.

Step 2

Measurable & meaningful

Determine how you will *measure* progress

- objective (tests, scans etc)
- subjective (resolution of symptoms)

and how *meaningful* this will be to the overall case:

- which leg of my journey will it help with?
- how far will it get me to my end point?

If you can't monitor progress then there is no way of knowing the value of treatment.

Step 5

Treatment alignment rating

Use *My Treatment Alignment Rating Template* and select the various treatments which may help, indicate how they may work/what they will do and what benefit they offer in helping you get to your end point. Make sure that the treatment can be monitored. Next rate each treatment and make your decision on which treatments will offer you the most value.

Step 3

Benefit/Risk assessment

Complete the *SWOT analysis* and the *Quadrant chart* when you need to factor in:

▸ the risks of treatment in your individual case;

▸ the risks of not doing treatment; or

▸ when the benefits of treatment are unknown.

These charts will facilitate decision-making when there is an absence of scientific proof or clinical data for a treatment, or when you need to make a decision based on a range of criteria which include how your condition and the potential treatment could affect your life. These charts are invaluable as they will provide a basis for collaboration and help clarify your position to all parties.

These charts can be completed with simple information provided at an appointment and require no medical expertise. They do not require reference to scientific data. The quadrant chart can be used as a visual platform to match the relative value of many therapies and/or treatments to the patient's end point.

Step 4

Scientific & Clinical Validation

Use *My value template* (column 4) to select your own criteria for validating treatments. Then use the simple steps from the *Evaluating scientific evidence* chart to determine how appropriate the treatment is to your case and its potential value in getting you to your end point.

3 Rating each treatment

We are now ready to rate each treatment using the *Treatment Alignment Rating Template*. Using this chart, like the Therapy Alignment Rating Chart, you can list all the potential treatments in the left column and from your research you can then state what each treatment will achieve (what it will do) and then align each treatment to your end point: those aligning the most closely will score the most highly. Keep it simple so that your core focus is on the journey and where you're heading rather than on the individual treatments.

Begin by referring back to your *Treatment Alignment Template* (pp126-127, 234). Using this template (example below) you would have already selected specific treatments on offer and matched the claims of each treatment against your end point and prioritized goals, and also determined the type of monitoring required for each treatment.

Treatment Alignment Template

TREATMENT					
My aspirational end point					
List of prioritized goals					
Tests for monitoring					

Review the template and select the treatments you feel will offer you the most value and list them in the left column of the *Treatment Alignment Rating Template (pp179, 235)*. By this time you will have hopefully researched each treatment option so that you can factor in both the pros and cons of the treatment. It may be that you have already discarded some of the recommended treatments on the basis that they offer little value or could take you in the opposite direction.

Use the *Tips on completing the Treatment Alignment Rating Template (p180)* before you complete the template to double check that you are clear on what the treatment claims to do, how this aligns with your end point and the monitoring required. Next you can rate each treatment on a score of 1-10, where the highest score represents the treatment/s that can take you the furthest to your end point.

Once this is completed you can fill in the relevant section on the *Full Alignment Template* under *Treatments* (pp181, 224).

Treatment Alignment Rating Template

Treatment options	What will the treatment do?	End point alignment	What is used to measure outcome?	Rating

Tips on completing the Treatment Alignment Rating Template

Treatment	What will it do	End point alignment	What is used to measure outcome	Rating
List each proposed treatment or product	For each product state exactly what it will do within the context of your case. For example, supplementing with a mineral may address a deficiency, but you would need to say how that would help you. Similarly, taking a herbal product may have specific actions, but you need to indicate how that would influence your case. Taking a liver tonic may be meaningless unless you know how it will help and what improvement you could expect within your individual case. So each product will have a specific action which you need to match to your case. Products may be specific to goals you need to achieve on your journey, so matching products to goals is also a good indicator of its value to you.	Return to your aspirational end points and match each product or treatment against one or more of these.	Ask each practitioner: ▸ what tests they will use to monitor if the treatment is working; ▸ what those tests will indicate; and ▸ how frequently you will be monitored. If a treatment cannot be monitored then you may be driving blind, or taking a product that has no measurable outcome on your case. Alternatively, the monitoring may be subjective "How do I feel, have my symptoms reduced....etc." This may be perfectly adequate, but you need to be sure which treatment is having the positive effect so seek clarification on what you can expect from each treatment in terms of outcome, symptom reduction etc.	Score each treatment from 1-10: those that are most closely aligned to your end point will score more highly. Your score for treatments may change on your journey. This is normal. For example, if you were to deteriorate then another treatment may become of greater value, and if you are improving, then drugs may be removed as they have less value.

Make sure the vehicle you choose will get you there!

Full Alignment Template

Prioritized list of Goals (measurables)	End point alignment	THERAPIES	TREATMENTS	MONITORING

Remember, treatments represent how you travel (the means) or the vehicle you use for each stretch of the journey. The vehicle has to be capable of getting you from A to B, it should not take you down a cul-de-sac nor in the opposite direction, and it may have to travel within a specific time frame. For example, if you have a deadline to meet then you are unlikely to travel the ocean by ship, but instead go by air; or if you have time on your hands you may well choose to travel by sea. In both these instances the destination remains the same, but the means of travel differs. Choose the means carefully and keep your eye on the end point.

Monitoring

With regard to objective monitoring remember to ask which type of test will be used (blood test, scan etc.) and what indicator or marker will be used for monitoring. For example, if you have anaemia and an inflammatory disease, then a blood test may be requested for the following markers: iron levels, haemoglobin, complete blood count, inflammatory markers (ESR and CRP) and specific antibodies. If you are having a scan then monitoring will be for progression/regression of lesions, the type of lesion, their position and size.

Pauline's treatment alignment rating

Treatment options	What will the treatment do?	End point alignment	What is used to measure outcome?	Rating
Corticosteroids	▲ Suppresses inflammation in my whole body	▲ Will stop disease progression within 3 months & there is an 80% chance I will get into remission	▲ Objective: blood tests ▲ Subjective: reduction in pain, better mobility	9
Vit D & Iron	▲ Resolve anaemia and increase energy (iron), support mineralization of bones (vitamin D)	▲ Reduce my future health risks ▲ Increase my capacity to heal	▲ Objective: blood test ▲ Subjective: more energy	7
Diet therapy *low allergy, alkaline diet*	▲ Help stop inflammation (anti-inflammatory/high alkaline) ▲ Address my digestive problems ▲ Resolve food intolerance/allergy ▲ Help me increase my weight ▲ Help restore menses	▲ Long term remission/drug free by addressing possible causes, risks and exacerbating factors; ▲ Increase my odds of pregnancy	▲ Objective: blood tests ▲ Subjective: reduction in pain, improvement in digestion, improved energy, menses	9
TCM herbs *name herbs each month*	▲ Suppress inflammation, support adrenal glands ▲ Help with side-effects of drugs ▲ May restore menses	▲ Help me come off the drugs ▲ Improve my chances for remission and stay in remission for longer ▲ Increase my odds of pregnancy	▲ Objective: pulse and tongue diagnosis ▲ Subjective: less drug effects, reduce inflammation/pain, restore menses	8
Physiotherapy	▲ Exercise and strengthen muscles, bones and joints ▲ Increase bone density	▲ Reduce future health risks (osteoporosis)	▲ Objective: bone densitometry ▲ Subjective: more mobility, less pain & stiffness	6

Pauline has scored the corticosteroid therapy and the diet therapy both highly, but for different reasons. The corticosteroids will bring her into remission quickly, but the diet therapy may keep her in remission and drug-free. Pauline has scored the herbs less highly as she puts it "a deficiency of herbs is not the cause of my condition", but she sees that they may have enormous benefit in helping her deal with the side-effects of the drugs, come off the drugs and perhaps help regulate her menstrual cycle. Most of the treatments can be monitored objectively (through tests), but with all treatments Pauline is looking for perceivable improvements. Pauline kept a record of which herbal formulae addressed which symptoms and which pattern of disharmony.

Pauline's full alignment template

Prioritized list of Goals (measurables)	End point alignment	Therapy	Treatment	Monitoring
reduce inflammation	▲ remission, reduce future health risks	▲ rheumatology, TCM, diet therapy	▲ corticosteroids ▲ high alkaline diet ▲ TCM herbs	▲ blood tests ▲ pulse & tongue
restore mobility	▲ reduce future health risks (osteoporosis)	▲ physiotherapy	▲ physical exercise	
resolve digestive problems	▲ remission, reduce future health risks	▲ diet therapy	▲ diet	
gain weight	▲ fertility, reduce future health risks	▲ diet therapy	▲ diet	
restore menses	▲ fertility (get pregnant), reduce future health risks (osteoporosis)	▲ TCM, diet therapy	▲ diet ▲ TCM herbs	
improve bone density	▲ reduce future health risks (osteoporosis)	▲ diet therapy, physiotherapy	▲ supplements ▲ diet ▲ physical exercise	▲ bone densitometry ▲ blood tests
improve energy	▲ reduce future health risks	▲ diet therapy	▲ supplements ▲ diet	
restore nutritional status	▲ reduce future health risks	▲ diet therapy	▲ supplements ▲ diet	▲ blood tests

When you fill in the treatment alignment section of your *Full Alignment Template* you are aligning the treatments with the prioritized list of goals and with the end point alignment: treatments must align with both. For example, in Pauline's case the corticosteroids (through suppressing inflammation) will help restore mobility but they won't reduce the future risk of osteoporosis; they will increase this risk. So physical exercise is the only treatment that aligns with both the end point and restoring mobility. By transcribing your treatments into this chart, you can see at a glance what each treatment addresses/achieves and its specific alignments.

On the following page you can see how Pauline has completed her Journey Road Map by placing where each practitioner can take her against a time line, and in terms of achieving her goals aligned with her aspirational end point. She has also entered her own three key goals (reduce inflammation, improve bone density and get pregnant) and she can see at a glance whether these are realistic from what others can offer. For example, Pauline has indicated that she wants to improve her bone density within 18 months, but her nutritionist has indicated that improvements may not be seen for 2 years, depending on how long she is on the corticosteroids.

Pauline's Journey Road Map: where treatments can take her

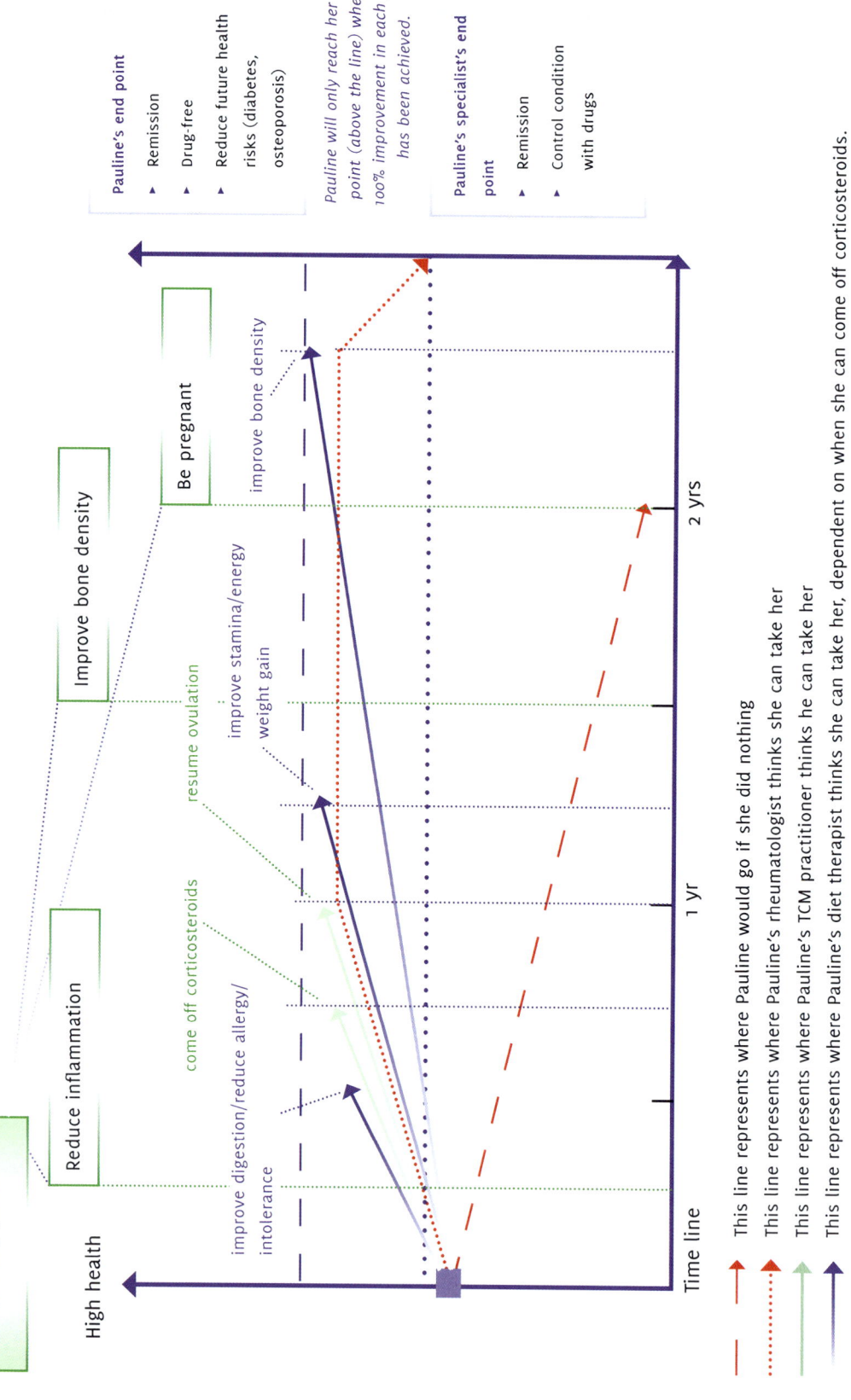

Pauline's way points

High health

Reduce inflammation

Improve bone density

Be pregnant

Pauline's end point
- ▲ Remission
- ▲ Drug-free
- ▲ Reduce future health risks (diabetes, osteoporosis)

Pauline will only reach her end point (above the line) when a 100% improvement in each goal has been achieved.

Pauline's specialist's end point
- ▲ Remission
- ▲ Control condition with drugs

improve bone density

improve bone density

come off corticosteroids

resume ovulation

improve stamina/energy weight gain

improve digestion/reduce allergy/intolerance

Time line

1 yr

2 yrs

This line represents where Pauline would go if she did nothing

This line represents where Pauline's rheumatologist thinks she can take her

This line represents where Pauline's TCM practitioner thinks he can take her

This line represents where Pauline's diet therapist thinks she can take her, dependent on when she can come off corticosteroids.

Andrew's treatment alignment

f you remember, Andrew is 45 years old, is overweight, has high blood pressure and high cholesterol and early signs of diabetes (high blood glucose). His father suffered from *a heart attack in his 50s* and also had *late onset diabetes*. Andrew is not given any specific advice other than he should try to reduce his weight and is offered cholesterol-lowering medication. His end point is to reduce his future health risks (heart disease, diabetes and stroke), improve his general health and be drug-free. In order to achieve this he needs to lose weight, reduce his blood pressure, cholesterol and blood glucose.

Andrew is not one to go to practitioners, nor does he like going on weight loss diets. He has tried these in the past and he has managed to regain all the weight lost within six months of achieving his goal. He has numerous weight loss books, most of the programs he has tried, and he likes to research products on the internet. He has found a good website *www.iherb.com* where he can research his condition and find out what products are recommended for his diagnosis, and even read reviews from customers who bought the products to see how effective they were for them.

Andrew decided to ask the gym's personal trainer if he could help him with his diet. The trainer recommends protein shakes and a low carbohydrate diet. Andrew knows that this will not be sustainable long-term and he could simply regain any weight lost, and it could exacerbate his kidney stones. He needs a sustainable long-term program that reduces his health risks and improves his general health. The high protein diet does not fit the bill. So he seeks the opinion of a nutritionist who comes highly recommended. She prepares a program that gives him the best of both worlds; it will reduce his cholesterol and his weight, and he should be able to gradually change his eating habits over the coming year.

Andrew has found a number of products that could help reduce his cholesterol: red yeast rice extract, which works like a statin and is combined with policosanol which helps inhibit the absorption of cholesterol, and niacin which helps in the removal of LDLs (and hence cholesterol) from the circulation by increasing its uptake by the cells. Many iherb customers also take CoQ10. Andrew

doesn't like the thought of being product-dependent for life and sees that CoQ10 may be outside his budget.

So he decides that he will see what the diet can do just with the minimum of supplementation (policosanol and red yeast rice extract) as this would be ideal and the red yeast rice would probably be the most effective supplement for reducing cholesterol within a short time frame (his doctor has given him 3 months).

However, it's the early symptoms of diabetes that really worry Andrew and this is where he is going to put most of his attention. Diet is the key treatment and he has found that various herbs may help, such as Goat's Rue, Cinnamon, Bitter Melon, Fenugreek and Gymnema. He is at a bit of a loss because there are so many products to choose from. He doesn't know enough about herbs and he doesn't want to see a herbalist as he is concerned about the expense and they may wish to treat him for other things that are not a high priority. So after more research he sees that doctors in Germany have been using alpha lipoic acid for many years as this seems to increase the cells capacity to take up glucose and hence lower blood sugar. The product is an excellent antioxidant which will also protect his arteries so it seems to Andrew that it will be good for his general condition.

The personal trainer at the gym has thrown another spanner in the works and said that he could be carrying a lot of heavy metals due to his work as mechanic. He says that heavy metals cause oxidative stress which could compound inflammation and cholesterol build-up in the arteries. Andrew is now concerned about this but unsure of how best to approach it, so the personal trainer recommends a naturopath who will do a hair analysis.

Andrew goes along and has the hair analysis which reveals high levels of heavy metals. He thinks about having chelation therapy with a GP who specializes in this. On research this he finds that any improvements only last a few months and that it is only generally given to people with existing heart disease. He sees that lipoic acid is also a good heavy metal chelator and as he wasn't convinced that heavy metal detoxification was core to his case he opted to concentrate on his other treatments which, hopefully, would give meaningful and measurable outcomes.

Andrew's treatment alignment rating

Treatment options	What will the treatment do?	How will it help me get to my end point?	What is used to measure outcome?	Rating
Red yeast rice extract	▲ Acts like a statin to reduce my blood cholesterol	▲ Reduce my risk factors for heart disease ▲ Help me stay drug-free	▲ Objective: 6 monthly blood tests ▲ Subjective: nil	5
Policosanol	▲ Inhibits the uptake and recycling of cholesterol	▲ Reduce my risk factors for heart disease ▲ Help me stay drug-free	▲ Objective: 6 monthly blood tests ▲ Subjective: nil	5
Alpha Lipoic acid	▲ Increases insulin sensitivity and reduces blood glucose ▲ Reduce oxidative stress especially in tissues damaged by glucose (eyes, nerves, arteries, brain)	▲ Reduce my risk factors for diabetes, cataracts, nerve degeneration, arterial degeneration, brain degeneration ▲ Help me stay drug-free	▲ Objective: blood test ▲ Subjective: more energy	7
Heavy metal detoxification	▲ Chelates and removes heavy metals that cause oxidative stress	▲ May help reduce future health risks	▲ Objective: urine challenge, hair analysis ▲ Subjective: nil	2
Diet	▲ Help me lose weight and keep it off ▲ Help me lower my BP & cholesterol ▲ Help me reduce my blood glucose	▲ Reduce my risk factors for heart disease and diabetes and so reduce future health risks ▲ Improve my general health ▲ Help me stay drug-free	▲ Objective: weigh-in; blood tests ▲ Subjective: feel better, more energetic	10
Exercise	▲ Help me lose weight ▲ Increase my cardio fitness ▲ Reduce cholesterol ▲ Reduce blood sugar	▲ Improve my general health and level of fitness ▲ Reduce future health risks ▲ Help me stay drug-free	▲ Objective: weigh-in ▲ Subjective: feel better, more stamina	8

Andrew ideally wants to be drug and product-independent so he has decided not to score the supplements highly as he knows that without making dietary changes and doing exercise then nothing much will improve even if he takes many supplements. He feels that if he can achieve results on as few supplements as possible then he will be able to see what his body is capable of achieving on its own. However, he feels that the alpha lipoic acid may be a good long-term supplement to take as he is getting older and his work place could be a hazard to his long-term health.

Andrew's full alignment template

End Point				
▲ reduce future health risks				
▲ improve general health				
▲ be drug-free				

Symptoms &/or diagnostics	Prioritized list of Goals (measurables)	End point alignment	Therapy	Treatment
BP 160/95	reduce blood pressure	▲ reduce future health risks (heart attack), be drug-free	▲ nutritionist	▲ diet ▲ exercise
BMI: 30	reduce weight	▲ reduce future health risks (heart, diabetes), be drug-free	▲ nutritionist ▲ fitness trainer	▲ diet ▲ exercise
fasting glucose: 8.3	reduce blood glucose	▲ reduce future health risks (diabetes), be drug-free	▲ naturopathy ▲ nutritionist	▲ diet ▲ lipoic acid ▲ exercise
cholesterol: 8.1	reduce cholesterol	▲ reduce future health risks (heart attack), be drug-free	▲ naturopathy ▲ nutritionist	▲ diet ▲ exercise ▲ red yeast rice ▲ policos-anol

When you cross check the treatments against the prioritized list of goals and the end point alignment you can see where each product fits and how important diet and exercise are to all aspects of the treatment. This tallies with the overall score for diet and exercise. So if you follow this model you will get a fairly accurate assessment of which treatments will take you the furthest and therefore how core they are to the case.

Andrew's Journey Road Map: where treatments can take him

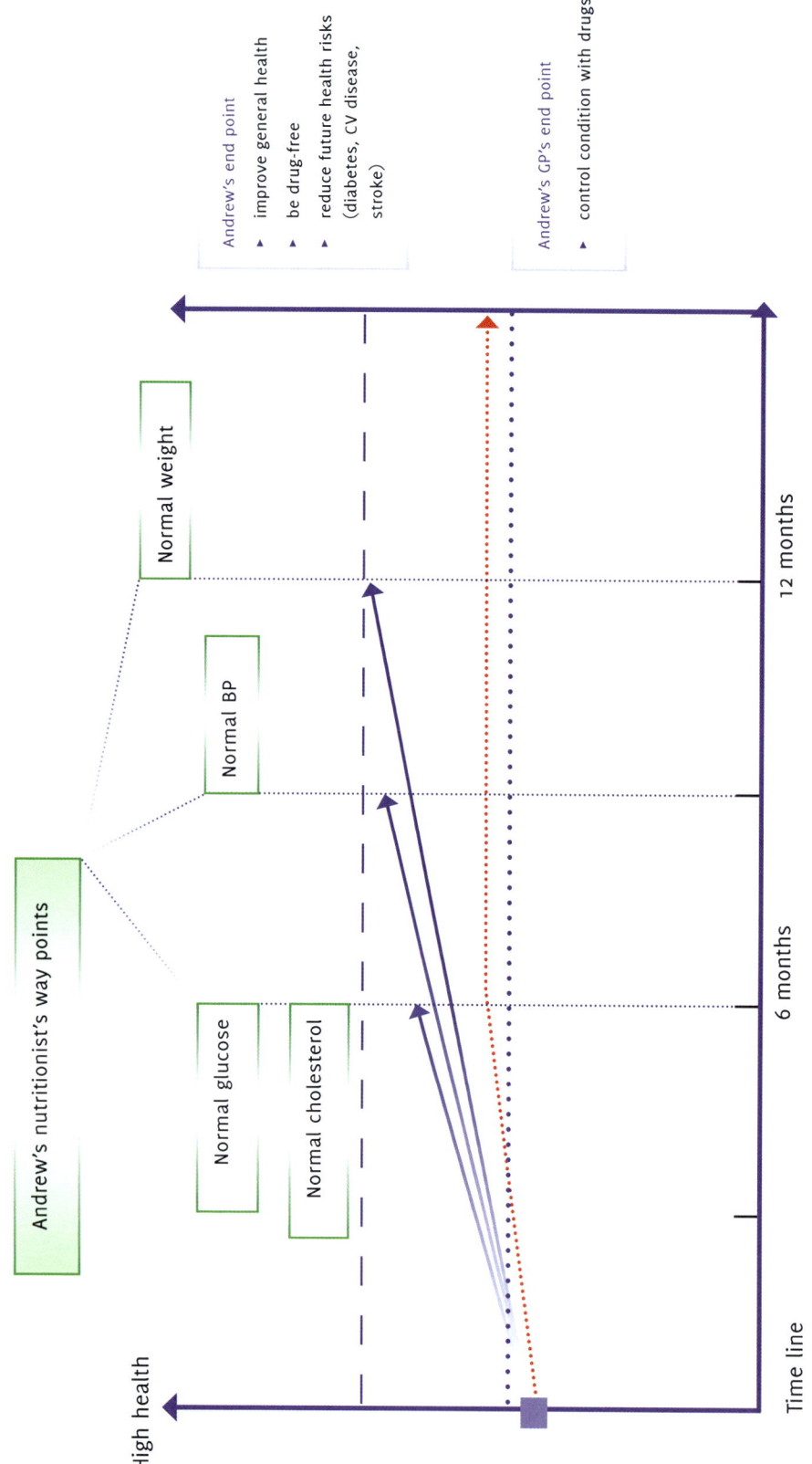

Andrew is working with his nutritionist's time line for monitoring and is happy to go at this speed. His doctor is delighted that Andrew has chosen this route and is happy to monitor him at 6 monthly intervals. Andrew has bought himself some weighing scales and also a blood pressure kit so that he can keep an eye on his blood pressure as this is his most serious risk for cardiovascular events.

Charlotte's Case

At 21 years Charlotte was diagnosed with chronic fatigue syndrome and fibromyalgia. At 24 years her condition had deteriorated and she developed chronic low grade ulcerative colitis which was managed with the drug mesalazine over the next 10 years. She was not able to attain remission and become drug-free during this period. By the age of 34 years she began to suffer acute episodes and required hospitalization. She was given cortisone to manage the flare-ups over the next 6 years. Her condition deteriorated and by the age of 40 she was on full time cortisone and mesalazine. Within 2 years she had developed inflammatory arthritis and was in considerable pain and greatly reduced mobility. She was started on methotrexate and amitriptyline along with the mesalazine. Cortisone was gradually withdrawn.

Charlotte drew a retrospective road map of where she had come from and what treatments she had received. These road maps tell it all and tell it once. They are an excellent way to present your case, particularly if it is long and complicated. They enable all your practitioners to be on the same page, and if patient quality of life is a priority they usually help to create an environment of collaboration.

By the time Charlotte came for treatment, at 42 years, she was unable to work, had two children under the age of five and the family budget was tight. With no hope of remission, and a future leading to greater drug-dependency and deteriorating health, Charlotte decided to investigate whether there was anything she could do to improve her outcome and help reduce her drug dependency. Her limiting criteria were cost and her capacity to undertake the program.

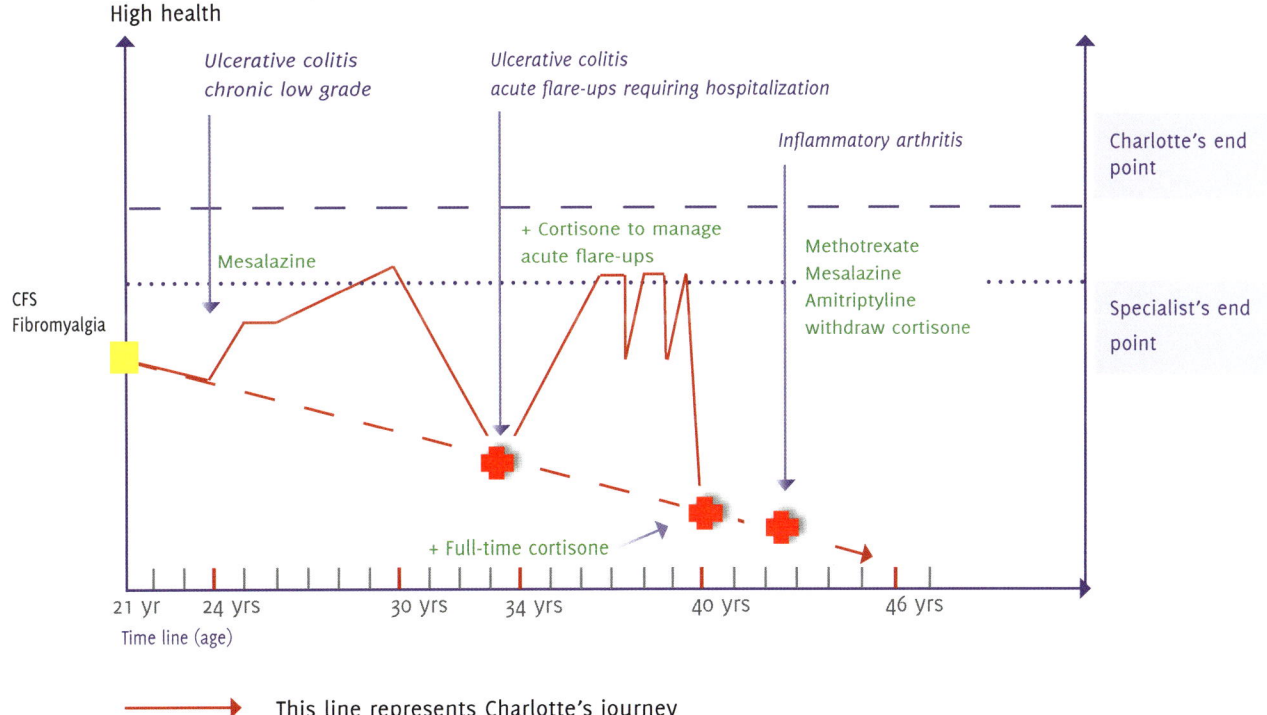

This line represents Charlotte's journey

Charlotte's Journey Road Map: where treatments took her

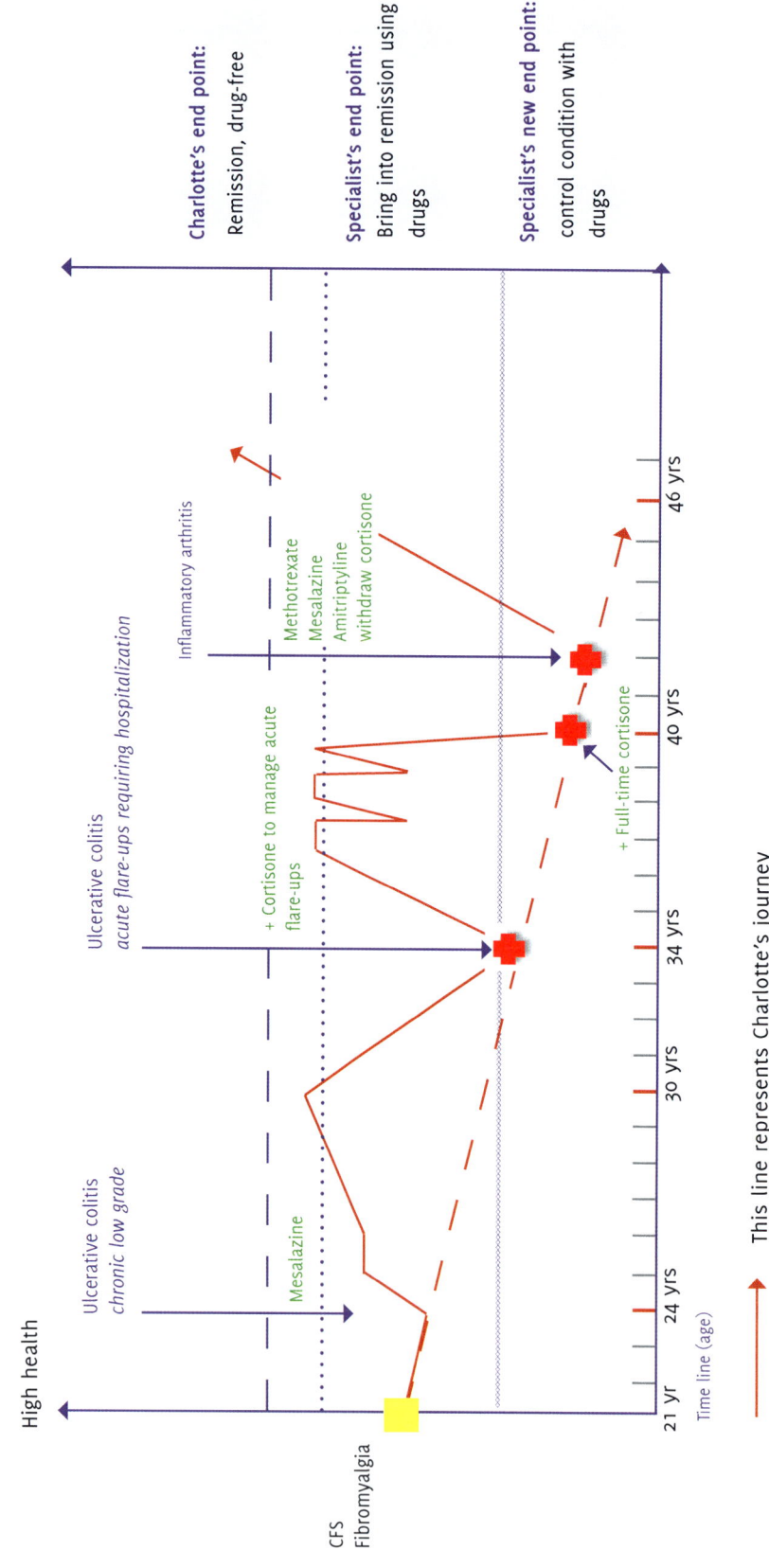

High health

CFS
Fibromyalgia

Ulcerative colitis
chronic low grade

Mesalazine

Ulcerative colitis
acute flare-ups requiring hospitalization

+ Cortisone to manage acute
flare-ups

Inflammatory arthritis

Methotrexate
Mesalazine
Amitriptyline
Withdraw cortisone

+ Full-time cortisone

Charlotte's end point:
Remission, drug-free

Specialist's end point:
Bring into remission using
drugs

Specialist's new end point:
control condition with
drugs

21 Yr   24 yrs   30 yrs   34 yrs   40 yrs   46 yrs
Time line (age)

This line represents Charlotte's journey

Charlotte decided on a dietary approach, a modified Gerson Therapy, and opted for a few supplements to reduce the highest risk factor, the chronic inflammation. The dietary regime knocked out many of the foods which would exacerbate the inflammation in the gut. Three years later she writes:

> "I am still going along on the modified Gerson (more than three years now) and doing very well. I have added a few more things into my diet (all natural and organic of course) and still do three juices and one coffee enema. I thought you would like to hear that people tell me I am looking SO WELL these days and that I look fantastic. I am feeling stronger with every passing year and there are less setbacks. I rarely get sick or get infections that everyone else gets! I have been off all colitis drugs for over one year now with no problems. I have less and less fibromyalgia. I have been back to studying part time for my Masters degree this year with no trouble (clear head at last) except a little fatigue. "

However, Charlotte's bowel was seriously damaged from years of chronic disease and eight years following her recovery she developed a mega-colon and had to have the bowel removed. There was no disease discovered in the removed bowel, and the surgeon was able to save part of the bowel which meant that Charlotte did not need a colostomy. She recovered well and continues to lead a good life, drug-free.

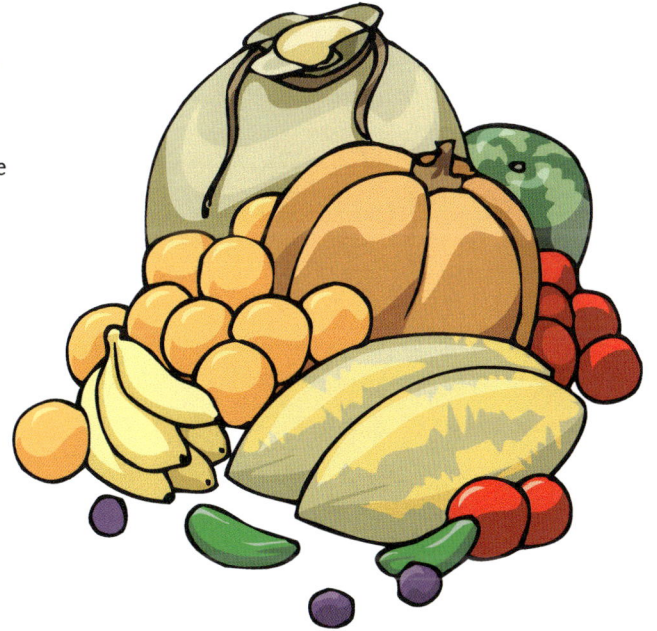

Charlotte's treatment alignment rating

Treatment options	What will the treatment do?	How will it help me get to my end point?	What is used to measure outcome?	Rating
Mesalazine	▴ Will control the inflammation/colitis which will control the diarrhoea and blood loss	▴ Offers some control of my condition without which I would suffer a faster deterioration of my general health	▴ Objective: blood tests ▴ Subjective: reduction in symptoms	7
Methotrexate	▴ Reduce over-activity of the immune system leading to less pain, swelling and damage to the joints	▴ Enables me to move around so that I can actually do the diet therapy	▴ Objective: blood tests ▴ Subjective: reduction in symptoms	7
Amitryptamine	▴ Reduce pain associated with the nerves	▴ It is helpful with the pain and I can sleep better so have more energy to do the diet therapy	▴ Objective: blood tests ▴ Subjective: reduction in symptoms	7
Gerson therapy (diet therapy)	▴ Reduce inflammation in my whole body ▴ Detoxify my body of all the drugs ▴ Increase my healing potential	▴ Reduce my risk factors (inflammation) ▴ Reduce my drugs ▴ Could bring me into remission ▴ Could offer cure	▴ Objective: blood tests ▴ Subjective: improvement/reduction in symptoms	10
Enzymes Antioxidants	▴ Pancreatin, Bromelain, Papain to reduce inflammation	▴ May help reduce my risk factors (inflammation) ▴ May help get me to remission	▴ Objective: nil ▴ Subjective: improvement/reduction in symptoms	6
Iron + B vitamins	▴ Help resolve my anaemia due to chronic blood loss	▴ Support my general health and level of fitness ▴ Reduce future health risks	▴ Objective: blood results ▴ Subjective: feel better, more stamina	7

Charlotte could not take the risk of stopping her medications as the consequences of relapse were too serious; it would take her backwards and also mean that she would be unable to undertake the program of her choice. So the drugs score highly. She was very anaemic, due to recurrent haemorrhage, and she needed supplemental iron. The Gerson Therapy scores the most highly as it is the only treatment that had the potential to take her to her end point, although at the time she did not know how far it would take her. This was a remarkable case and Charlotte was both tenacious and brave. It took around 18 months to come off all the medications, and then a further 18 months to fully stabilize and regain her health.

Monitoring

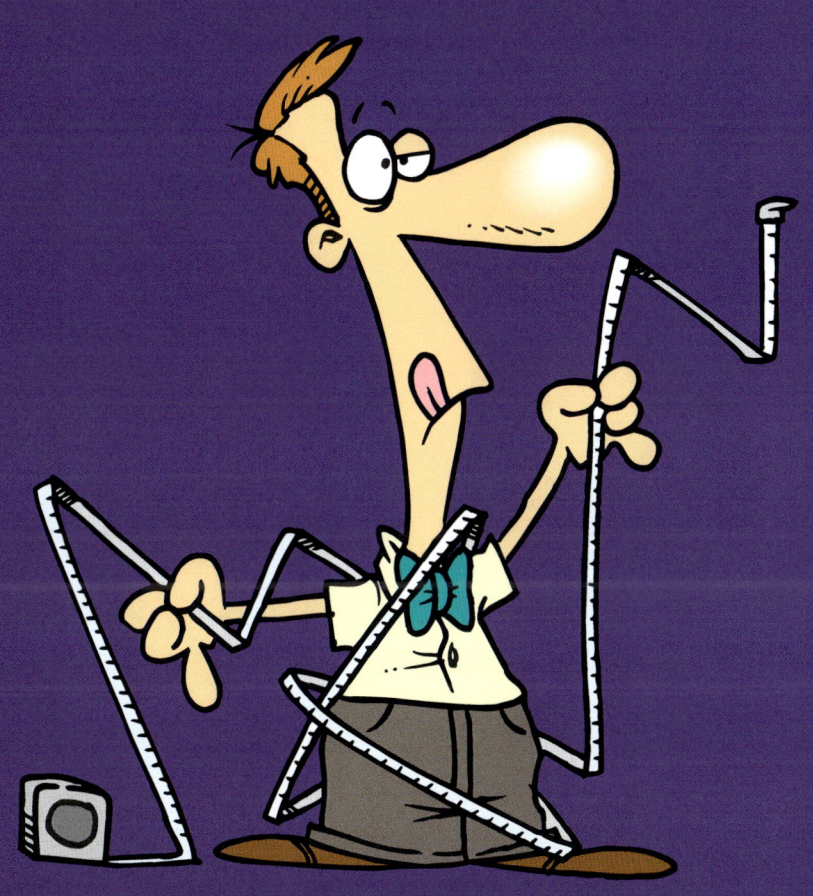

To do

1   Qualify tests for monitoring progress

Select a range of questions from *A conversational approach: how will we monitor my progress?*

2   Set up your charts for monitoring

View the chart examples and choose the ones that will suit your monitoring. Enter your starting and end point measurements and plot your way points for monitoring.

3   Your Journey Road Map

Use your charts for monitoring the progress of high, medium and low risk goals. Combine the results and calculate your overall progress.
Enter this as a progress line on *My Journey Road Map.*

Why do I need to monitor my progress?

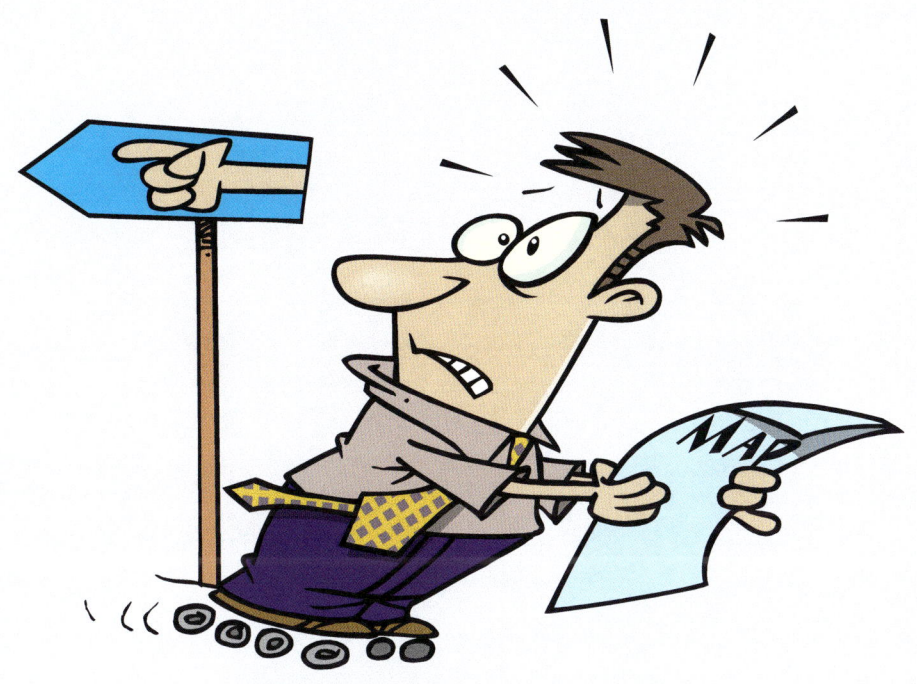

Because you won't know if, or by how much,
the treatment is working.

If you don't monitor then you may. . . . .

forfeit an opportunity should you need to change treatments for more effective ones

leave things for too long and narrow your options on treatment

waste time and money on treatments that don't get you anywhere

increase your risks if treatment is ineffective

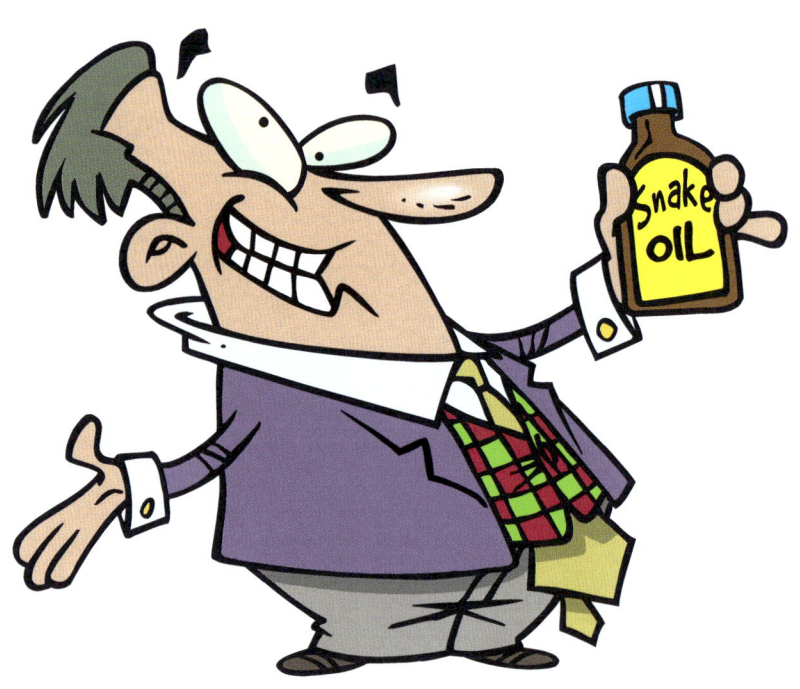

1 Qualify tests to monitor your progress

Following a treatment plan without monitoring to make sure you are on track is like going on a journey without a map. So choosing tests to monitor treatments will tell you if the treatment is working and within the estimated time frame. By monitoring you can change or add to the treatment if progress is not as expected.

So we need to monitor progress over time where we are able to measure improvement (or deterioration) against:

▶ a time line; and

▶ your end point.

The main pitfall of monitoring is that it is easy to end up monitoring the test result in isolation of where you want to go. Test results always monitor the treatment, they will tell you *if the treatment is doing what it says it will do*. However, it's up to the patient to determine how relevant the results are to where they are trying to get to. For example, if you take a drug to correct an abnormal test result, say that of reducing your cholesterol, but your end point is to be drug-free and in better health, then you could end up going backwards if you become drug-dependent and experience negative health effects. So you have to make sure that any tests and the results of treatment are relevant to your condition, your progress and your end point.

Jonathan has been diagnosed with bowel cancer. His specialist has found that he has normal/low levels of cortisol and has prescribed Cortrate 25mg. Jonathan feels better on this treatment and his blood results show that his cortisol levels have increased. Jonathan sees another practitioner as he wishes to improve his overall outcome and undertake a natural treatment for his cancer. This practitioner points out that although his cortisol test results may improve, that Cortrate is a corticosteroid and may become a risk factor for his condition. Jonathan realizes that the cortisol test result may not be relevant for monitoring his progress on his journey.

Measurable and meaningful

There are two distinct parts to monitoring: the results need to be *measurable* and the outcome needs to be *meaningful*. Meaningful means that the outcome should relate to your end point, not just the test result itself.

Measurable progress

Whether you are using objective tests (blood tests, scans) or a "how do I feel" (subjective) barometer you will be measuring treatment outcomes. There are different types of graphs to choose from to monitor your progress but you will need to give a starting value and an end point value. Use estimates given by your practitioner on predicted time frames for achieving your goals, and then plot way points against these time frames to monitor your progress.

Subjective measuring

When measuring "how do I feel" you may either rate your symptoms on a scale of 1-10 and then monitor improvement, or measure improvement as a percentage (for example, I am 25% or 50% better). Progress is then measured as improvement or deterioration against a base line (starting point) for each symptom.

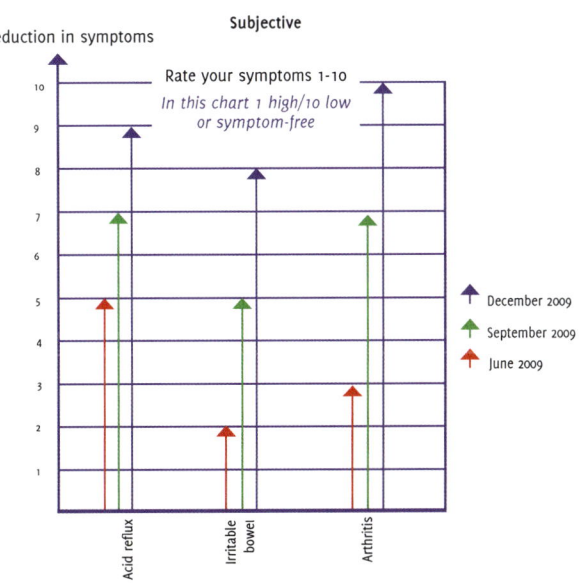

Objective measuring

This aspect relates to using objective tests which will give the starting point value to the readings you are monitoring, such as cholesterol levels, weight or blood pressure, size of lesion etc. Subsequent tests will allow you to do comparative readings to make sure you are heading in the right direction. There are many tests available, such as blood tests, live blood analysis and medical imaging (X-ray, ultrasound, MRI, CT or PET scans) which can be used to monitor change or the outcome of treatment. In order to monitor treatment accurately you will need to use the same test or type of scan to compare the progress.

Again you will need to plot your starting test results, and use estimates given by your practitioner on predicted time frames for achieving your goals.

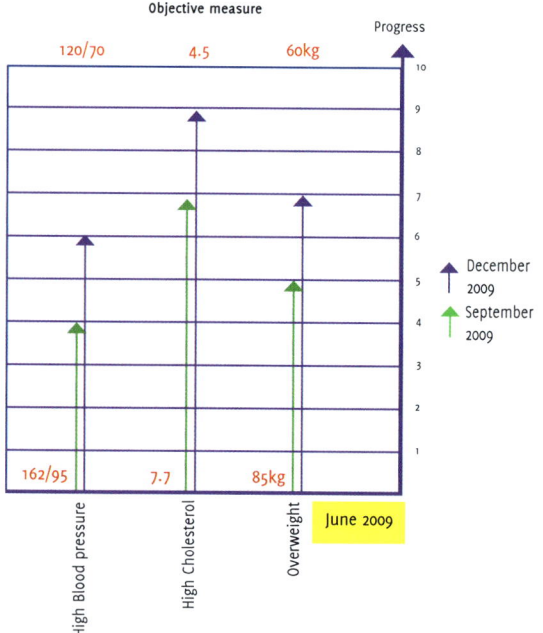

Meaningful progress

This aspect relates to measuring progress with reference to your end point rather than just referencing changes to the test result. *Is the progress shown by the tests relevant to my end point?* or *Of what benefit is this test and its results to me?* Here you will need to cross-check whether the tests recommended for monitoring are relevant to your outcome.

If a treatment can be seen to produce results that are bringing you to better health and not simply producing changes that may have no impact on the case, then the treatment and test are integral to delivering and measuring outcome, respectively.

Unlike the simple graphs we create to monitor the results of treatments, the journey road map makes sure you are on track. It is used to enter way points for monitoring your progress (and to remind you of when to monitor) and it is used to plot a general progress line which represents how well you are travelling in relation to your end point.

For example, a patient may see a positive result in their blood tests, but in other areas their general health may be declining. Sometimes the blood test result may be less meaningful than other health indicators. The journey road map will depict the total clinical outcome or the general direction you're heading as a result of your treatment.

Resolving the high priority risks will take you the furthest, so keep your eye on these as it will focus you on the core rather than lesser problems. It will also inhibit you from being enticed down a cul-de-sac of treatments that will take you nowhere and expensive tests that will tell you nothing about your overall progress.

In short, the progress line represents the sum total of all the treatment outcomes, but in truth is more reflective of resolving the highest to intermediate health risks.

Monitoring the treatment and not the patient

If you remember, Andrew was diagnosed with high cholesterol, was overweight and had a family history of heart disease and diabetes. He was recommended to address the causes of his condition by changing his diet, losing weight and taking up some exercise. He was told that these steps would lower his cholesterol and reduce future health risks. Let's suppose that Andrew has decided *not* to follow this advice but has opted to go for a cholesterol-lowering medication. His destination end point is to reduce his risk of heart attack using drugs. His criteria are that he doesn't want to make any lifestyle changes, nor does he want to spend any time, energy or money on other treatments which may help. As he is not treating the cause of his condition we could expect his condition to deteriorate even though he is taking the drugs which, he is told, will reduce his relative risk of heart attack by 19%.

Andrew is taking medications in the belief that he will not only reduce his risk of heart attack but that the drugs will keep him healthier for longer. Andrew and his GP place a heavy reliance on the test results for monitoring progress. The GP is monitoring to make sure the drugs are working, and Andrew thinks that if the test results are good then this is an indication of increased health. Andrew is clear that these are the improvements he wishes to see, and he imagines that he is going in the right direction.

You can see from Andrew's progress chart (below) that his condition is deteriorating and that he is heading in the opposite direction to where he thinks he is heading. Two years after his initial diagnosis he is diagnosed with high blood pressure and a year later with diabetes. The next year he suffers a heart attack. By this time he is on various medications to manage his condition. His doctor and specialist are monitoring the results of the drug medication through blood tests and blood pressure readings, making sure that each drug is achieving its outcome. This is a clear example of monitoring the treatment rather than patient outcome. Needless to say the outcome is a deterioration of Andrew's health and that unless he takes steps to try and improve this then his health will continue to decline.

This is also a clear example of a treatment producing a measurable outcome, where the result is meaningless to the patient's outcome and may play little to no role in where the patient wishes to go.

High health

Blood tests at 6 monthly intervals

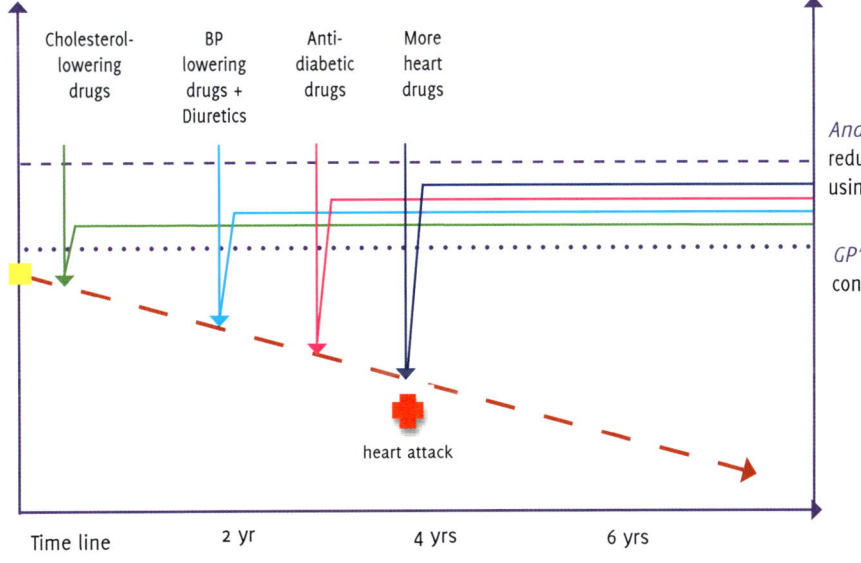

Cholesterol-lowering drugs

BP lowering drugs + Diuretics

Anti-diabetic drugs

More heart drugs

Andrew's destination end points
reduce risk of heart attack & diabetes using drugs

GP's destination end points
control of disease markers with drugs

heart attack

Time line   2 yr   4 yrs   6 yrs

However, if Andrew had achieved the same test results on his diet therapy, then the results would be measuring meaningful progress as he would have been treating the cause of his condition. Although the test results would still be a consequence of treatment, they would also be an indicator of his general health improving.

When seeing a number of specialists be mindful that each one may be singularly focused on their field of expertise, monitoring their own treatment and may fail or be unwilling to factor in the impact of another treatment on your case. Under these circumstances it is vital that you monitor yourself and become aware of any potential contraindications or health risks that the mixing of medications may cause. Be vigilant in monitoring any adverse reactions, particularly symptoms that have arisen since starting any treatment and don't be too quick in accepting assurances as your case may be unique. It will pay to do your own research.

Journey Road Map: the sum total of all treatment outcomes

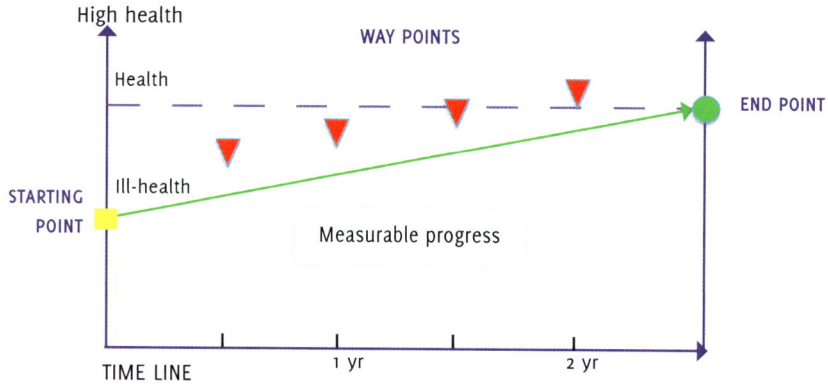

Way points are the estimated time frames for monitoring where you are matching the claims of treatment against your end point. They are the sign posts on the journey, making sure you are on track.

Is the treatment taking me to where I want to go and within the predicted time frame?

Marketing tests

*W*hether for diagnosis or measuring treatment outcome, testing is evolving into a market within its own right. We now have better imaging techniques and the capacity to test for a broader range of individual markers either in tissue, blood, saliva or stool samples. These tests can facilitate diagnosis and lead to a more tailored treatment.

This emerging market of testing services is often used as a tool for the promotion and sale of products. As more products become available then so too do tests that measure the very markers that relate to or match the claims of specific products or product ranges. Many products are sold on the basis that they can increase/ reduce specific blood markers associated with various health risks, or alter test profiles to reflect those of a younger person, and these changes, by default, will "improve" your health. In an industry that is product-centric this approach increases the amount of sales to a single consumer, but in a patient-centric model the basis for determining treatment is "what works".

With each test proposed, you will need to go back to the drawing board to determine:

▸ *what will the test tell me;*

▸ *what treatment will be recommended; and*

▸ *is this relevant to my end point?*

and with each product proposed you need to determine its value:

▸ *does the product address the cause or a known/ proven risk factor for my condition; and*

▸ *what are my odds of reducing my risks if I take this product?*

For many products there are no scientific studies, so mostly these products are taken on faith (sounds good), or because the practitioner recommending the treatment has had "good" results where *good* should be defined in terms of "meaningful".

So health consumers need to determine which tests may prove the most value in indicating which treatments or products are most likely to take them the furthest.

*S*arah was in reasonable health but had a few food allergies herself and a family history of heart disease and arthritis. She decided to find out about genetic testing and how this could help her protect her future health. Sarah did a search on the internet and found a practitioner near to home who offered this testing service which would profile her individual DNA and the practitioner would then be able to "tailor a customized program of lifestyle choices for optimal health and well-being and bypass any roadblocks on her way to health." Sarah asked what sort of treatment would be offered in addition to common-sense advice on lifestyle and diet. She was told that this very exciting field of nutrigenomics (of applying the human genome to nutrition and personal health) enabled practitioners to offer individualized dietary recommendations and products specific to the individual's DNA profile. She was told that our genes determine our health and that although they cannot be changed they can be compensated for through a growing range of products and new functional foods (foods or dietary components that may provide a health benefit beyond basic nutrition). Her practitioner indicated that she would be able to tell her exactly what dietary changes she should make and which supplements to take that would enable her to take greater control of her health.

Sarah asked what the science was based upon and whether any clinical studies had been done to prove that these programs actually worked. She didn't get a satisfactory answer to this other than the technology and treatments were new, so Sarah could not make any determination of whether, or by how much, the treatment program would help. Sarah still decided to go ahead with the test through curiosity and thought that she would keep an eye on this growing science rather than commit to taking a multitude of products indefinitely, as although her end point was to reduce her future health risks, it didn't involve being product-dependent for life.

Monitoring progress

*M*onitoring your outcome and progress is key to ensuring that treatments are effective in getting you to where you want to be. If you use the questionnaire guide you will be able to ascertain from your practitioner how and what you will monitor, and how frequently. Cross-check that the outcomes are relevant to your end point, then draw your time line and enter way points for monitoring.

If you're unsure of any test and its value, ask what the test is, what it's for, what treatment it measures and what it's value would be to you. Then you can identify how it fits into your overall plan and how critical it is for monitoring.

Most tests are fairly obvious, but occasionally a practitioner may push for a test for where you cannot see the relevance or how it would benefit your outcome, particularly if the test is costly and may lead to the recommendation of yet another treatment or range of products. Alternatively, some tests, such as scans, carry inherent risks and you may decide that any of the perceived benefits are not worth the risks, particularly if you have no intention of progressing with treatment.

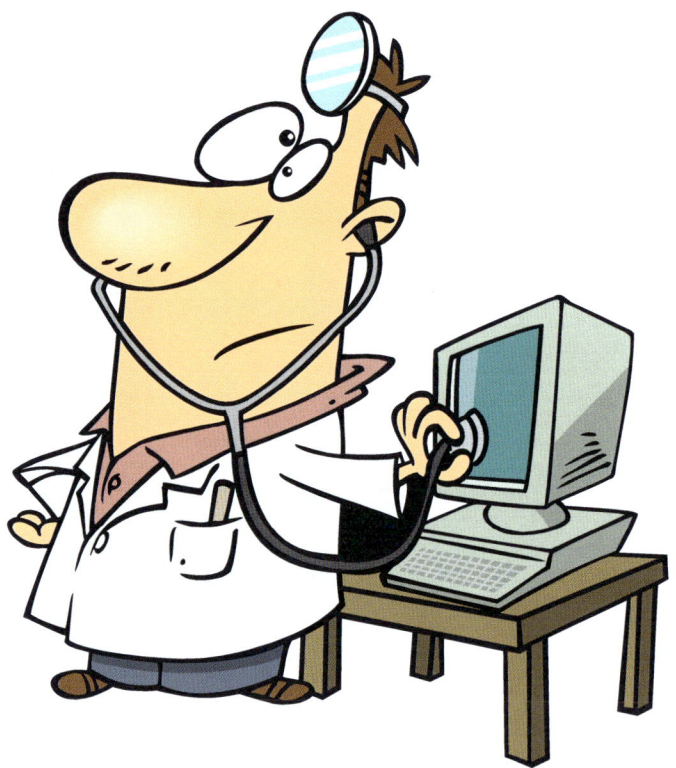

"I went to the GP today to pick up my blood test results. I haven't been feeling well for about a year now so I asked him if he would run some tests. The *tests came back normal* and he told me there was *nothing wrong* and that I should *go and see a counsellor*. I burst into tears and ran out of the room."

A conversational approach: how will we monitor my progress?

QUESTIONS	What tests will be used to monitor progress?	How does the test align with my end point?
Why ask these questions?	You need to qualify what the practitioner is monitoring and whether the tests are appropriate.	You need to know how far the test results are aligned to your end point.
Questionnaire Guide	▸ What is the test? (Name of test.) ▸ What will the test measure? ▸ What treatment is the test measuring? ▸ What aspect of my case is the test monitoring? (cause, risk factors, future health risks) ▸ How frequently will we test to make sure that the treatment is working?	▸ What benefits will I experience as a consequence of improved test results? ▸ Are these improvements core to getting me to my end point? ▸ Are these improvements core to me achieving my goals, and if so, which goals?
Professional criteria for monitoring	▸ to measure the efficacy of the product or protocol (treatment outcome) they prescribe which may not factor in other treatments or conditions that the patient has that are outside their field of expertise; *(monitoring the product and not the patient)* ▸ to monitor the disease progression/regression which may not factor in other risk factors or conditions that the patient may have that are outside their field of expertise *(monitoring the disease and not the patient)* ▸ to interpret the test results in isolation of the patient's general condition *(monitoring the test results and not the patient)* ▸ to rely and base recommendations on the test results rather than the clinical condition of the patient *(treating the test result and not the patient)*	

Sally's Case

WHY			NOW		FUTURE HEALTH RISKS
Causes/Risks		Tests	Diagnosis	Prognosis	
▸ gender ▸ age ▸ inherited predisposition ▸ peri-menopause ▸ stress ▸ alcohol ▸ dietary intolerance/allergy	Medical	▸ blood test ▸ blood pressure	▸ hypertension (BP 130/90) ▸ overweight (BMI 27) ▸ high cholesterol (7.2) ▸ IBS ▸ arthritis	▸ heart disease ▸ diabetes, heart disease ▸ heart disease ▸ General deterioration of health ▸ lose mobility	
▸ stress ▸ poor eating habits ▸ poor diet (too many "heating" foods)	TCM	▸ pulse & tongue diagnosis	▸ Heart Blood & Heart Qi deficiency ▸ Liver & Kidney Yin deficiency ▸ Liver over-acting on stomach & spleen		
▸ peri-menopause ▸ dietary intolerances ▸ stress	Naturopathy	▸ blood tests	▸ oestrogen dominance ▸ insulin-resistance ▸ + GP's diagnoses		
	End Point		▸ reduce future health risks ▸ improve general health ▸ become drug-free ▸ become pain-free		

Symptoms &/or diagnostics
▸ BP 130/90
▸ BMI 27
▸ Cholesterol 7.2
▸ insomnia, waking in the early hours & unable to get back to sleep
▸ digestive pain with griping spasms, diarrhoea & constipation
▸ sore joints in hands, feet, hips and lower back ache
▸ heart palpitations, anxious feelings, unable to cope, emotional & irritable, poor concentration, feels low at times
▸ headaches

"I am 48 years old and have been recently diagnosed with high blood pressure and high cholesterol for which I have been recommended to take medication. I already take medication for arthritis and irritable bowel. I would like to address my health, reduce my future health risks and preferably become drug-free before I hit menopause as I have already noticed other health changes, including some depression and anxiety."

*S*ally is peri-menopausal and although she has had some arthritis and irritable bowel issues, for which she takes medication, she is suddenly finding herself with a range of other health concerns. She has recently gained weight which is proving difficult to shift, she is suffering from moods, irritability, depression, anxiety, heart palpitations and recent migraines - and she can't sleep, finding that she is waking in the early hours of the morning and unable to get back to sleep. She has family health risks for heart disease and diabetes, and is therefore disturbed to find that her blood pressure and cholesterol have shot up. She knows that if she wants to improve her prognosis then she needs to lose weight and she also knows that her diet can exacerbate her digestive symptoms and her arthritis.

Sally's end point is to become pain and drug-free, to improve her overall general health and reduce her future health risks. When she looks at all the risk factors she can change she realizes that she could have a big impact on her case. However, she can see that her GP is not going in the same direction as she is so she will need to find additional help. She sees a TCM practitioner who confirms some of the causes for her condition and gives her a TCM diagnosis. Stress is a major player in her case, but Sally can't see how she can reduce this at present. She also seeks the help of a naturopath to assist with dietary issues.

*S*ally has completed all her alignments (see Sally's Alignment Template p206) and is confident that the tests she will use to monitor her progress are appropriate and will indicate that the treatments are delivering outcomes that are core to her case. However, her naturopath has just thrown in another test, a bioimpedance analysis. Sally asks what will the test tell me and what is it used for? The naturopath says that the test *measures body composition*, such as how much fat and muscle you have in your body and that this will help her to plan a diet and supplement strategy to improve her health. She will then use the test to measure changes in Sally's body composition on the program. Sally then asked what is the benefit of changing her body composition to her overall health. The naturopath says that the changing of her body composition is an indication in itself of improved health but she could not tell her specifically which symptoms she would see an improvement in. On reflection Sally decided that the program was tailored to the test results rather than to her end point, and that although she could see her naturopath's rationale of the program she was proposing, she didn't feel that it addressed her irritable bowel nor her arthritis. So she elected to seek the help of another naturopath, one that was more aligned to her end point.

Sally's full alignment template

End Point					
reduce future health risks					
improve general health					
be drug-free					
be pain-free					

Symptoms &/or diagnostics	Prioritized list of Goals (measurables)	End point alignment	Therapy	Treatment	Monitoring
BP 130/90	reduce blood pressure	reduce future health risks (heart attack), be drug-free	naturopathy	diet, exercise	BP test
BMI: 27	reduce weight	reduce future health risks (heart, diabetes), be drug-free, improve general health	naturopathy, fitness trainer	diet, exercise	weigh-in, bioimpedance analysis
cholesterol: 7.2	reduce cholesterol levels	reduce future health risks (diabetes), be drug-free	naturopathy	diet, supplements, exercise	blood test
insomnia, waking in the early hours & unable to get back to sleep	improve sleep	improve general health	TCM	herbs, acupuncture, diet	subjective, pulse/tongue
digestive griping pain, spasms, diarrhoea and constipation	reduce IBS	improve general health, be drug-free	TCM, naturopathy	herbs, acupuncture, diet	subjective, pulse/tongue
sore joints in hands, feet and hips, lower backache	reduce arthritis	improve general health, reduce future health risks, be drug-free & pain-free	TCM, naturopathy	herbs, acupuncture, diet	subjective, pulse/tongue
heart palpitations, anxious feelings, unable to cope, feeling emotional and very irritable, poor concentration, feels low at times	reduce stress, depression & anxiety	improve general health, reduce future health risks	yoga, TCM	meditation/yoga, herbs	subjective, pulse/tongue
headaches	reduce headaches	improve general health, reduce future health risks	TCM, naturopathy	herbs, diet	subjective, pulse/tongue

Troubleshooting tests

What will the test tell me?	▸ my diagnosis, and if so, what specific aspect of my condition will it help diagnose; ▸ the cause/risk factors for my condition; ▸ the treatment I should have; ▸ will the test provide sufficient proof of my condition (is it diagnostic enough), of my progress or for the recommended treatment?
What will the test monitor?	▸ the efficacy of treatment (is the treatment working?); ▸ progress on a specific treatment (improvement or deterioration); ▸ a specific aspect of my case (using specific markers as indicators); ▸ my general condition.
How relevant is the test?	▸ Are the changes it measures key to my end point (where I would like to be); ▸ Are the changes it measures key to my specific goals (what I need to achieve); ▸ Are the changes it measures key to indicating treatment; ▸ Will the test result make any difference in my choice of treatment/s? (Is it worth having?)
Risk	▸ Are there any health risks associated with the test that apply to me?

Tips

▸ Use the same test for monitoring progress for an accurate comparison of your progress.

▸ Match the test to your goals and end point to determine how relevant the test is for monitoring. *(What do the test results mean and how does this relate to my case and where I want to go?)*

▸ Make sure that the test is a true and accurate indicator of its claims.

▸ Make sure that the interpretation is correct, or treatment may be inappropriate and you may have to pick up the health cost.

▸ Make sure that the interpretation of the results relates to your case and where you want to go.

▸ Make sure you are in agreement for the test to go ahead. Unnecessary tests are costly and may carry risks.

▸ Avoid falling into the trap of monitoring the test results instead of your progress. This can occur when a practitioner is testing to see whether the product or drug they have prescribed is "doing the job". Although a product or drug may be scientifically proven to have a specific action, producing a "good" result does not necessarily mean that you are travelling in the right direction.

▸ Adjunct therapies often have their own range of tests which may or may not relate to where you are trying to go, but are used to determine a treatment program or product. These tests tend to be tailored to the program rather than the patient.

▸ Beware of the practitioner who loves to diagnose, but for all the tests can't offer you a meaningful outcome.

Focus on the journey rather than the individual test results.
Make sure they indicate overall improvement.

2 Setting up your charts for monitoring

There are many different types of charts for monitoring progress and sometimes patients come up with quite unique ways to "tell it all at a glance".

Firstly, you have to decide what you want to measure and how you want to depict this. Simple charts will just show improvement or deterioration of specific symptoms or test results over time using units of measurement (objective) or giving symptoms a value on a scale of 1-10 (subjective). These charts measure the achievement of goals on your journey.

In setting up your chart you need to establish:

▸ your starting measurement;

▸ your desired end measurement; and

▸ a time line.

For objective results, work out where you would like to get to and the time line with your practitioner (where they think they can get you and within what time frame). The way points for monitoring will be entered onto your Journey Road Map.

The easiest type of graph is the linear one where you can measure incremental progress against the time line. If you have your starting measure and end measure, then you simply create progress lines so that you can see where you are in relation to your goal.

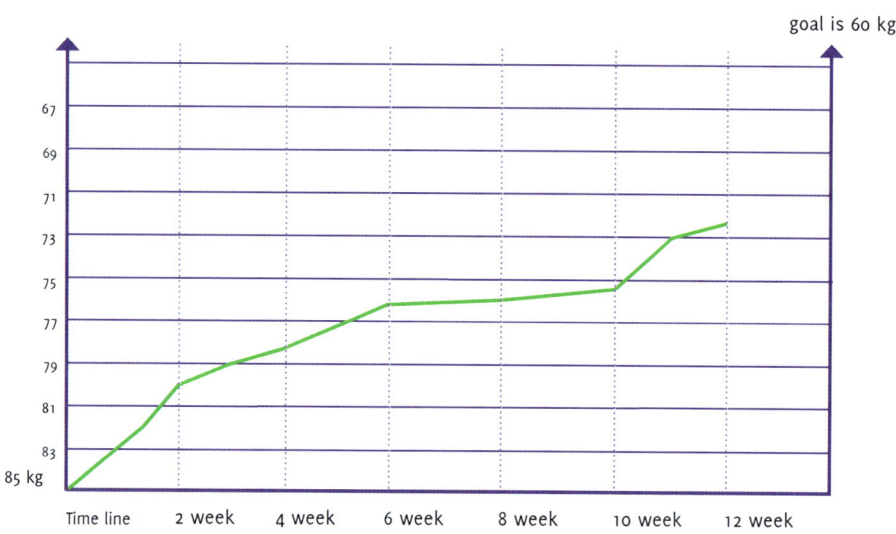

goal is 60 kg

These graphs are more traditional and useful if a patient is monitoring just one or two outcomes. The time line is the horizontal base line, and the vertical line represents improvement. You can either place units of measure along the vertical bar (as seen above where kilograms are used), or the degree of improvement using a score of 1-10 or a percentage (opposite chart). Both these charts apply to the same person who is trying to lose weight

and reduce blood pressure. By measuring improvement as a percentage it is easy to depict multiple progress lines on the one graph. Improvements in blood pressure were measured against a starting point of 160/95 and a desired end point at 120/70. Improvements for a desired 25 kg weight loss indicate that after 3 months he is 50% there (loss of 12.5 kg), and by 6 months, 70% there.

Monitoring graph for objective readings

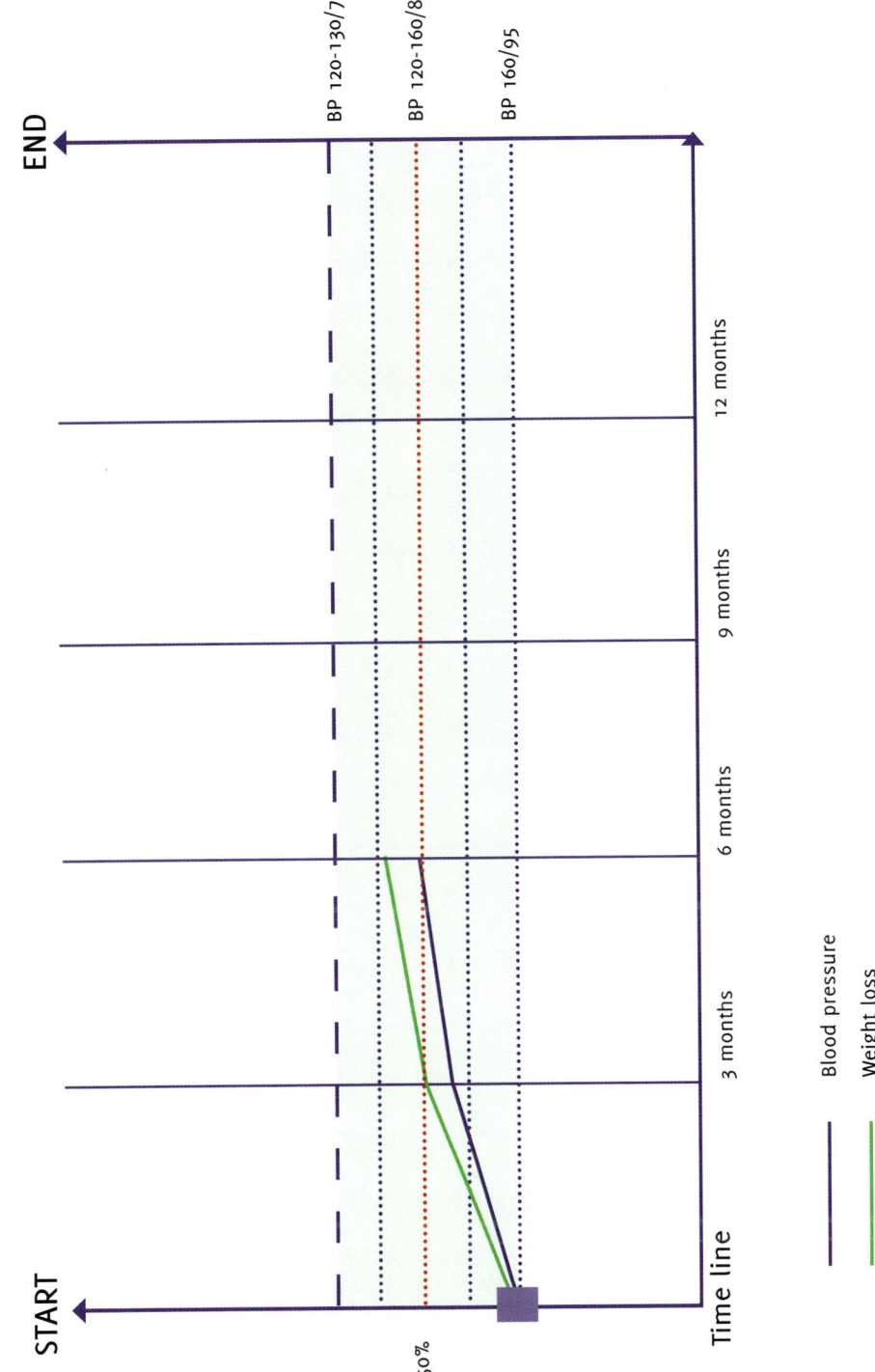

This graph can be used to measure both objective and subjective scores by measuring improvement on a scale of 1 to 10. So for patients who are monitoring both it is easy to see at a glance how well they are progressing on all fronts. The base line represents worst case for subjective symptoms, and the starting measure for objective measures. Geoffrey has scored his subjective symptoms out of 10. The pain of his arthritis is scored as 3 out of 10, with 3 being high (if you normally rate pain as say 7/10 for high, then you would reverse this to 3/10 for the purposes of this graph), the irritable bowel syndrome as 2/10 and the acid reflux as 5/10. It is often easier to measure symptoms by grading them on a scale of 1-10 but if you wish to translate this onto the road map, it is better if you can start from a base line of 0% and monitor the improvement of symptoms as a percentage of the total improvement required, 100% (see example pp 211, 212.)

The right side of the graph, which measures the objective results also uses the scale of 1 - 10 but the starting point at the base line represents the starting weight, blood pressure and cholesterol, and the finishing line (10) the desired goal. The patient can then measure the incremental improvements represented as a fraction of ten with five representing the halfway mark. For example, this patient needs to reduce their cholesterol by 3.2 points; if we divide this by 10 then each incremental loss is 0.32. By September, this patient's cholesterol is 5.46 which means that they have dropped 2.24 points. If you divide this loss by 0.32 then you will see that this represents 7 or they are 70% of the way there.

We are using colour coded arrows to track progress, with each colour representing a specific month/date. There is no requirement for a red arrow for the objective results as the base line represents the starting point.

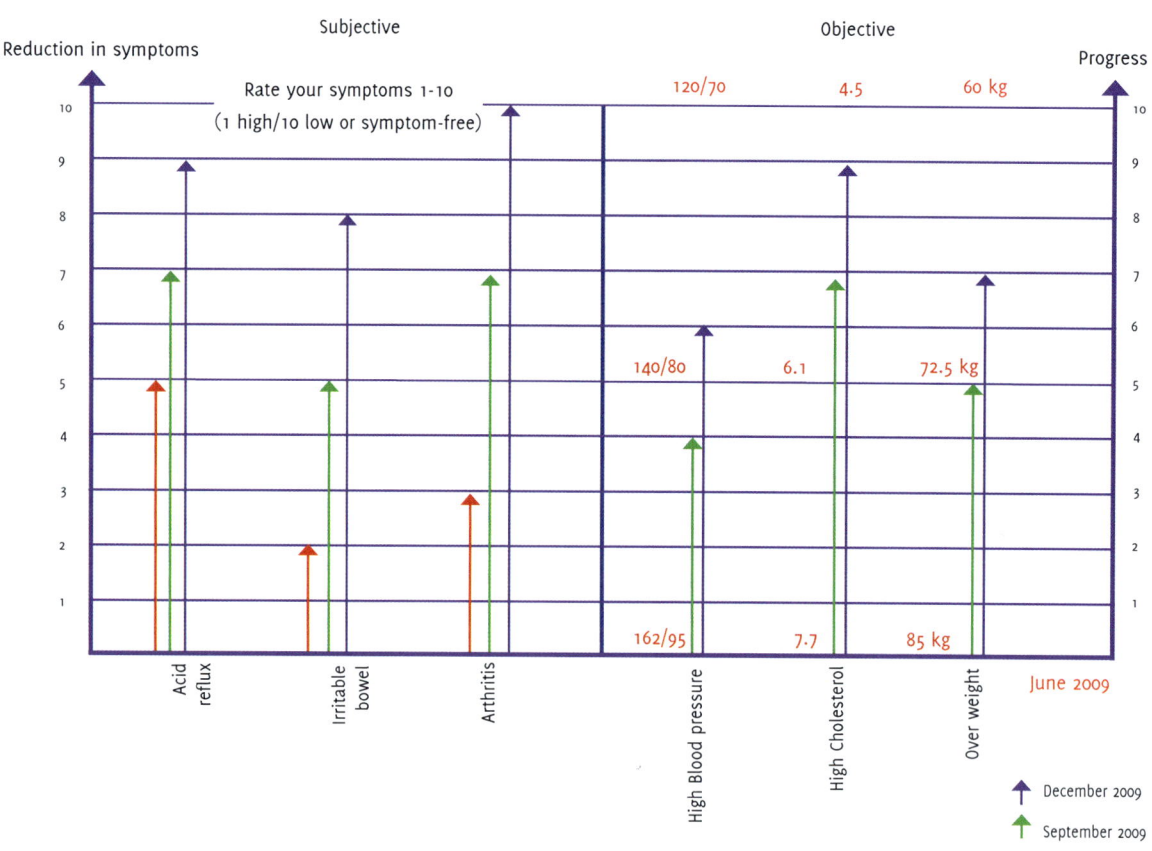

This is a useful graph for patients who do not have major health risks but reduced quality of life, or for patients that need to monitor their category 2 or 3 symptoms (medium or low risk) along the basis of "how do I feel" or subjective monitoring. The symptoms on this graph (Hilary's symptoms) would all fall into categories 2 and 3.

This graph represents improvement as a percentage, or by how much the symptoms have improved, with 100% representing total resolution. The base line is the starting point. In this case Hilary started in November 2008 and the first monitoring was recorded by the red arrows in May 2009. By colour coding the arrows for each monitoring it is easy to see where the improvements are (and by how much) and where the case may have slipped back. In addition, you can relate any changes (beneficial or detrimental) to any recorded changes in the prescription.

Your practitioner may be monitoring signs which may bear little relationship to your experience of your condition. For example, a practitioner of Chinese medicine may monitor the pulse and the tongue for measuring progress and determining treatment. You would need to ask which of your specific symptoms relate to the pulse or tongue diagnosis, so that you can understand where the treatment is focused and how you can tell whether the treatment is working. If your practitioner says that you have a "deficient Spleen" and "the liver is over-acting on the Spleen", then you can enquire which symptoms indicate this and what you could expect from treatment and within what time frame. You can then set up your monitoring of the specific groups of symptoms to measure progress.

Hilary was 42 years old and had been struggling since her mid-20s with chronic fatigue syndrome (CFS). She had been vegetarian for many years and had gone on a raw food diet for a year as she believed that his would help. Her health worsened and she developed lichen planus with unsightly lesions in the mouth. Her doctor did not know how to help as her as most of her blood tests came back normal, except that she was chronically anaemic. Despite iron supplementation, Hilary's iron levels did not improve. With her general condition worsening she decided to seek further help. When she came for treatment her list of problems was very long. In addition to the chronic fatigue, anaemia and lichen planus she was suffering from burning mouth syndrome with red, dry, puckered and peeling lips, night sweats, red eyes, skin rash and skin welts, nausea, period pain, pre-menstrual tension, anxiety, food cravings and low blood sugar.

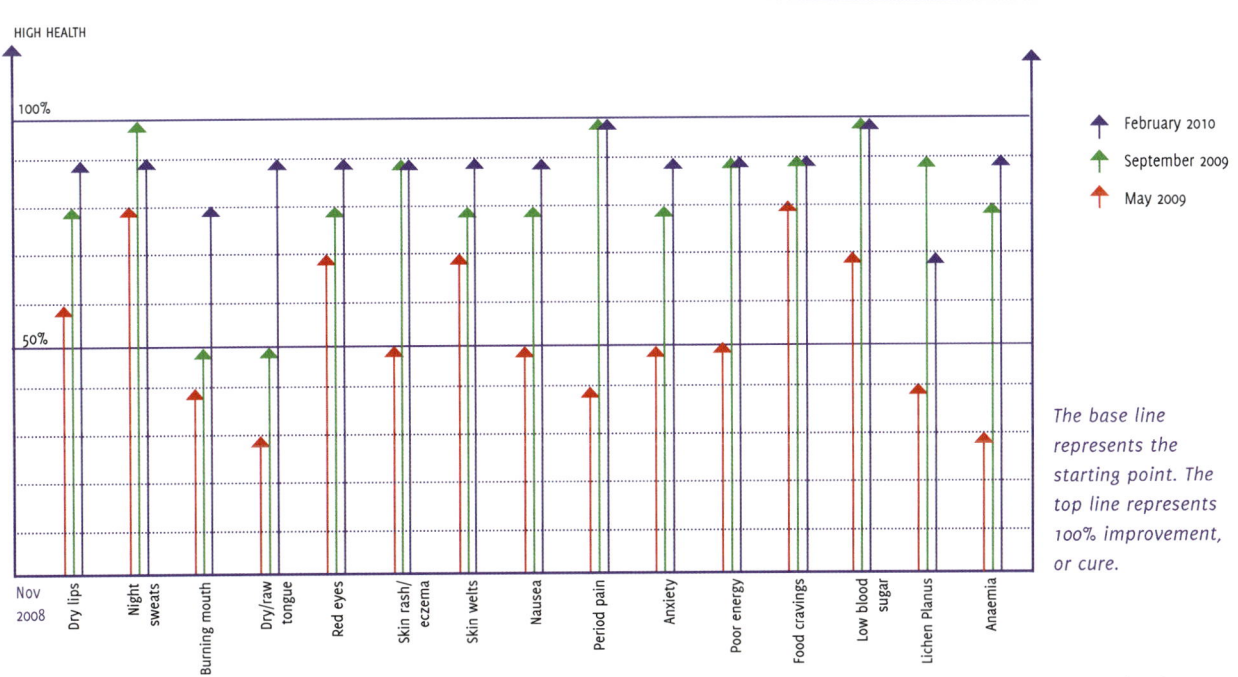

The base line represents the starting point. The top line represents 100% improvement, or cure.

Hilary's monitoring graph for subjective symptoms

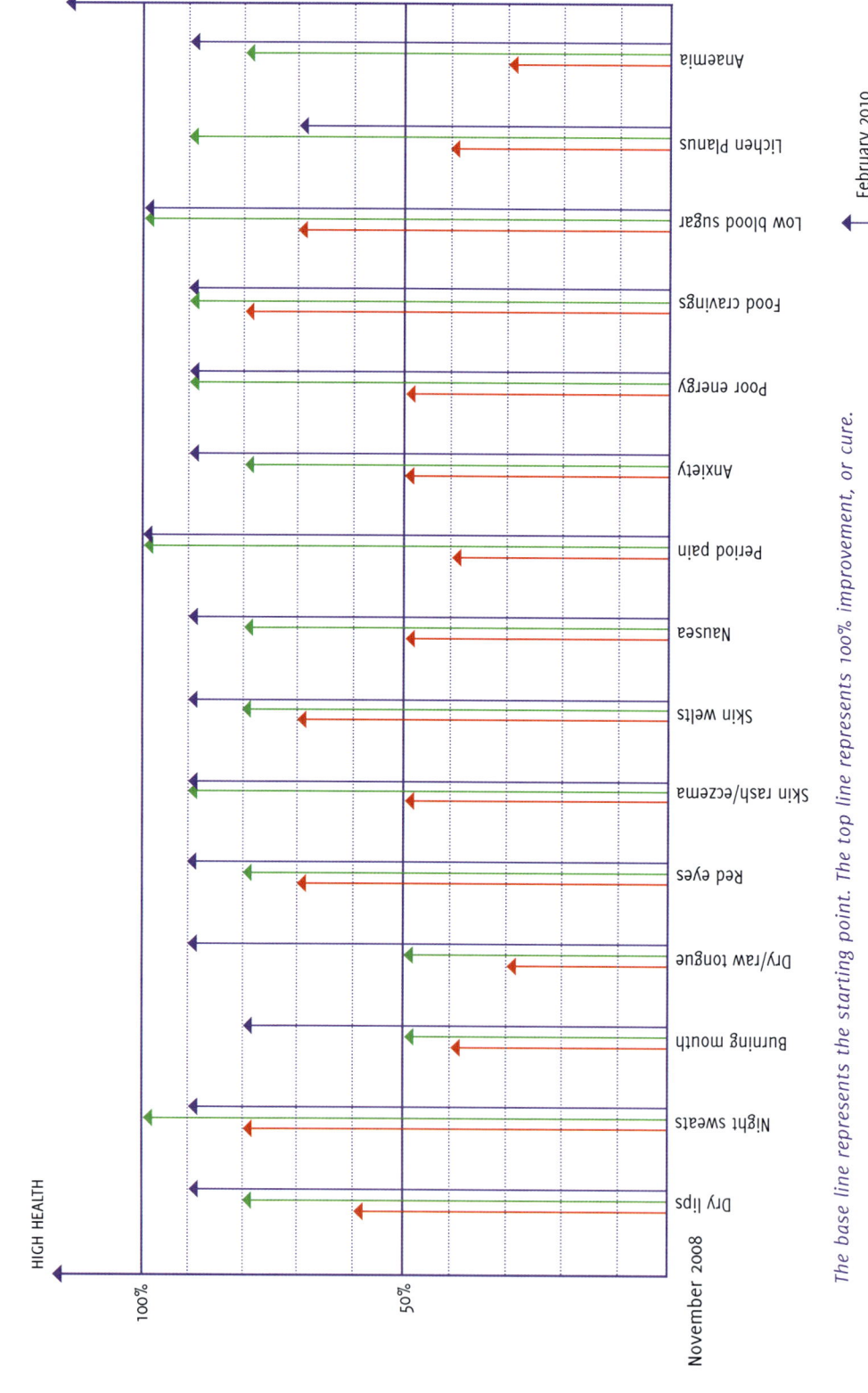

HIGH HEALTH

100%

50%

November 2008

Dry lips

Night sweats

Burning mouth

Dry/raw tongue

Red eyes

Skin rash/eczema

Skin welts

Nausea

Period pain

Anxiety

Poor energy

Food cravings

Low blood sugar

Lichen Planus

Anaemia

February 2010

September 2009

May 2009

The base line represents the starting point. The top line represents 100% improvement, or cure.

Hilary had two main destination end points: to resolve the lichen planus and to increase her energy. She sought the help of her acupuncturist who had helped her in the past and he assured her that he could help her with many of her symptoms and warned her against nutritional supplements and said that she should be careful with herbs. She sought the advice of a nutritionist who advised on a diet to rebuild her deeply deficient body and indicated that she needed some supplements and that she should take herbs as, in her opinion, the acupuncture alone would not help build her stamina nor resolve some of the deeper patterns of disharmony. The nutritionist said that although the acupuncture could help rebalance her energy, it would not build what she described as a deficient Yin. Hilary needed to not only rebuild her "capital" with diet and some supplementation but she also needed to take herbs for their pharmacological properties. The nutritionist, who was also qualified in Chinese herbal medicine, said that her pattern of disharmony was Liver stagnation caused by Liver Yin and Liver Blood deficiency with Empty Heat Flaring indicated by heat, sweating, redness and itching, and liver Qi stagnation indicated by premenstrual syndrome with painful periods.

You can see that Hilary has a problem. She trusts her acupuncturist, but he seems to be giving opposing advice to that of her nutritionist. So for Hilary there is conflict as she needs to determine who is correct, or which practitioner offers the most appropriate treatment for her individual case and can take her the furthest.

In the end Hilary decided to take the dietary advice from the nutritionist and work with her acupuncturist. She did not ask the acupuncturist which symptoms he could help with and within what time frame as she trusted his judgement and that he would "get her there". She assumed that he knew where he was going and that it was where she wanted to go.

Hilary started her program in November 2008. Progress was painfully slow as at that time she opted for diet alone in conjunction with the acupuncture. She was advised to monitor her progress by her nutritionist by creating a chart where the base line was her starting point and then to measure month by month the percentage to which she improved in each symptom.

By May 2009 (red arrows) you can see that none of her symptoms are fully resolved and that the lichen planus and poor energy still remain her chief complaints. She agreed to start some supplements and herbs. Her nutritionist gave her high dose vitamin A for the lichen planus and her anaemia and the improvement was dramatic for the lichen planus. In September, she halved the dose of vitamin A but the problem started to resurface by February 2010, so she increased the amount back to the original dose. The vitamin A also helped with the dietary iron uptake but the anaemia still required iron supplementation. Herbs were given for the liver Qi stagnation and empty heat and so most of the other problems resolved quite rapidly, except the burning mouth syndrome with the dry and raw tongue. The nutritionist recommended activated forms of B12, B6 and folic acid and the improvement, again, was dramatic.

You can see that problems arise either when practitioners do not explain how their treatment works in terms of what outcome they can expect and within what time frame, or when patients fail to clarify what it is that they want fixing. Sometimes this is difficult for patients as they do not want to put their practitioner on the spot. Our culture has instilled in us that this could be viewed as being disrespectful. Whilst it may be true that some practitioners could take offence, particularly if they cannot give absolute guarantees, practitioners need to understand that the patient simply needs to know if the practitioner can help and by how much, whether they have had experience and helped others with a similar condition and how long it will be before they see improvement. This is not only reasonable but also necessary, particularly if you are a smart patient and you want to form a collaborative relationship, or if you are dealing with more than one practitioner at the same time. If a treatment can't be qualified or monitored then it may be unwise to act in good faith, particularly if time is not on your side.

If your practitioner is monitoring signs that you do not understand the relevance or relationship to your experience of your condition you will need to ask which of your symptoms relate to the monitoring. For example, a practitioner of Chinese medicine may monitor the pulse and the tongue for measuring progress and determining treatment. You would need to ask which symptoms relate to the pulse or tongue diagnosis, so that you can understand where the treatment is focused and how to tell whether the treatment is working. If your practitioner says that you have a "deficient Spleen" and "the liver is over-acting on the Spleen", then you can enquire which symptoms indicate this and what you could expect from treatment and within what time frame. You can then set up your monitoring of the specific groups of symptoms to measure progress. In Hilary's case it was fairly easy for her to see the "heat" symptoms and understand which treatments were focusing on what symptoms. She could then be more discerning about her improvements, as symptoms that she may have felt were unimportant or unrelated suddenly assumed greater relevance to her overall progress.

3 Your Journey Road Map
calculating your improvement

Although you may be monitoring several conditions or aspects of the case you need to be able to represent your achievements on the Journey Road Map as a single progress line. The progress line represents the combined improvement of all your goals.

However, not all your goals will carry the same weighting as some goals will be more important to your success than others. When prioritizing your goals you will have divided them into high, medium and low risk where the high risk goals would carry the greatest weighting:

▸   **1:** high risk (not much time on your side);

▸   **2:** medium risk (some time on your side, symptoms that will lead to chronic health); and

▸   **3:** low risk (time on your side, or minor symptoms).

If the progress line is going to reflect your overall progress it's important to combine the goals within each category and work out the average improvement for each category separately. So if you have 4 goals in the high risk group and you have made a 70%, 60%, 20% and a 30% improvement respectively, then by adding the improvements together (180%) and then dividing by 4, you will get the mean average rate of improvement for that group which, in this case, will be 45%. You can then do the same for the other groups.

Next we need to weight the improvement. The 45% improvement in the high risk group is going to be worth more, in terms of getting to your end point, than a 45% improvement in the medium or low risk category. To reflect this we simply weight each group thus:

▸   multiplying the high risk average by 3;

▸   multiplying the medium risk average by 2;

▸   leave the low risk average as is; and

▸   then divide the total number by 6.

If any of your groups are vacant, that is you either have no high risk goals or no low risk goals, or no medium risk goals, you simply adjust the calculation. For high risk and medium risk goals divide the total number by 5, for high risk and low risk divide the total number by 4 and for medium and low risk divide the total number by 3.

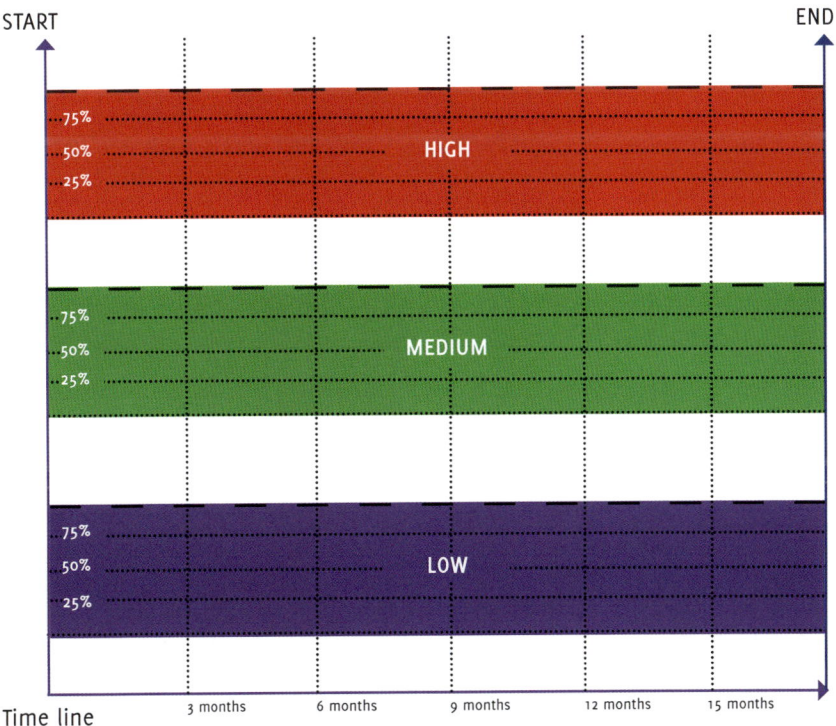

START   END

HIGH — 75% 50% 25%

MEDIUM — 75% 50% 25%

LOW — 75% 50% 25%

Time line   3 months   6 months   9 months   12 months   15 months

If you use this type of chart for mapping progress for your high risk, medium risk and low risk conditions, you may draw a mean average for each group and then convert this to a single progress line for your Journey Road Map by using the calculation method described above.

Geoffrey has categorized his symptoms into high risk (high blood pressure and overweight) and medium risk (acid reflux, IBS, arthritis and high cholesterol) and has used the chart opposite to measure his progress. He adds together the percentage improvements for each group on a 3 monthly basis and works out the mean average improvement by dividing the total by the number of complaints he is monitoring for each group. You can see that the mean average progress for the high risk group is 45% and 65% progress at 3 and 6 months, respectively. In the chart (opposite, below right) Geoffrey has plotted each monitored complaint as a percentage improvement against a time line. He has placed the high risk conditions in the red chart and the medium risk conditions in the green chart.

You can see that the mean average improvements for the medium-risk group (90%) are higher than those for the high risk group (65%). But as improvements in the high risk group are more core in getting Geoffrey to his end point, they will be given a higher weighting. Geoffrey will multiply the high risk mean average by 3 (65 x 3 = 195), and the medium risk mean average by 2 (90 x 2 = 180), and then add both these results together and divide by 5 (195 + 180 = 375 ÷ 5 = 75) to give the overall average progress which can then be entered on the Journey Road Map as a progress line.

HIGH RISK ↓   MEDIUM RISK ↓

high risk	3 months	6 months	medium risk	3 months	6 months
high blood pressure	40%	60%	acid reflux	40%	80%
overweight	50%	70%	irritable bowel syndrome	45%	85%
			arthritis	55%	100%
			high cholesterol	70%	90%
mean average (total ÷ 2)	45%	65%	mean average (total ÷ 4)	55%	90%
weighting (x 3)	135%	195%	weighting (x 2)	110%	180%
Average Progress					
3 months	135 + 110 = 245 ÷ 5 = 50%				
6 months	195 + 180 = 375 ÷ 5 = 75%				

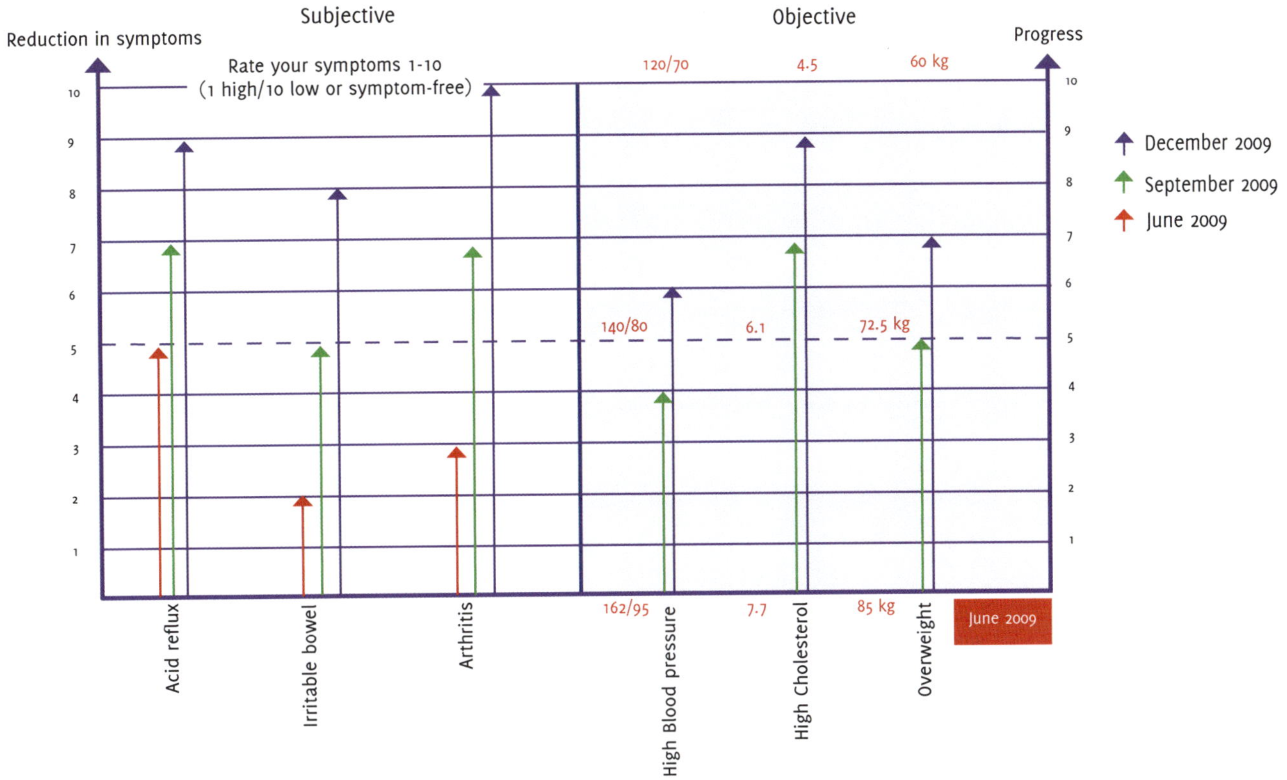

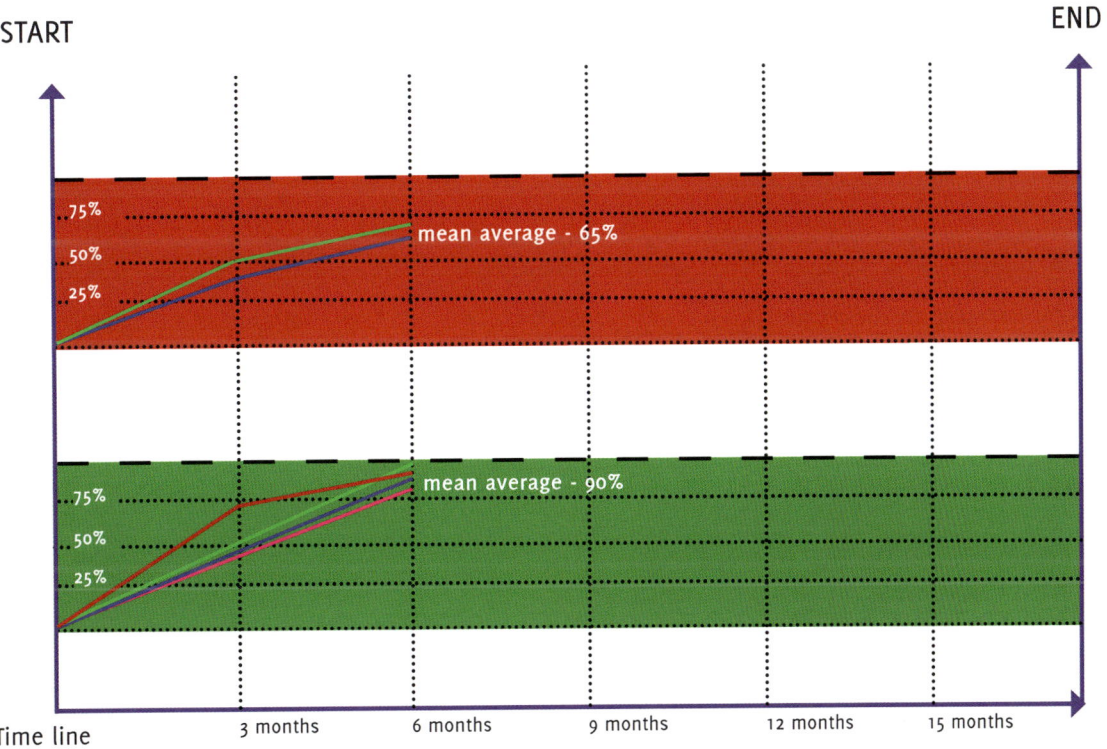

Subjective   Objective

Reduction in symptoms   Progress

Rate your symptoms 1-10
(1 high/10 low or symptom-free)

120/70   4.5   60 kg

140/80   6.1   72.5 kg

162/95   7.7   85 kg

↑ December 2009
↑ September 2009
↑ June 2009

Acid reflux

Irritable bowel

Arthritis

High Blood pressure

High Cholesterol

Overweight

June 2009

START   END

75%
50%
25%

mean average - 65%

75%
50%
25%

mean average - 90%

Time line   3 months   6 months   9 months   12 months   15 months

Geoffrey's Journey Road Map

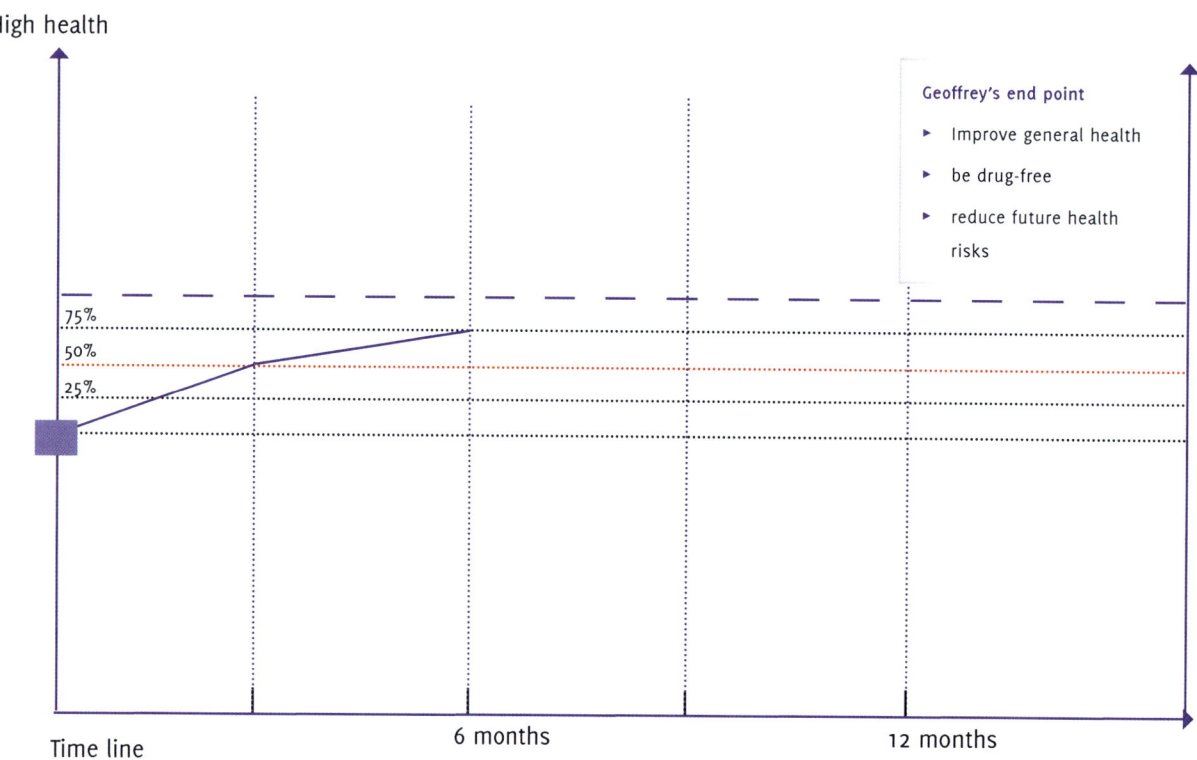

high risk	3 months	6 months	medium risk	3 months	6 months
high blood pressure	40%	60%	acid reflux	40%	80%
overweight	50%	70%	irritable bowel syndrome	45%	85%
			arthritis	55%	100%
			high cholesterol	70%	90%
mean average (total ÷ 2)	45%	65%	mean average (total ÷ 4)	55%	90%
weighting (x 3)	135%	195%	weighting (x 2)	110%	180%
Average Progress					
3 months	135 + 110 = 245 ÷ 5 = 50%				
6 months	195 + 180 = 375 ÷ 5 = 75%				

*H*ilary's practitioner has helped her categorize her symptoms into medium and low risk. Although Hilary initially came for treatment for the lichen planus, her practitioner has indicated that many of her symptoms have arisen through the long-term nutritional depletion and general loss of health and would therefore resolve as her health improved. As a TCM practitioner she diagnosed Hilary with Liver & Kidney Yin deficiency, Liver Blood deficiency, Liver Qi stagnation with Liver Yang/Empty Heat rising and treated her with herbs, diet and some supplements. By checking the improvement of symptoms in this way, the practitioner was able to see which groups of symptoms were improved and where the next focus should be. You can see that the lichen planus showed marked improvement, then deteriorated suddenly. This was due to a change in prescription which was subsequently remedied. As Hilary has many symptoms she has simply worked out the mean average for each group, then weighted each group accordingly and from this worked out her average progress.

medium risk	May 2009	Sept 2009	February 2010	low risk	May 2009	Sept 2009	February 2010
low energy	50	90	90	lichen planus	40	90	70
anxiety	50	80	90	skin rashes	50	90	90
low blood sugar	70	100	100	skin welts	70	80	90
anaemia	30	80	90	period pains	40	100	100
night sweats	80	100	90	food cravings	80	90	90
				dry lips	60	80	90
				red eyes	70	80	90
				dry/raw tongue	30	50	90
				burning mouth	40	50	80
				nausea	50	80	90
mean average (total ÷ 5)	280 ÷ 5 = 56	450 ÷ 5 =90	460 ÷ 5 = 92	mean average (total ÷ 10)	530 ÷ 10 = 53	790 ÷ 10 = 79	880 ÷ 10 = 88
weighting x 2	112	180	184		53	79	88

Average Progress	
6 months	112 + 53 = 171 ÷ 3 = 55%
10 months	180 + 79 = 268 ÷ 3 = 85%
15 months	184 + 88 = 272 ÷ 3 = 90%

Hilary's Journey Road Map

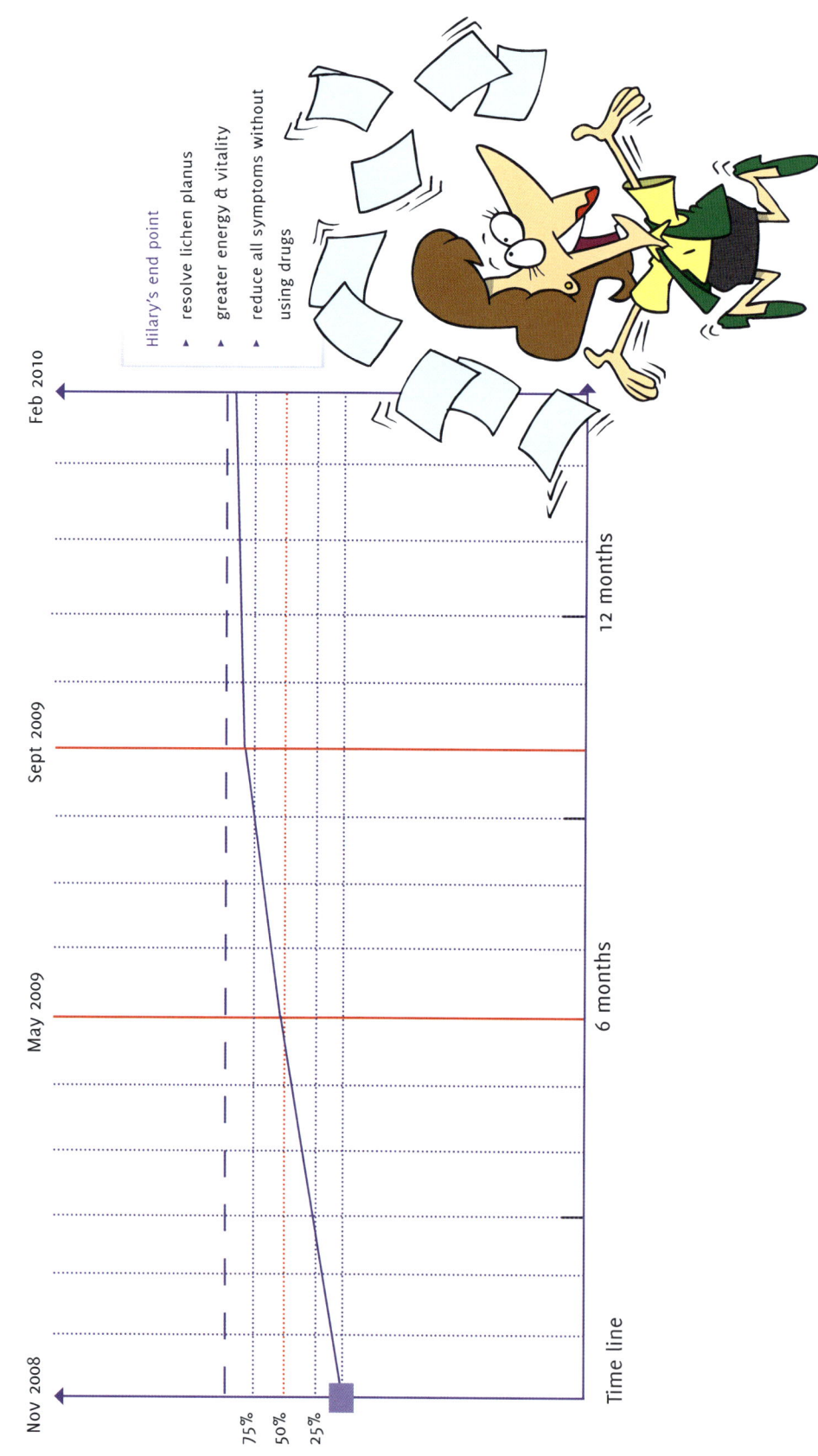

Templates & Charts

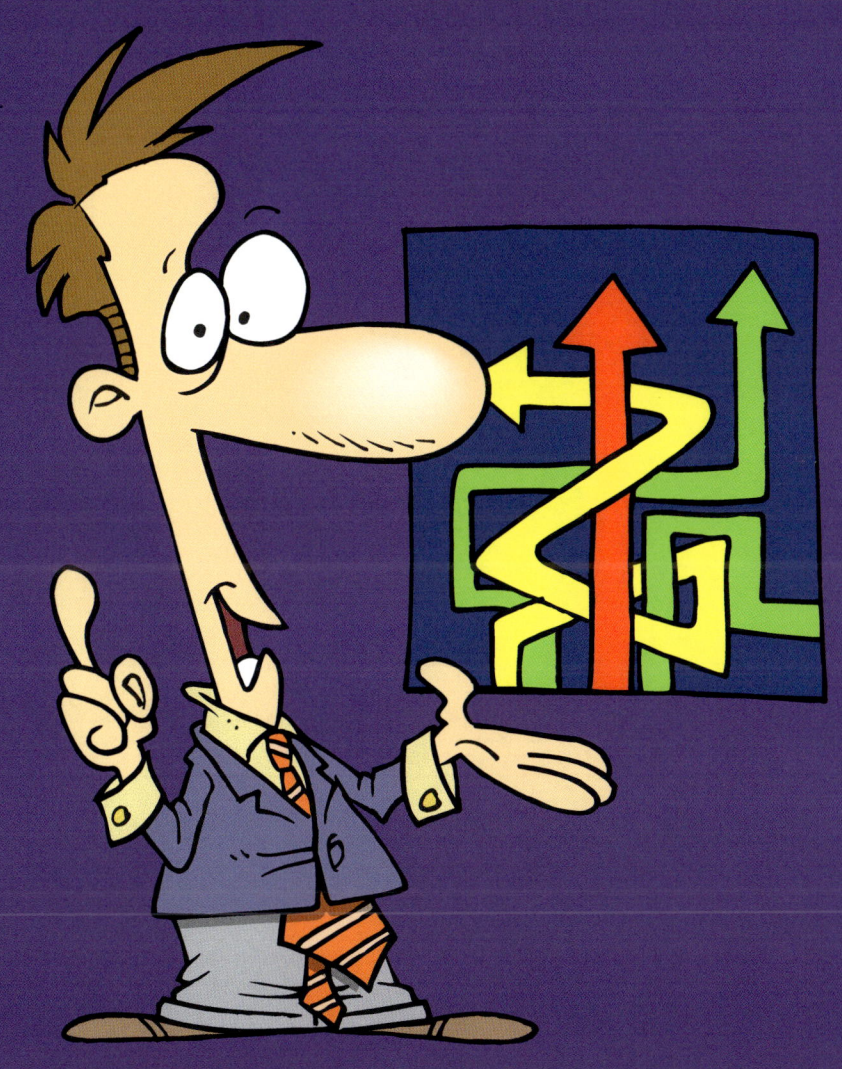

The Diagnosis Pathway

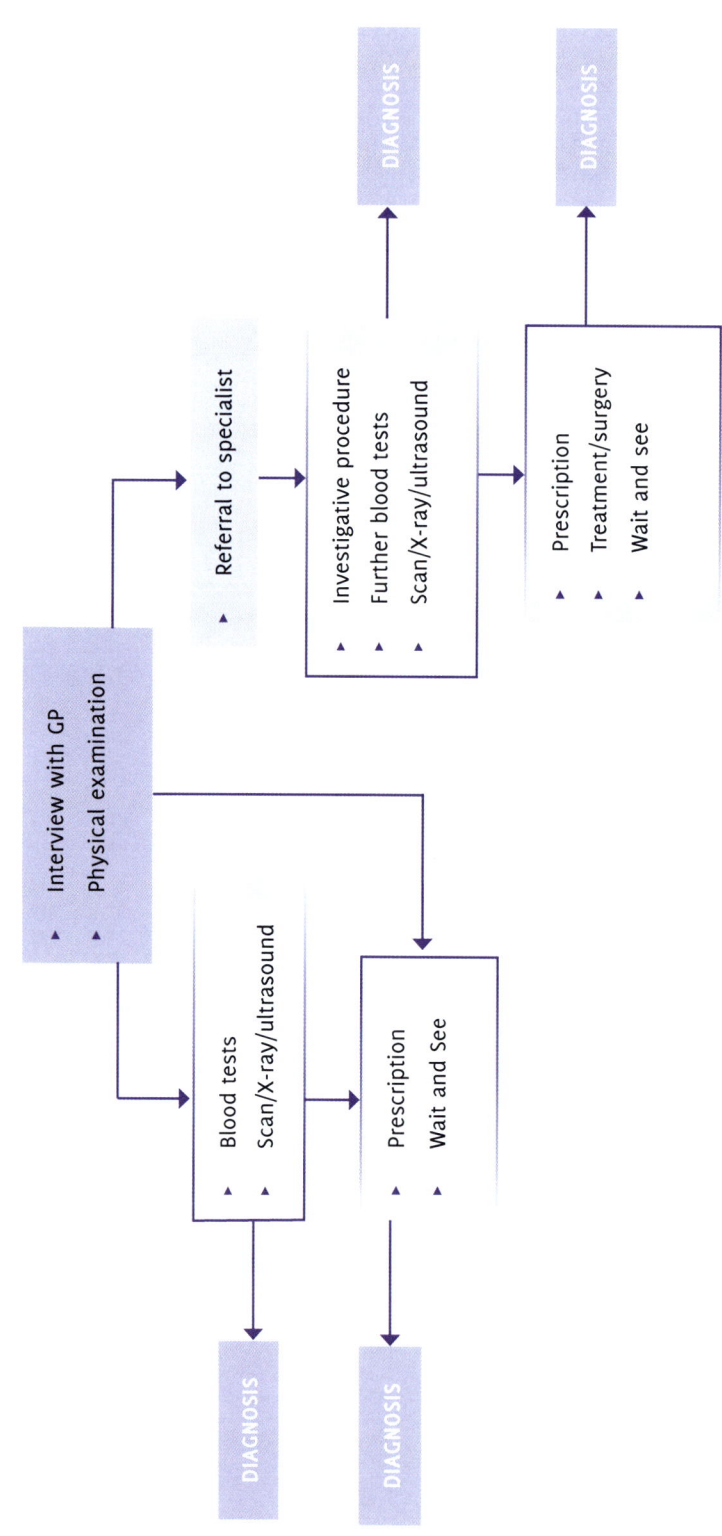

Interview with GP
- Physical examination
- Interview with GP

Referral to specialist
- Referral to specialist

Investigative procedure
- Investigative procedure
- Further blood tests
- Scan/X-ray/ultrasound

Prescription
- Prescription
- Treatment/surgery
- Wait and see

DIAGNOSIS

DIAGNOSIS

Blood tests
- Blood tests
- Scan/X-ray/ultrasound

Prescription
- Prescription
- Wait and See

DIAGNOSIS

DIAGNOSIS

Useful websites:

- http://www.uptodate.com
- http://www.nhs.uk/conditions
- http://www.netdoctor.co.uk/
- http://www.rightdiagnosis.com
- http://www.virtualmedicalcentre.com
- http://www.medicinenet.com/
- http://health.usnews.com/health-conditions
- http://www.omnimedicalsearch.com/conditions-diseases/index.htm
- http://www.omnimedicalsearch.com/forumsearch.html
- http://www.cancer.net/patient/Cancer+Types
- http://www.macmillan.org.uk/Cancerinformation
- http://news.cancerconnect.com/
- http://www.cancernetwork.com/
- http://www.cancer.gov/cancertopics/alphalist/
- http://www.cancerhelp.org.uk/index.htm
- http://www.cancer.org/Cancer/
- http://www.chemocare.com/
- http://www.medbroadcast.com
- http://www.patient.co.uk
- http://www.drugs.com/drug-classes.html
- http://www.health.harvard.edu/diagnostic-tests/
- http://www.labtestsonline.org.au

Strategy Flow Template

Symptoms → Tests → The Diagnosis → Future health risks

How serious is my condition?

How much time do I have to address my condition, or aspects of it, before the risks of the disease/condition outweigh the risks of the recommended treatment? (Which symptoms or risks are the worst and could land me in the most trouble?)

Causes

- genetic
- environmental exposure (toxins/allergens)
- Primary nutrient deficiencies
- lifestyle (diet, smoking, alcohol, sedentary life, stress)

Your Risk factors

(increases the risk for the development of a condition, worsens the prognosis or compounds the problem)

- age
- gender
- ethnicity
- inherited susceptibility
- initiating factors (infection, sunlight, surgery, pregnancy)
- weight
- lifestyle (diet, smoking, alcohol, sedentary life, stress)
- correlative factors (nutrient deficiency, alcohol, smoking, exposure to toxins, specific disease markers, weight, age at menopause/menarche)
- other health conditions
- specific drug medications

Exacerbating factors

(aggravates an existing condition)

- diet
- exposure to toxins/allergens
- lifestyle (as above)
- hormonal shifts
- stress etc.

Full Alignment Template

WHY	NOW			FUTURE HEALTH RISKS
Causes/Risks	Tests	Diagnosis		Prognosis
Medical				
risks you can't change				
risks you can change				
Non-medical				
End Point				
Symptoms &/or diagnostics	Prioritized list of goals/ measurables	End point align- ment	THERAPY	TREATMENTS	MONITORING

Health Statement Template

	My starting point	My end point	My criteria
Why state this		You need to tell the practitioner where you want to get to and match where the practitioner can take you against your own aspirations.	You need to measure how much synergy the practitioner and their treatments share with your values, convictions and criteria.
	You need to give a concise account of your diagnosis and treatment to date to allow the practitioner to judge whether they feel they can help you.		
Statement Guide	▲ I have been diagnosed with _____ and I have _____ (symptoms)	▲ I would like to achieve _____ (remission/cure, improved outcome/slow progression)	▲ Do you have experience & success in treating people with similar conditions to myself? (i.e. can you help me and with what aspect of my case?)
	▲ I have had this condition for _____ (length of time)	▲ I would like to reduce my drug/product/treatment dependency	▲ Can you tell me how long the therapy/treatment will last?
	▲ I have received medical treatment/am not on medication (indicate treatment, when you received it & length of time on treatment)	▲ I would like to reduce the risk factors for my condition (name these)	▲ What lifestyle changes may I need to make?
	▲ I have been given a time frame (months/years) before my condition becomes serious	▲ I would like to reduce my future risk/s of _____ associated with this condition	▲ Can you give any indication of the costs involved?
	▲ I have these known allergies/inherited risks	▲ I need help in addressing _____ (symptoms)	▲ Are you open to working with me if I use a mix of conventional and alternative treatments?
		▲ I would like to see improvement in _____ within (a specific time frame)	▲ Are you open to collaboration or liaising with other practitioners?
			▲ Are you open to working with me if I refuse any medical intervention?
			▲ My religion/culture forbids specific treatments, can you still work with me?
What the answers mean to me	▲ If the practitioner can help me;		
	▲ What, specifically, the practitioner may be able to help me with;		
	▲ How far they can take me/how long the benefits of their treatment will last;		
	▲ Whether I can undertake the treatment (afford it, lifestyle limitations); and		
	▲ Whether I will "get on" with the practitioner.		

My Value

will help me filter out all the things that will not work for me

Any choice of treatment	Any choices
must work for me	**must fit my lifestyle**

Prerequisites

Clinical outcome	Cost
Time frame	**Capacity to embrace lifestyle changes**

Criteria for measuring value

Cure

Reversal of condition

Remission/slow the disease process

Longer survival

Improved health/recovery potential

Maintain my health

Give me better quality of life

Reduce exacerbating factors (list these)

Reduce risks associated with my condition & prognosis (list these)

Reduce future health risks associated with my condition (list these)

Reduce drug/product dependency

Be symptom-free (name these)

Improved symptom-management/symptom relief (name these)

Specific goals: eg. to increase my fertility, reduce weight etc.

Cost (within my specified budget)

I need to be able to do at home

It must fit with my family

I can/cannot travel for treatment

I must be able to carry on working/education

I can/cannot take time off work

I have/have no physical impairments

I require a specific diet

I can change my diet

I can/cannot make lifestyle changes (name these)

Must work within my time frame

Template

so I can look more closely at what might work best for me

Any choices
must fit with my own values
& convictions

Any practitioner/product/service
must demonstrate a value
in helping me with my journey

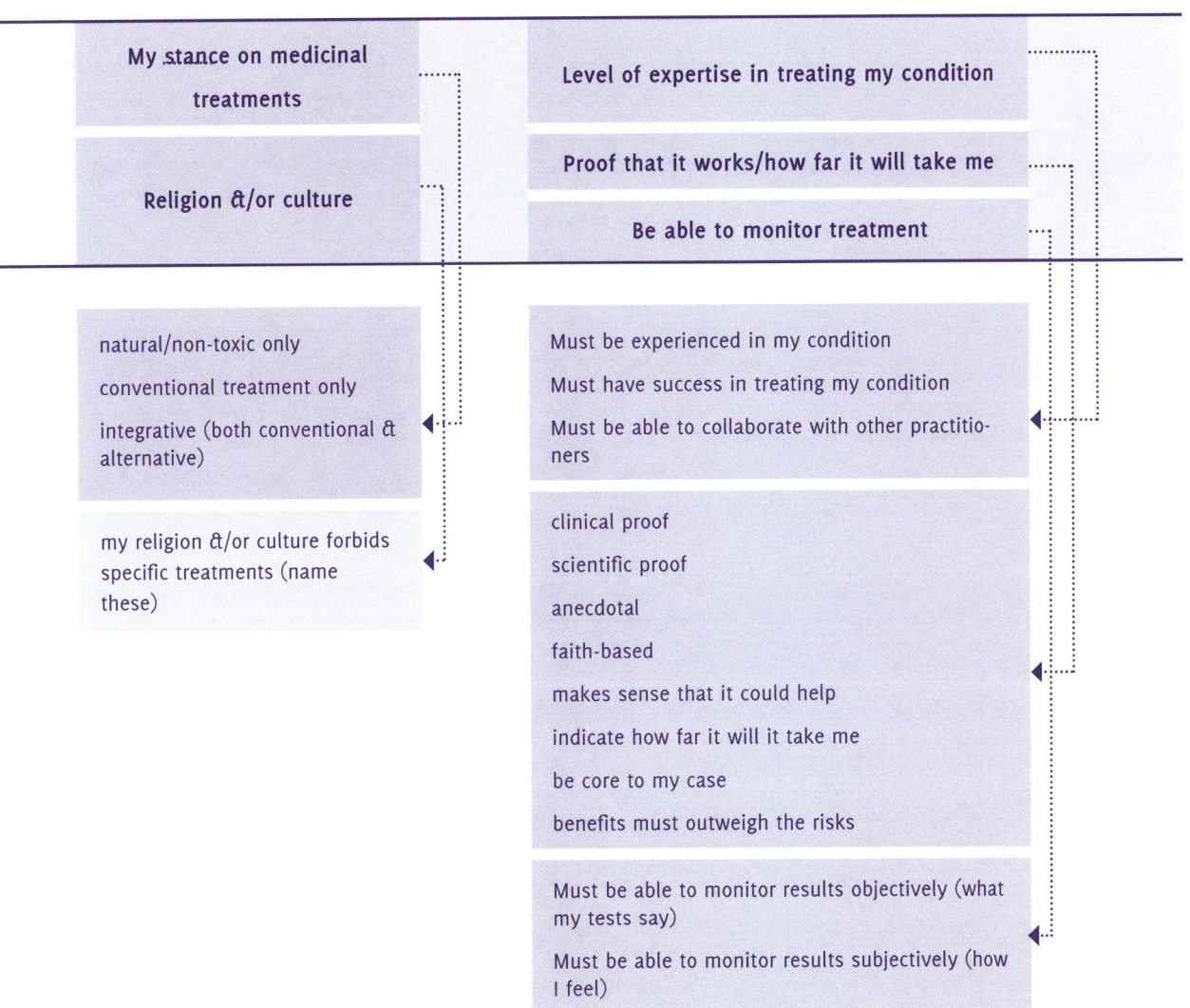

My stance on medicinal treatments

Religion &/or culture

Level of expertise in treating my condition

Proof that it works/how far it will take me

Be able to monitor treatment

natural/non-toxic only

conventional treatment only

integrative (both conventional & alternative)

my religion &/or culture forbids specific treatments (name these)

Must be experienced in my condition

Must have success in treating my condition

Must be able to collaborate with other practitioners

clinical proof

scientific proof

anecdotal

faith-based

makes sense that it could help

indicate how far it will it take me

be core to my case

benefits must outweigh the risks

Must be able to monitor results objectively (what my tests say)

Must be able to monitor results subjectively (how I feel)

A conversational approach

QUESTIONS	About my diagnosis	About my prognosis (How will my condition affect me?)
Why ask these questions?	You need an accurate diagnosis in order for you and others to know what needs to be fixed.	You need to know where you are heading (what to expect) in the short and long-term in order to set goals and time-frames.
Questionnaire Guide	▸ What is my condition/diagnosis? ▸ Which of my symptoms relate to this condition? ▸ What are the causes of my condition? ▸ What things may worsen my condition or are associated with a poorer prognosis? ▸ Is my condition reversible/curable with treatment; and ▸ Is my condition reversible/curable without treatment? If you don't have a proper diagnosis then you need to ask: ▸ What tests could I have or which person should I see in order to get a diagnosis? ▸ What will these tests tell me?	▸ What could happen to me and within what time frame if I do nothing? (complications of disease; acute events) ▸ How great is this risk? (What are the odds of this happening to me?) ▸ What are the health risks for my condition if left untreated? (related health risks) ▸ If I take treatment, am I likely to experience any adverse or medical events related to my condition? If so, what are these and when, in your opinion, could these occur? (Events against a time-line which will give me my time frame.) ▸ Could I narrow my options on treatment if I leave my decision for too long?

What the answers mean to me	
▸	How advanced my condition is (how far away am I from where I would like to be?)
▸	How quickly it may progress (how quickly am I going in the opposite direction?)
▸	If there are any immediate, medium or long-term health risks (where could I end up if I do nothing?)
▸	What I need to do, and how quickly I need to act in order to make sure that I am heading in the right direction and do not narrow my treatment opportunities

Factor in their professional criteria	
▸	They can only work within their field of expertise
▸	Their end point may be aligned to part of your journey, but not to your end point
▸	Their end point may not be aligned to your journey or your end point

Where can you take me?

You need to find out what stretch of your journey they can help you with.

- ▸ What is the aim of your therapy/program?
- ▸ Which aspects of my condition will your program address?
- ▸ What sort of improvement/s can you offer me?
- ▸ What results can I expect on this program? (worst, median, best case scenario)
- ▸ Within what time frame will I see an improvement?
- ▸ Will the improvement last and how long will it last?
- ▸ How long will I need to be on your program?
- ▸ Could the program fail in my case (produce little or no response) or is there any chance that it could worsen my condition?
- ▸ In your clinical experience how effective do you think your program will be for me? (clinical outcome)
- ▸ If I require additional treatments on your program later on when would this likely be? (If yes, then the same questions will apply for each program: how successful would it be and how long would the improvements last?)
- ▸ What would you advise if your program doesn't work?
- ▸ How will we monitor the program, and how frequently, to make sure that it is working as predicted?

- ▸ How core is the practitioner in getting me to my end point?
- ▸ Which part of my journey can they help me with?
- ▸ How far can the practitioner take me on my journey?
- ▸ What goals can the practitioner help me with?
- ▸ How fast can they take me there?

A conversational approach (cont'd)

QUESTIONS	What value are your treatments to me?	Research: Is the treatment suitable for me?
Why ask this question?	You need to know how effective the treatment will be in your case or how far it will get you to your end point.	You need to know the risks of the treatment and if there are any additional individual risks for you.
Questionnaire Guide	▸ How does the treatment work? (scientific basis) ▸ What aspect of my case will it treat? (cause, risk factors, symptoms) ▸ In your clinical experience how effective do you think this treatment will be for me? (clinical outcome/what are my odds?) ▸ Within what time frame will I see an improvement? ▸ Will the improvement last and how long will it last? ▸ How long will I need to be on this treatment? ▸ Will you be able to monitor my progress and, if so, how will you do this and how frequently?	▸ Is the treatment recommended appropriate for my condition/symptoms? ▸ Does the treatment match my profile? ▸ Are there any specific contraindications for the treatment that would apply to me? ▸ Are there any health risks for the treatment, both in the short and long-term and, if so, what are they and how great are those risks? ▸ Are there any side-effects/adverse reactions and, if so, what would these be and how would we monitor for them? ▸ Could this treatment fail in my case (produce little or no response) or is there any chance that it could worsen my condition?
Factor in their professional criteria	▸ to only prescribe treatment procedures endorsed by their medical body & based within their field of expertise ▸ to recommend treatment based on medical risk/benefit criteria which may not factor in long-term or individual risks, or a range of variables that have not been scientifically proven ▸ to follow procedures for monitoring treatment, the results of which may not have a bearing on the patient's overall clinical condition ▸ to prescribe only the products from their own retail range	

What tests will be used to monitor progress?	How does the test align with my end point?
You need to qualify what the practitioner is monitoring and whether the tests are appropriate.	You need to know how far the test results are aligned to your end point.

▸ What is the test? ▸ What will the test measure? ▸ What treatment is the test measuring? ▸ What aspect of my case is the test monitoring? (cause, risk factors, future health risks) ▸ How frequently will we test to make sure that the treatment is working? ▸ What markers are you looking for and what will these tell you?	▸ What benefits will I experience as a consequence of improved test results? ▸ Are these improvements core to getting me to my end point? ▸ Are these improvements core to me achieving my goals, and if so, which goals?

▸ to measure the efficacy of the product or protocol (treatment outcome) they prescribe which may not factor in other treatments or conditions that the patient has that are outside their field of expertise;

(monitoring the product and not the patient)

▸ to monitor the disease progression/regression which may not factor in other risk factors or conditions that the patient may have that are outside their field of expertise

(monitoring the disease and not the patient)

▸ to interpret the test results in isolation of the patient's general condition

(monitoring the test results and not the patient)

▸ to rely and base recommendations on the test results rather than the clinical condition of the patient

(treating the test result and not the patient)

Therapy Alignment Template

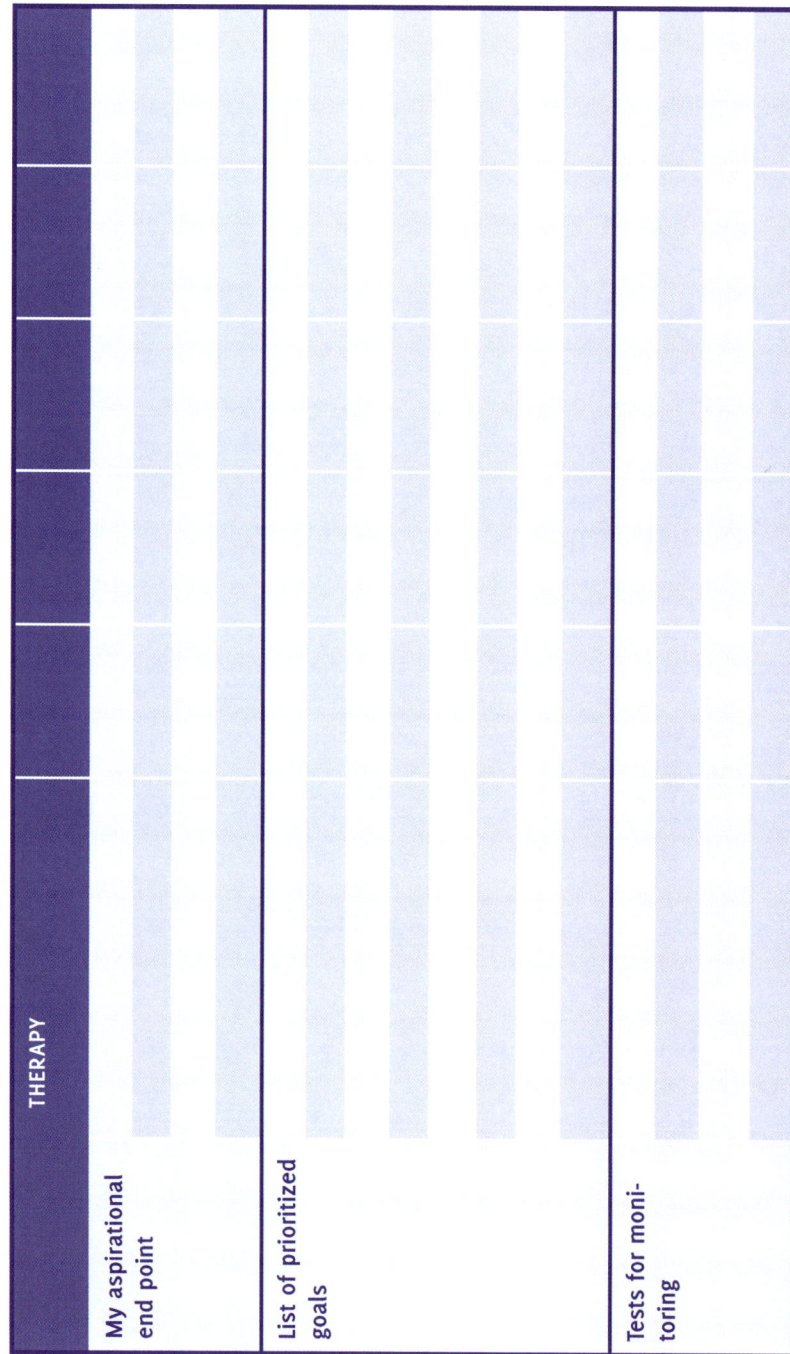

THERAPY			
My aspirational end point			
List of prioritized goals			
Tests for monitoring			

Therapy Alignment Rating Template

Therapy options	What is it?	What is its end point?	How does this align to my end point?	Rating

Treatment Alignment Template

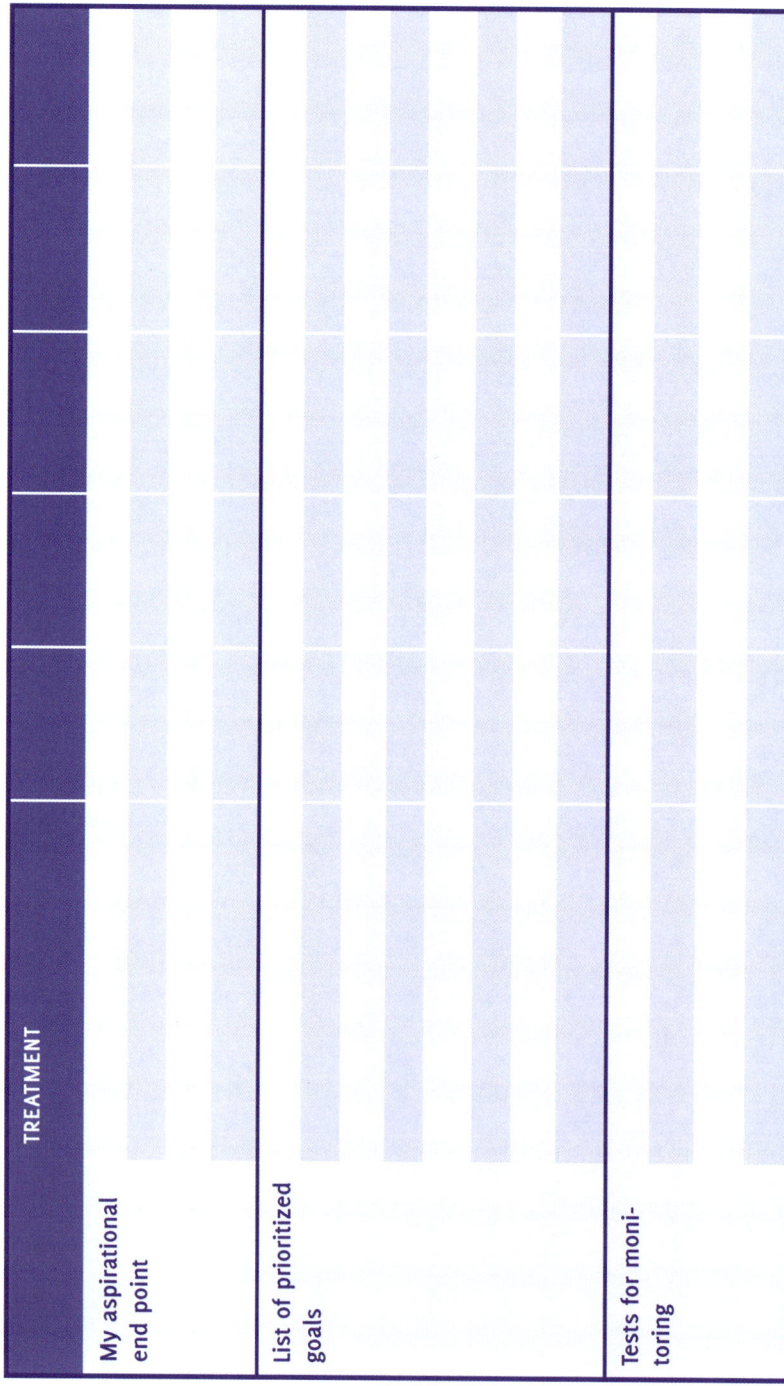

TREATMENT						
My aspirational end point						
List of prioritized goals						
Tests for moni-toring						

Treatment Alignment Rating Template

Treatment options	What will the treatment do?	How will it help me get to my end point?	What is used to measure outcome?	Rating

Monitoring Chart

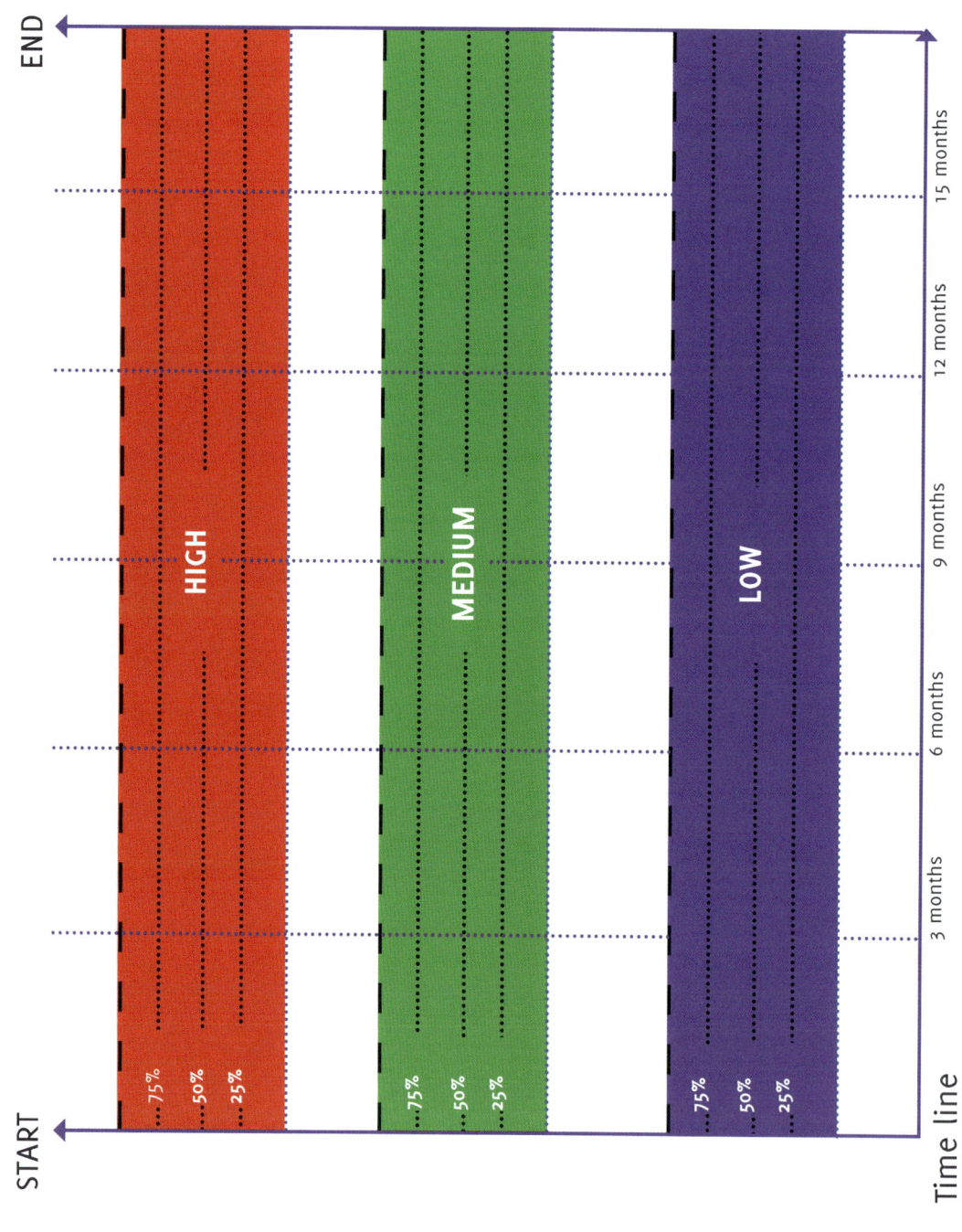

Journey Road Map

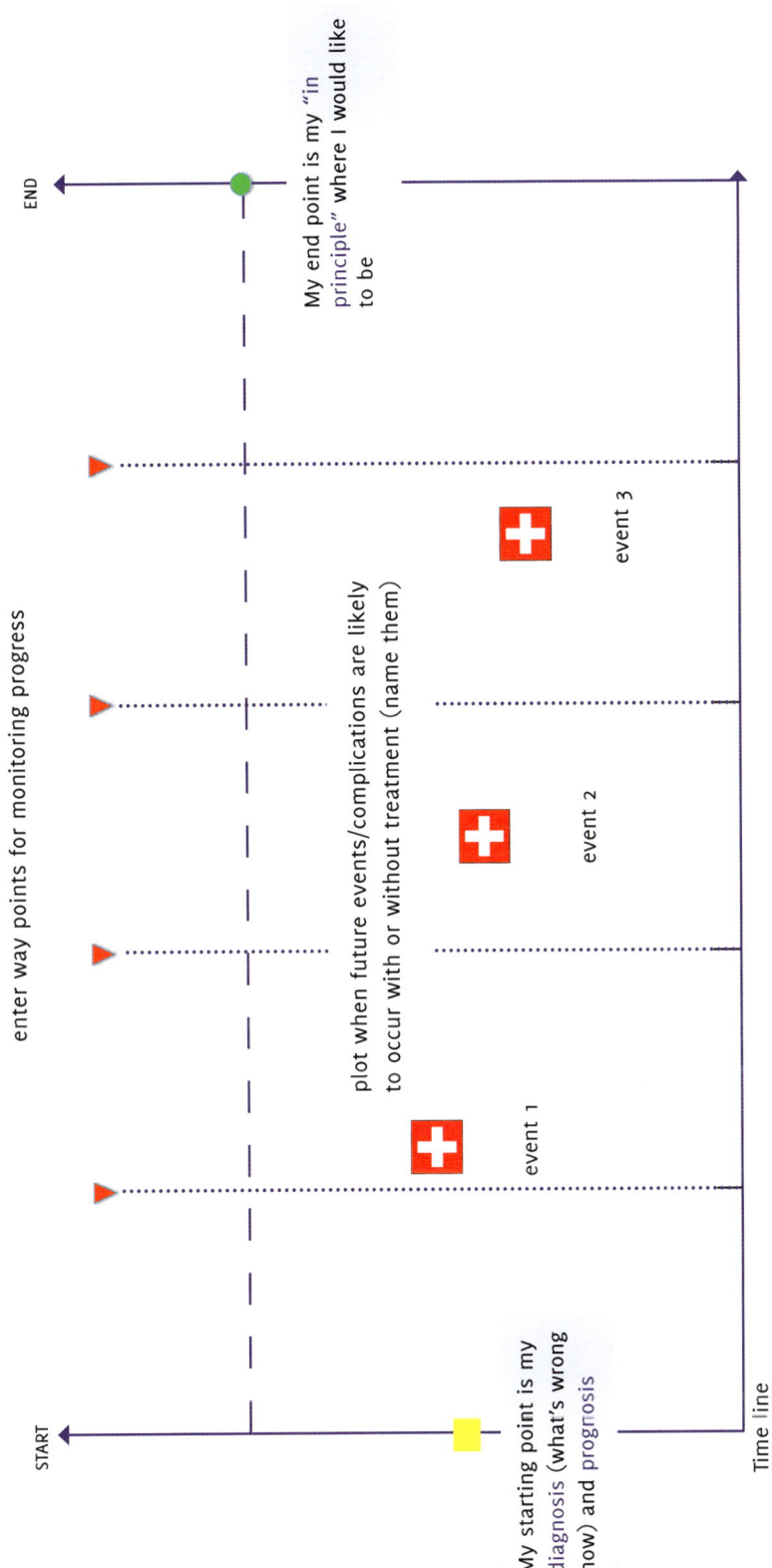

START

My starting point is my diagnosis (what's wrong now) and prognosis

enter way points for monitoring progress

plot when future events/complications are likely to occur with or without treatment (name them)

event 1

event 2

event 3

My end point is my "in principle" where I would like to be

END

Time line

Prevention saves you "the labor of being sick".

Thomas Adams
1583 - 1623

Case Studies

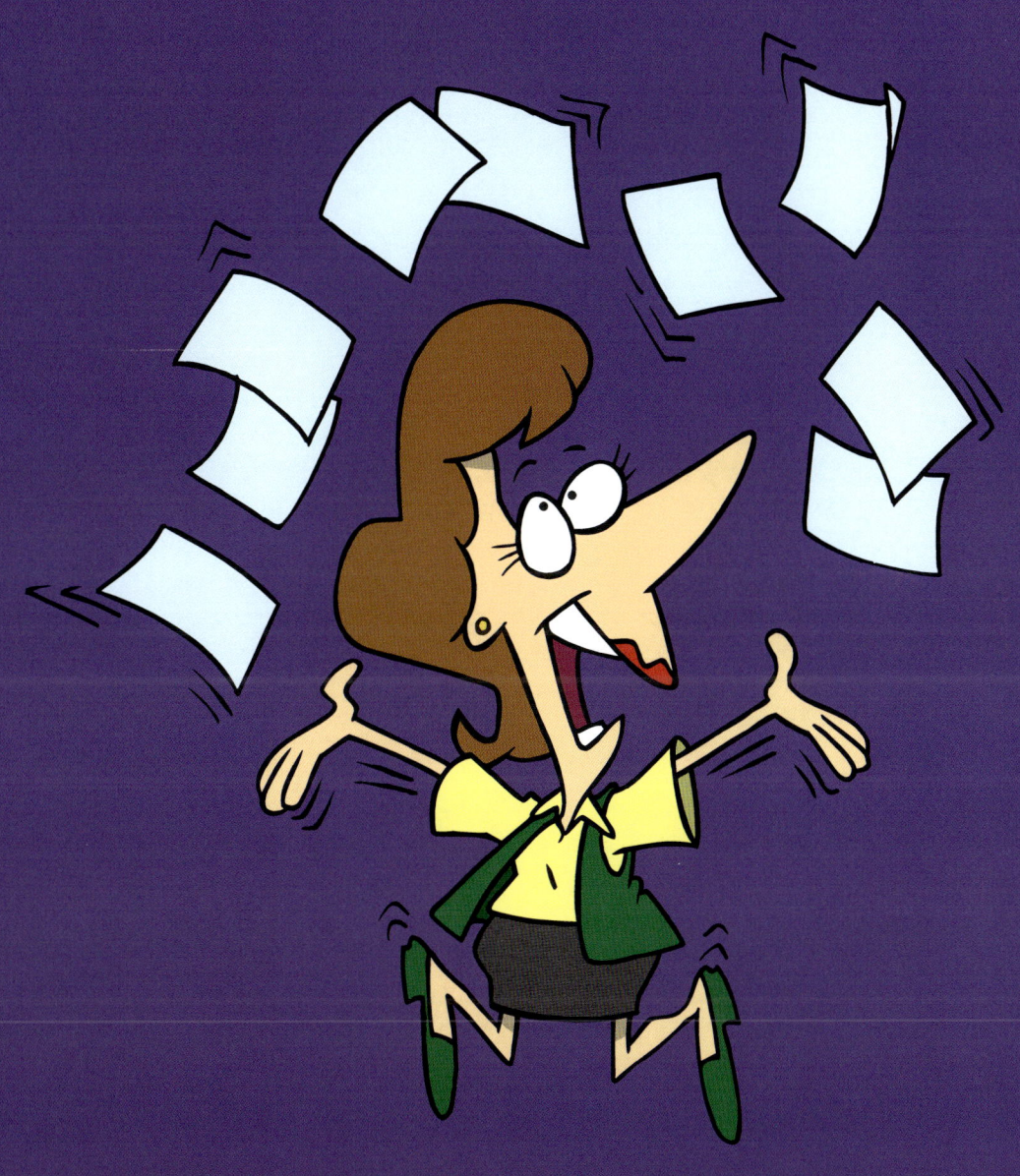

Natalie's Journey
2003-2009

Natalie is 21 years old and has been diagnosed with polycystic ovarian syndrome with haemorrhagic ovarian cysts. Her problems started at 20 with surgery for a ruptured haemorrhagic cyst and following this blood tests revealed PCOS. Her GP said that her condition was incurable that she would need to take some form of hormonal medication to control her condition. Over the next year she was prescribed a bio-identical progesterone cream to try and control her symptoms, but this aggravated all her symptoms especially the jaundice, nausea and vomiting. Natalie's ongoing problems were painful & flooding periods, premenstrual mood swings, bloating, fluid retention, migraines, vomiting, unwanted hair growth, acne and depression. Natalie decided to seek further help from alternative therapies to try and reduce her symptoms so that she could have a life.

Natalie's Strategy Flow Template

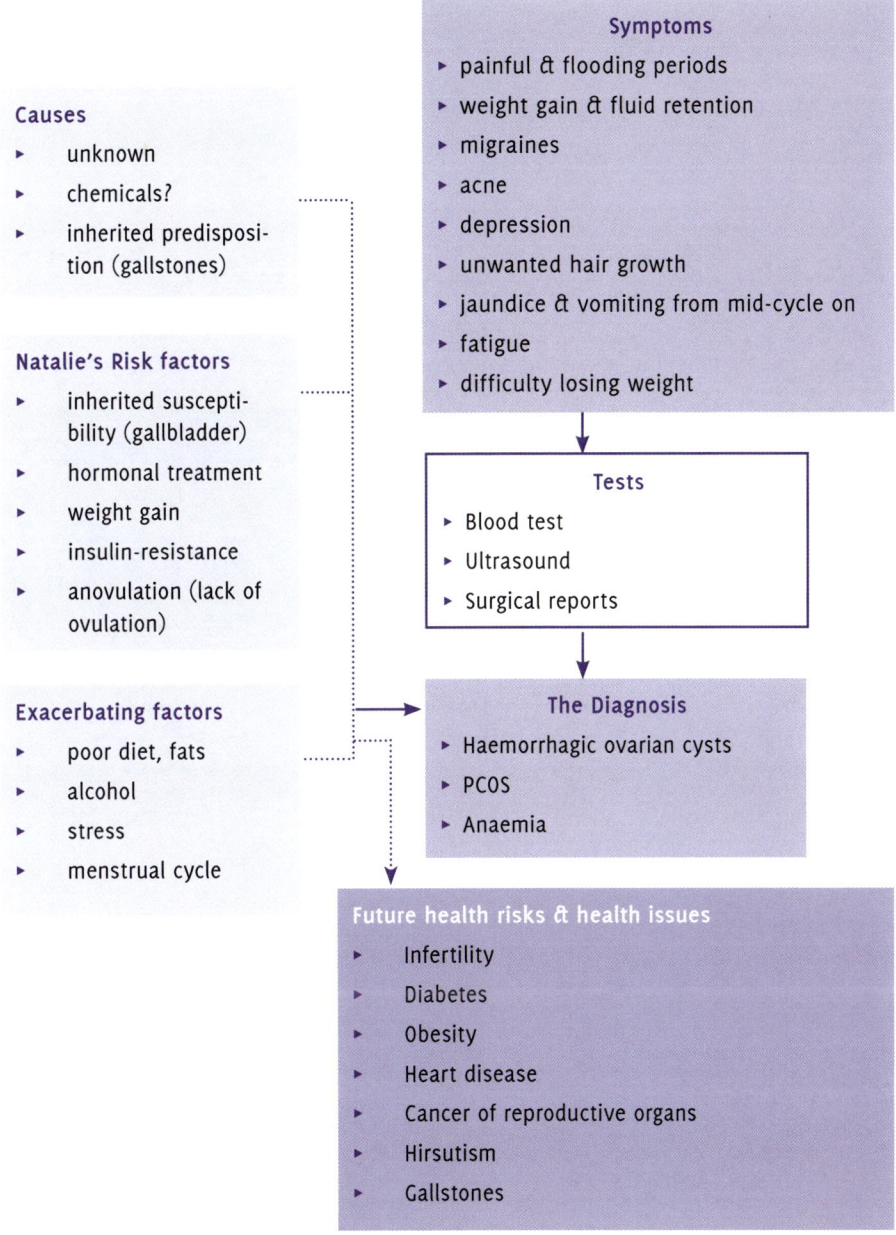

Symptoms
- painful & flooding periods
- weight gain & fluid retention
- migraines
- acne
- depression
- unwanted hair growth
- jaundice & vomiting from mid-cycle on
- fatigue
- difficulty losing weight

Causes
- unknown
- chemicals?
- inherited predisposition (gallstones)

Natalie's Risk factors
- inherited susceptibility (gallbladder)
- hormonal treatment
- weight gain
- insulin-resistance
- anovulation (lack of ovulation)

Exacerbating factors
- poor diet, fats
- alcohol
- stress
- menstrual cycle

Tests
- Blood test
- Ultrasound
- Surgical reports

The Diagnosis
- Haemorrhagic ovarian cysts
- PCOS
- Anaemia

Future health risks & health issues
- Infertility
- Diabetes
- Obesity
- Heart disease
- Cancer of reproductive organs
- Hirsutism
- Gallstones

How serious is Natalie's condition?
- My condition may be controlled with medical treatment, but not cured
- I may prejudice my health if I don't have treatment to slow its progression
- My condition may become serious without treatment and monitoring, and I may prejudice my outcome or narrow my treatment options if I don't accept treatment now
- I need 6 monthly regular check-ups with my gynaecologist

Natalie's Journey Road Map

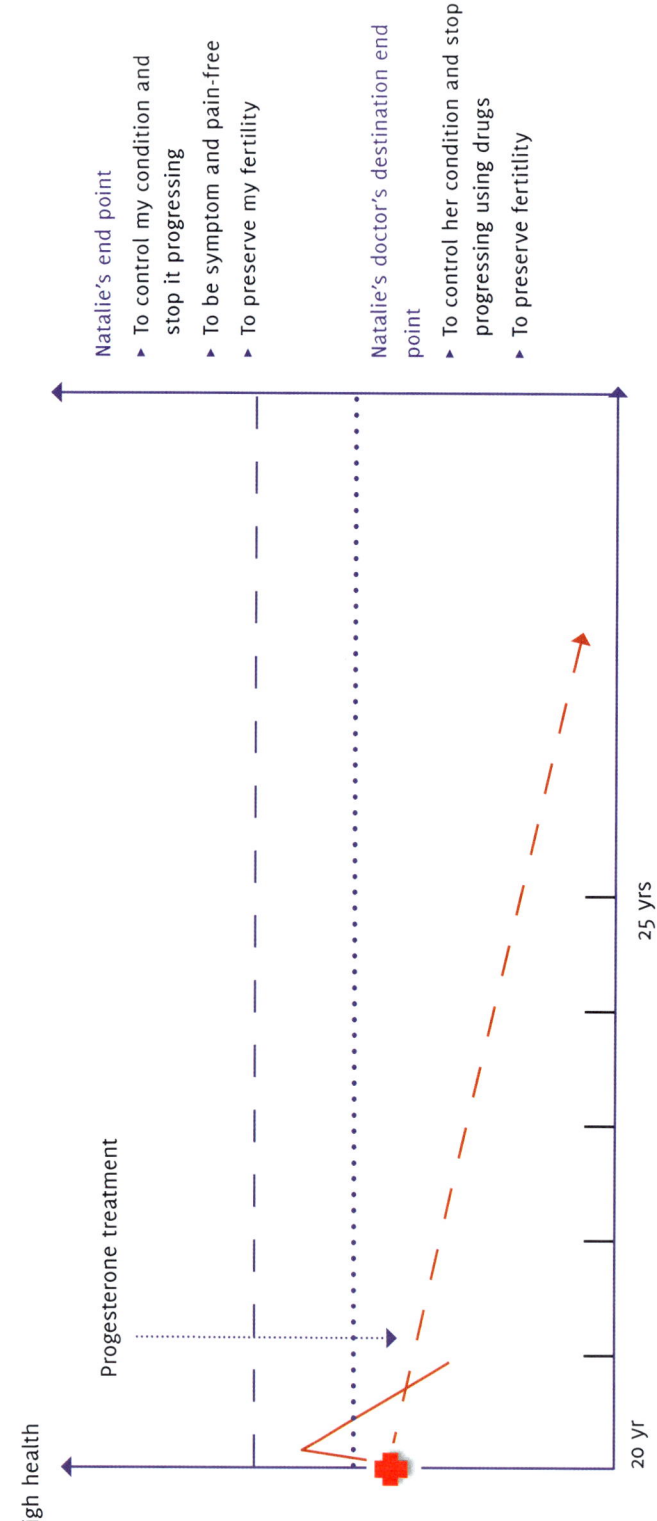

Natalie's end point

- To control my condition and stop it progressing
- To be symptom and pain-free
- To preserve my fertility

Natalie's doctor's destination end point

- To control her condition and stop it progressing using drugs
- To preserve fertility

High health

Progesterone treatment

20 yr

25 yrs

You can see from Natalie's journey road map the brief improvement after surgery but she was unable to remain symptom-free. It was at this time that she saw a doctor who specialized in female complaints and prescribed bio-identical hormones. She ran blood tests which showed that Natalie had PCOS and so she prescribed a bio-identical progesterone cream. Natalie's symptoms worsened dramatically on the treatment, especially with the nausea and vomiting. Her premenstrual symptoms were also aggravated with severe bloating during the second half of each cycle.

Natalie did further research and found that several lifestyle factors could make her situation worse. She found that PCOS usually involved other endocrine disturbances, such as insulin-resistance, which would not only aggravate her current hormonal imbalance of high testosterone and failure to ovulate (and hence threaten fertility), but had inherent risks for later onset diabetes and heart disease. Natalie also discovered that weight gain was not only a consequence of insulin resistance but could also perpetuate this, so it would be necessary to keep this in check. She also found that she had an hereditary susceptibility for gallstones which explained the nausea and vomiting during the second half of her cycle and why this intensified when taking any hormonal treatment.

Natalie's Full Alignment Template

WHY	NOW			FUTURE HEALTH RISKS
Causes/Risks	**Medical**			
		Tests	**Diagnosis**	**Prognosis**
Hereditary gallbladder problems		Blood test	▲ haemorrhagic ovarian cysts	potential for multiple surgeries with risk of adhesions
Hormonal imbalance/anovulation		Transvaginal ultrasound	▲ PCOS	Insulin-resistance/diabetes
Being overweight/insulin-resistance		Surgical reports		Heart disease; infertility
Alcohol			▲ endometriosis (suspected)	endometriotic implants in pelvic organs, possible removal of parts of organs (such as bowel), cancer
Fatty foods				
Stress			▲ anaemia	worsening general health/fatigue
High carbohydrate diet				
Sedentary lifestyle				
Heavy menstrual cycle				
Dietary iron deficiency				
	End Point		**Prioritized list of goals/measurables**	**End point alignment**
			▲ control condition & stop progression	
			▲ symptom & pain free	
			▲ preserve fertility	
	Symptoms &/or diagnostics			
	▲ painful & flooding periods			
	▲ migraine			
	▲ vomiting, jaundice			
	▲ bloating & swelling			
	▲ unwanted hair growth			
	▲ acne			
	▲ overweight			
	▲ fatigue			
	▲ depression			

Natalie's End Point

*N*atalie was told that her condition was incurable but that it could possibly be controlled with drugs and surgery. She did her research and found some risk factors that she could change that may improve her outcome, such as not gaining weight, doing regular exercise and being careful with her diet.

It was easy for Natalie to make her "in principle" end point - she just wanted to have a life without all the debilitating symptoms that lasted two out of every four weeks, often having to take time off work, and she wanted to be able to have children in the future. She was under no illusion that her condition would need careful monitoring but hoped that her end point was realistic. Although a key treatment to halt the progression is an oral contraceptive pill Natalie knows that this may be unsuitable in her case and she would have to weigh the risks carefully due to the underlying problem with her liver and gallbladder.

Natalie will be looking primarily at reducing her risk factors and for symptom-management as she has been told that her main risks cannot be changed.

DESTINATION END POINT

Control my condition & stop it progressing;

To have a life (i.e. be symptom & pain-free); and

To preserve fertility

SPECIFIC GOALS

get ovulation happening,

reduce heavy periods & pain, bloating &

abdominal swelling

reduce nausea, vomiting & migraines

improve skin, reduce unwanted hair growth

reduce weight

Group 1:

Natalie wants to *control* her condition and stop it progressing

Group 2:

She would like to be *drug-free*, but if there was a drug that could help she would prefer this over surgery.

Group 3:

Her biggest health risks are the consequences of uncontrolled *endometriosis & haemorrhagic cysts* as so many future health risks will be aggravated by this.

Group 4:

Her main objective is to become *symptom-free* and *pain-free*. She would like to preserve her *fertility*.

Time-frame: She needs to hold the condition and monitor every 6 months.

End Point	control condition & stop progression	
	symptom & pain-free	
	preserve fertility	
Symptoms &/or diagnostics	**Prioritized list of goals/measurables**	**End point alignment**
▸ painful & flooding periods	stop painful and flooding periods *(get ovulation happening)*	▸ be symptom and pain free, control condition
▸ migraine	stop migraines	▸ be symptom and pain free, control condition
▸ vomiting, jaundice	stop vomiting and jaundice	▸ be symptom free
▸ bloating & swelling	reduce weight	▸ help control condition
▸ unwanted hair growth	resolve anaemia/improve energy	▸ be symptom free
▸ acne	address unwanted hair growth	▸ be symptom free
▸ overweight	address acne	▸ be symptom free
▸ fatigue	reduce stress, depression & anxiety	▸ be symptom free
▸ depression	address bloating & fluid retention	▸ be symptom free

Natalie's Summary

❝ I am 22 years old and have been diagnosed with polycystic ovarian syndrome, haemorrhagic ovarian cysts and suspected endometriosis. I have had one surgery two years ago for a ruptured haemorrhagic cyst. I have tried progesterone to try and control my symptoms but this aggravated them, particularly the migraines and vomiting. I may have to have further surgery but I need help with my current symptoms of painful & flooding periods, migraine, vomiting, unwanted hair growth, acne and depression as at the moment I don't have a life, I have to take a lot of time off work and I look five months pregnant for two weeks out of each month. I am looking for better control of my symptoms. ❞

Natalie's Therapy Alignment Template

		GP	Naturop-athy	Chinese medicine	Surgery
Natalie's end point	To control my condition and stop it progressing		?	?	√
	To be symptom and pain-free	?	?	√	√
	To preserve fertility		?	√	√
List of prioritized goals	painful and flooding periods	x	?	√	√
	migraine	x	?	√	x
	vomiting, jaundice	x	?	√	x
	reduce weight	x	√	x	x
	resolve anaemia/improve energy	√	√	√	x
	address unwanted hair growth	x	x	√	x
	address acne	x	√	√	x
	reduce stress, depression & anxiety, mood swings	√	√	√	x
	address bloating/fluid retention	x	√	√	x
Tests for monitoring	Transvaginal ultrasound scan	√			√
	Blood tests	√			√

Natalie selects various therapies and asks each specialist their opinion of her case and what they can do to help her. She is clear about what she wants fixing (goals) and where she wants to end up. She definitely wants children in the future, and she needs a life in the meantime. Her GP has recommended an anti-depressant to help with the depression, but fundamentally Natalie would like to be as drug-free as possible. Surgery, if required, is the most closely aligned to her end point, but she realizes that surgery will not fix the underlying causes and therefore she will need to take other steps and make lifestyle adjustments that will address her risk factors and future health risks which will, in turn, assist her with her goals and reaching her end point.

Natalie's Therapy Alignment Rating

Therapy	What is it?	What is its end point?	What is the core benefit to me?	Rating
Surgery	Surgical removal of diseased parts, prescribing of drugs and monitoring conditions using medical tests	Control my condition with surgery so that I don't go into acute	Could offer a five year remission I will be drug-free I will be pain-free Reduce my risks for other organ involvement Preserve my fertility	10
General practice	Diagnose, advise, prescribe drugs, monitor my chronic condition with tests, refer	Control symptoms and abnormal test results with drugs	Monitor my condition, order tests Refer if condition becomes acute	7
Naturopathy	The promotion of health using natural products, supplements & diet	Improve my general health, reduce future health risks and address current risk factors	Will help reduce risk factors (weight) Will address anaemia Will address future health risks (diabetes, heart disease)	7
Traditional Chinese Medicine (herbal)	The promotion of the correct function of organs using herbs	To restore ovulation and support menstruation; support the liver	Will support my healing after surgery May give me a longer remission Support my fertility; stop pain Stop unwanted hair growth Stop the nausea and vomiting	8

Scoring rationale:

Natalie has given the top score to the surgeon as she realizes that no-one else could fix her problem if it becomes acute. The surgeon also suspected that Natalie may have underlying endometriosis but he said that she should only consider surgery if her condition deteriorated. He was also very positive about her seeking alternative treatment as he could not address any of the chronic underlying health issues, particularly as she cannot take the contraceptive pill. Natalie decides to follow the advice of a naturopath as a preventive measure and also seek Chinese herbal treatment as this seems to offer the best outcome in terms of symptom management. She has a really good relationship with her GP and wants her in on her treatment strategy, so she gives her a relatively high score, even though she cannot prescribe her any treatment.

Natalie's Therapy End Point Alignment

End Point				
control condition and stop progression				
symptom and pain-free				
preserve fertility				

Symptoms &/or diagnostics	Prioritized list of Goals (measurables)	End point alignment	Therapy
painful and flooding periods	stop painful & flooding periods	▲ be symptom and pain-free, control condition	▲ Surgery ▲ TCM
migraine	stop migraines	▲ be symptom and pain-free	▲ TCM
vomiting/jaundice	stop vomiting & jaundice	▲ be symptom-free	▲ TCM
bloating, swelling	reduce weight	▲ help control condition	▲ Naturopathy
unwanted hair growth	improve energy	▲ be symptom-free	▲ Naturopathy ▲ TCM
acne	address unwanted hair growth	▲ be symptom-free	▲ TCM
overweight	address acne	▲ be symptom-free	▲ Naturopathy ▲ TCM
fatigue	reduce stress, depression & anxiety	▲ be symptom-free	▲ TCM ▲ GP
depression	address bloating/fluid retention	▲ be symptom-free	▲ Naturopathy ▲ TCM

Natalie's Treatment Alignment Template

	TREATMENT	Contraceptive pill	Iron, Mg, B vitamins	Diet	Surgical excision	TCM Herbs
Natalie's end point	Control condition & stop progression	√	x	?	√	?
	Be symptom & pain-free	?	x	?	√	√
	Preserve fertility	√	x	?	√	√
List of prioritized goals	painful & flooding periods	?	x	?	√	√
	migraine	x	x	?	x	√
	vomiting, jaundice	x	x	?	x	√
	reduce weight	x	x	√	x	x
	resolve anaemia/improve energy	x	√	√	x	√
	address unwanted hair growth	x	x	x	x	√
	address acne	?	x	?	x	√
	reduce stress, depression, anxiety & mood swings	x	?	?	x	√
	address bloating & fluid retention	x	?	√	x	√
Tests for monitoring	Blood tests	x	√	√	√	x
	Ultrasound	√	x	x	√	x
	Pulse & tongue diagnosis	x	x	x	x	√

Natalie's Treatment Alignment Rating Template

Treatment	What will the treatment do?	How will it help me get to my end point?	What is used to measure outcome?	Rating
Surgery	Surgically remove diseased parts/endometriosis/adhesions	Offer me remission Control disease progression Preserve my fertility	Objective: transvaginal ultrasound Subjective: reduction in symptoms	10
Iron, Mg & B supplements	Resolve my anaemia, improve my energy	Improve my energy and my healing capacity	Objective: blood tests Subjective: more energy	6
Diet	Help me lose weight Help reverse insulin-resistance Help with detoxification of oestrogen	Reduce future health risks and current risk factors (weight) May help reduce disease progression	Objective: weigh-in Subjective: feel better, less symptoms	7
Herbs (TCM) formulae according to symptoms	Reduce pain Reduce heavy blood flow Reduce unwanted hair growth Improve skin (acne) Stop nausea, vomiting and jaundice Reduce depression and mood swings, bloating & fluid retention	Could slow progression I will have a life by being symptom-free	Objective: pulse & tongue diagnosis Subjective: feel better, improved symptoms	8
Oral contraceptive pill	Reduce pain and heavy blood flow Increase jaundice, vomiting & migraines Increase my weight May aggravate insulin-resistance May increase premenstrual symptoms	It may take me further away from my end point I may have less of a life (from past experience)	Objective: blood tests, TVUS Subjective: progression or remission of symptoms	0

Scoring rationale:

Natalie has given the top score to surgery, based on the fact that this would represent an acute and technically life-saving treatment if her condition was allowed to progress. The next score goes to the TCM herbs as these products can manage the majority of her symptoms. However, she will need to be carefully monitored by her medical team, and if she requires surgery in the future then herbs can be offered to speed the healing. The next rating goes to diet. Natalie has been on a weight loss program that was recommended for her condition: a high protein, low carbohydrate diet. However, she found that although she lost weight the program worsened many of her premenstrual symptoms and so she elected to follow a different approach that was more balanced, but paying attention to the type of carbohydrate consumed. The iron supplements are not critical to her end point and an iron deficiency is not the cause of her anaemia, but they will support her iron status which gets severely knocked due to the heavy periods. The contraceptive pill is clearly out of the question for Natalie, and when she evaluates it against her symptoms and end point she can see just how detrimental this medication may be to her overall health.

Natalie's Health Flow chart

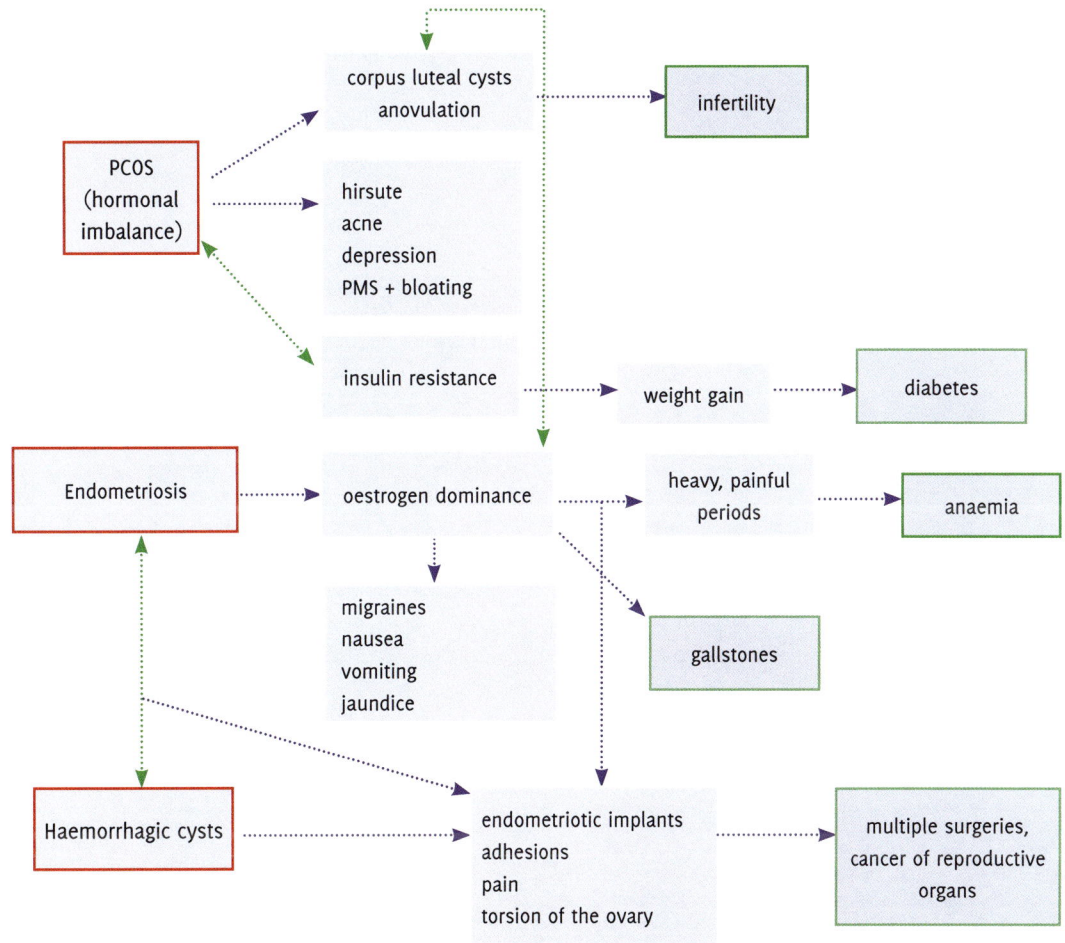

Natalie's Treatment End Point Alignment

End Point
- control condition and stop progression
- symptom and pain-free
- preserve fertility

Symptoms &/or diagnostics	Prioritized list of Goals (measurables)	End point alignment	Therapy	Treatment	Tests
painful and flooding periods	stop painful & flooding periods	▲ be symptom and pain-free, control condition	▲ Surgery ▲ TCM	▲ surgery ▲ herbs	▲ subjective ▲ hormone tests ▲ pulse diagnosis
migraine	stop migraines	▲ be symptom and pain-free	▲ TCM	▲ herbs	▲ subjective ▲ pulse diagnosis
vomiting/jaundice	stop vomiting & jaundice	▲ be symptom-free	▲ TCM	▲ herbs	▲ blood test ▲ subjective ▲ pulse diagnosis
bloating, swelling	reduce weight	▲ help control condition	▲ Naturopathy	▲ diet	▲ weigh-in
unwanted hair growth	resolve anaemia, improve energy	▲ be symptom-free	▲ Naturopathy ▲ TCM	▲ diet ▲ supplements	▲ subjective ▲ blood test ▲ pulse diagnosis
acne	address unwanted hair growth	▲ be symptom-free	▲ TCM	▲ herbs	▲ subjective
overweight	address acne	▲ be symptom-free	▲ TCM ▲ Naturopathy	▲ herbs ▲ diet	▲ subjective
fatigue	reduce stress, depression & anxiety, mood swings	▲ be symptom-free	▲ TCM ▲ GP	▲ herbs ▲ drugs ▲ supplements	▲ subjective
depression	address bloating/fluid retention	▲ be symptom-free	▲ Naturopathy ▲ TCM	▲ diet ▲ herbs	▲ subjective ▲ pulse diagnosis

Although Natalie's condition was stabilized for over a year, mostly through TCM treatment with herbs and by adhering to a strict diet, she did eventually deteriorate and returned to her surgeon who specialised in laparoscopic surgery for women with her condition. He assured her that she could expect at least a 2 year remission from symptoms and at best a 5 year remission, although he indicated that her chances of remaining symptom-free would be increased if she could take some form of hormonal treatment. Natalie was very hopeful and saw that her surgeon's end point was very closely aligned with her own and therefore she opted to go with this treatment with careful monitoring. Natalie underwent laparoscopic surgery which revealed extensive endometriosis. The surgeon said that although her condition was incurable, she should continue to monitor, have more surgery when required and that they would "meet the issue of children" when the time came. Natalie decided to continue with help from alternative therapies to try and get the best outcome and to be symptom-free for as long as possible.

Natalie's journey road map

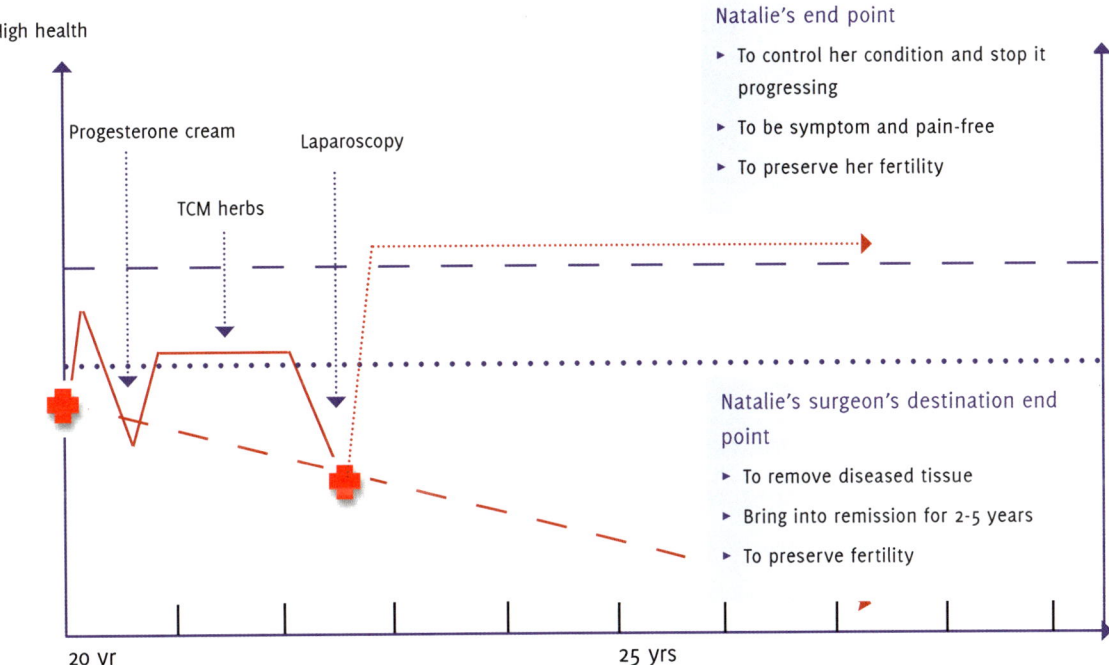

2005-2008

22-25 years old

Natalie was free from pain and many symptoms for a year following surgery. She travelled to the UK and started working in hospitality and joined a band where she performed in gigs and wrote her own songs. However, a year following surgery she was admitted to hospital in great pain and with a swollen abdomen and a scan revealed a large haemorrhagic cyst. Over the next 6 months Natalie had jaundice with vomiting every month from mid-cycle on, with heavy and painful cycles. Six months later she was again admitted to hospital for observation with a ruptured haemorrhagic cyst. Over the next few months Natalie had pelvic ultrasounds to monitor her condition and then she decided to return to Australia for further treatment. She contacted her surgeon to seek his advice but he indicated that in his opinion it could not be a recurrence of her condition so soon after his surgery.

Natalie had an appointment and was booked in for further surgery, just 2 1/2 years after the previous surgery. Following surgery the report indicated that there was severe endometriosis, level 4 or 5, and the biopsies showed either inflammatory tissue, normal peritoneum or endometriosis. No atypical features were seen.

Natalie decided to seek the opinion of a gynaecologist who recommended that she try Synarel for 6 months, which was a drug that would put her into chemical menopause. He said there was a 12% chance that she could be cured with this treatment. The treatment made Natalie very ill and resulted in chronic arthritis. However, she finished the treatment and was persuaded by the gynaecologist to try the Nuva ring, a low dose contraceptive treatment. Natalie reacted badly to the treatment with daily vomiting and migraines. She lasted just 2 months on this treatment before she was rushed to emergency with torsion of the ovary and widespread ascites. She was monitored in hospital over the next 5 days before being released.

Natalie was now facing some major decisions where retaining her fertility was fast becoming a non-option if it meant that she could have a life. So she embarked on a journey of finding a specialist who could help her make an informed decision on the best way forward.

Natalie's journey road map

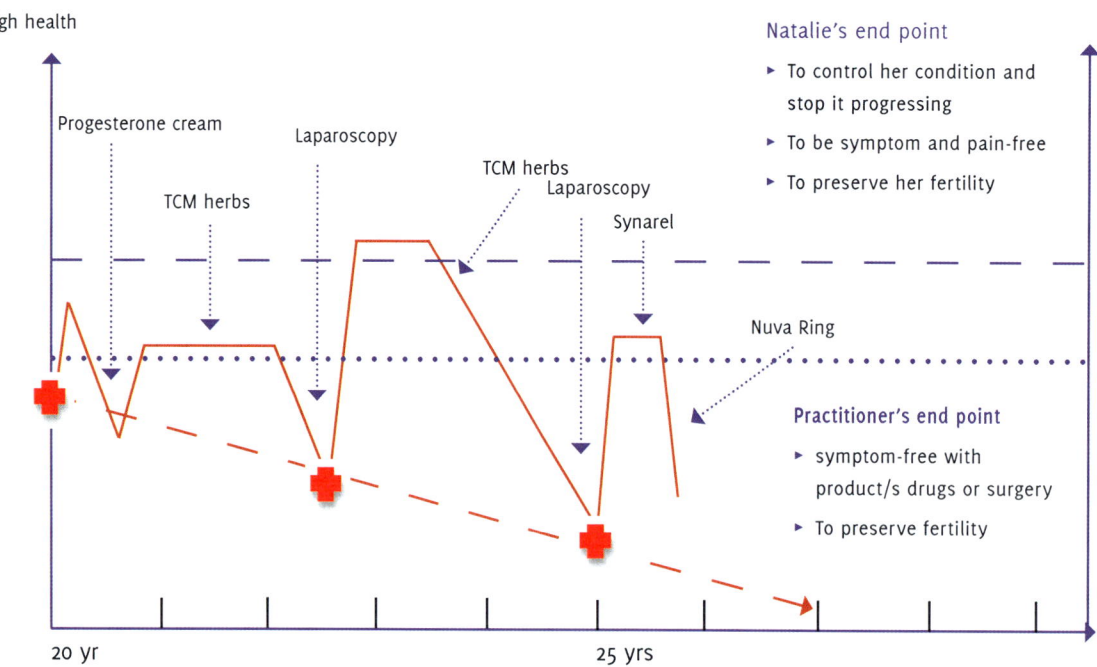

Natalie's SWOT analysis

Natalie had been to see several gynaecologists before she made her decision to have a total hysterectomy. Each one asked her to wait until she was in her 30s; one indicated that he could cut the nerves so that she wouldn't feel pain, another offered her anti-depressants, but none were willing to listen to her story and what her condition meant to her. So she decided to do the SWOT analysis in order to be really clear and lay out her position so that all parties could begin to appreciate what her condition truly meant to her and also give an opportunity for a decision to be made based on humanitarian grounds, rather than medical peer pressure. After much asking around Natalie was recommended a gynaecologist by a medical friend and she was offered an appointment. Prior to the appointment she wrote a letter which she sent with her medical notes to explain her situation (p256).

STRENGTHS	WEAKNESSES	OPPORTUNITIES	THREATS
Benefits or strengths of my preferred medical treatment (total hysterectomy): ▲ nil - the medical profession were unanimous in their opinion that this treatment was out of the question for someone of my age and were unwilling to discuss it. Several specialists asked me to wait as a drug may become available in the next 10 years.	Risks or weaknesses of my preferred treatment: ▲ I will not be able to have children ▲ I will get osteoporosis ▲ I will go into menopause and suffer hot flushes ▲ Inherent risk of any surgery ▲ The endometriosis may regrow with HRT	If I have this treatment I will be able to: ▲ Continue in my day to day life without pain ▲ Fulfill my singing ambitions and have a career ▲ Be able to have a partner and a sexual relationship without pain ▲ Find joy and happiness and be healthy to adopt a child in the future ▲ Reduce my risks for cancer in the reproductive area and the spread of endometriotic implants into the various organs ▲ No drug-dependency (I will not be able to take HRT)	The possible consequences for me: ▲ I would need to take steps to guard against osteoporosis as I won't be able to take HRT ▲ If I have a partner who wants their own children then this may pose a problem

Natalie's letter

2009: 27 years old

"My symptoms now are that I am in constant pain in my abdomen especially when any pressure is applied either from touching it, when I have eaten, or when my bowel and bladder are full. There is pain there all the time. Most importantly, I am unable to have any sexual relations as it is too painful and the heightened pain will last for five days after intercourse.

Because I am unable to have sex, as it is too painful, I have found that it pushes men away. I have, on a few occasions, had to go to hospital after having sex from the pain which occurred when there were ovarian cysts present. This created a lot of problems in the partnership which eventually became insurmountable. So I feel that a future relationship may become impossible if my condition isn't resolved. I have been single for 2 years now due to my condition.

For me, if my future means that I am unable to have a relationship, and that means being alone and celibate, then I have no quality of life and no future of building a good family environment for possible adoption, or if I meet a man who already has children, to care for these. No man wants to be with a woman who cannot be intimate and vice versa, problems always arise down the track no matter how hard they try.

The second major problem for me is that I am unable to commit fully to a career pathway as my health issues make me too unreliable. Singing is my passion and my aim is to make a career in this field. In fact, due to my condition I have already had two starts which have been suddenly curtailed which is not good in this profession. It has been acknowledged by my manager that I may become too much of a liability if my condition remains unresolved. The reason for this is that for 2 weeks of every month I am unable to sing properly as my diaphragm presses down and creates pain and when my period comes I may be in so much pain that I am unable to walk or stand. If my condition follows the same path that it has previously, this progressively worsens as each month goes by until I can no longer even pass stools. My condition will prevent me from touring, from performing and earning a living.

You can imagine that without treatment my future looks very bleak from a relationship and career standpoint. I would have to fall back on casual hospitality work which is very low paid and very depressing. As you will see I have tried everything that has been suggested but progesterone and the Nuva ring both exacerbated my condition, particularly triggering rapid growth of ovarian cysts making me look 6 months pregnant every month, not to mention the pain.

I am coming to see you hoping that we can review my case and find a way forward. Ideally, I would like to have a complete hysterectomy. I haven't come to this decision lightly. I have researched and thought about this for a long time but I know that by having this procedure done that the opportunities for me, my quality of life and happiness, considerably outweigh any negatives.

Last year I looked into freezing eggs, but decided not to go ahead with this as I felt the risks were far too high for me with my condition which involve a personal and family history of blood clots and liver problems as well as the recurrence of large cysts and torsion of the ovaries. I had an appointment with a specialist from the Sydney IVF clinic in October last year and she highlighted that I would be in the high risk category and I might not even be successful in harvesting eggs, let alone seeing the process through until the end.

Having my own child is no longer a priority of mine. For me to be able to live a healthy life is. I am very comfortable and happy at the thought of adopting a child in the future if I decide to have a family and feel this would be an incredible act as a human being to become a mother to a child who needs a mother.

Thank you for taking the time to look over my history. I look forward to our appointment and I hope we can work together to come to a solution."

Natalie's Journey Road Map

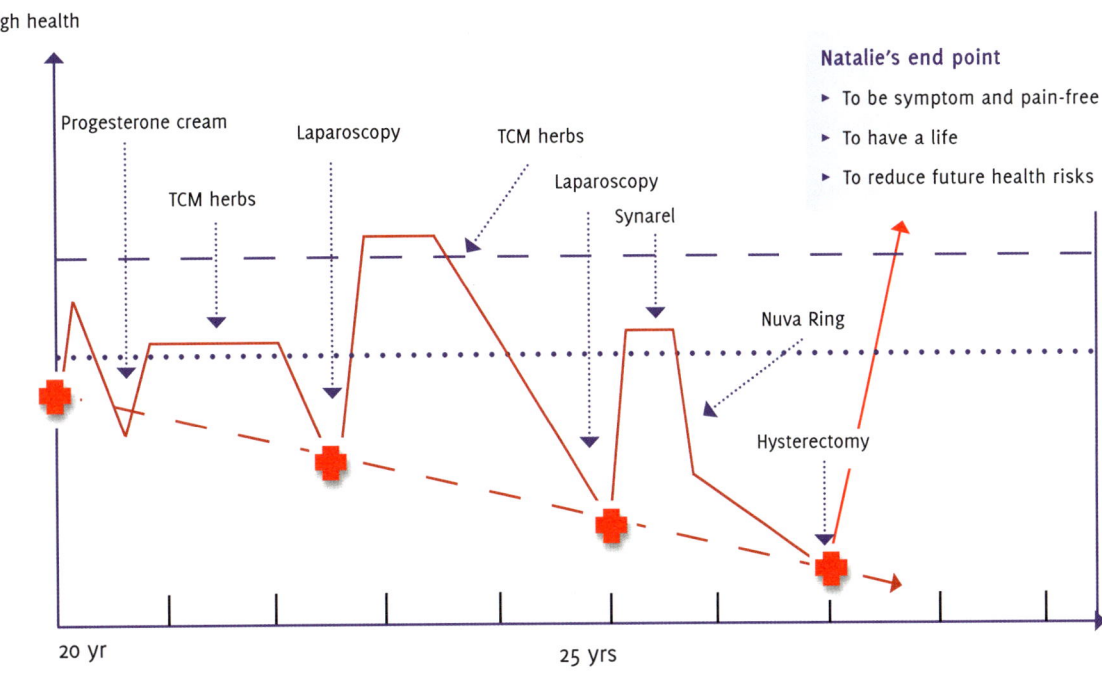

High health

Natalie's end point
▸ To be symptom and pain-free
▸ To have a life
▸ To reduce future health risks

Progesterone cream

Laparoscopy

TCM herbs

TCM herbs

Laparoscopy

Synarel

Nuva Ring

Hysterectomy

20 yr

25 yrs

Natalie had a very honest and fruitful exchange with the recommended gynaecologist. He paved the way for surgery on condition that she had a psychiatric assessment first. The psychiatrist was so impressed with all her journey road map charts and her SWOT analysis that he asked if he could keep a copy.

The surgery was agreed and Natalie was able to regain her life and embark upon her career. She is now successfully pursuing her singing and has done much research into adoption from around the world. She is confident that when the time comes she will be able to adopt and become a loving mother.

Linda's Journey
2010-2012

Linda is 35 years old and had just given birth to her first child four months before she was diagnosed with invasive ductal breast carcinoma, stage 2, triple positive and grade 3 (aggressive). She immediately had some eggs harvested as she wished to have more children and was concerned that the treatment may leave her infertile. Her oncologist recommended surgery and chemotherapy (ACT) as a first line treatment to be followed by radiotherapy, herceptin (H) and tamoxifen + goserilin as targeted treatments. There are some additional risks with the recommended ACT chemotherapy (such as heart damage, toxicity and a small risk of leukaemia further down the track) but the advantages, in terms of overall survival (OS) and disease-free survival (DFS), are worth it, according to her oncologist.

Linda, who is concerned about her future fertility, asks if there are any studies to compare the chemotherapy treatment proposed, against just having surgery, radiotherapy and the targeted treatments and her oncologist says - no. Linda asks whether she has any patients who have opted for this, and if so, how are they doing. The oncologist says, yes she does and they are going fine, but if Linda chooses this option then she would have to pay for all the drugs as only the full protocol is available under Medicare.

Linda decides to undertake the treatment recommended as she cannot afford to pay for the targeted treatments and to do nothing would pose a greater risk than any from the treatments themselves.

Linda's Strategy Flow Template

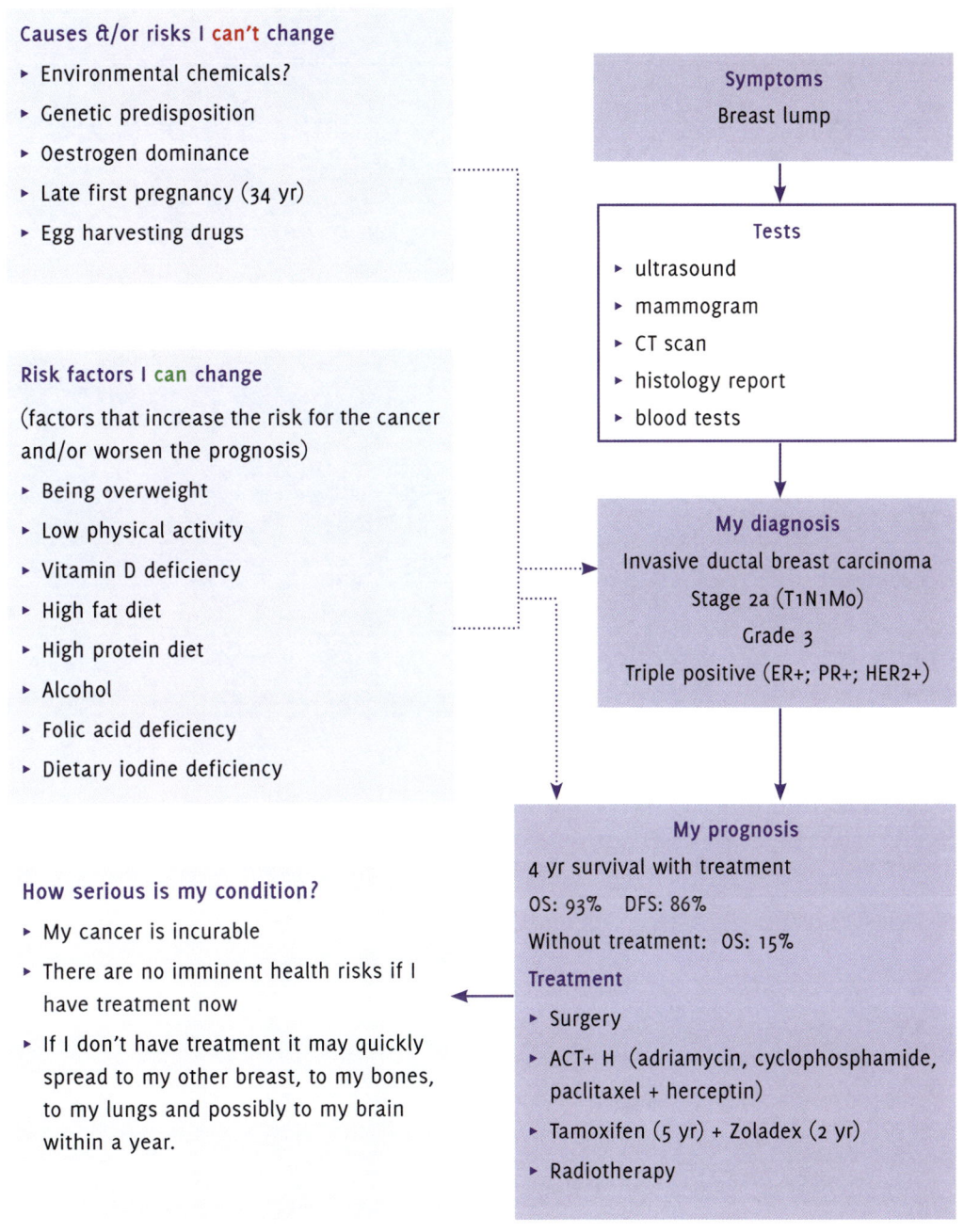

Causes &/or risks I can't change

- Environmental chemicals?
- Genetic predisposition
- Oestrogen dominance
- Late first pregnancy (34 yr)
- Egg harvesting drugs

Risk factors I can change

(factors that increase the risk for the cancer and/or worsen the prognosis)

- Being overweight
- Low physical activity
- Vitamin D deficiency
- High fat diet
- High protein diet
- Alcohol
- Folic acid deficiency
- Dietary iodine deficiency

How serious is my condition?

- My cancer is incurable
- There are no imminent health risks if I have treatment now
- If I don't have treatment it may quickly spread to my other breast, to my bones, to my lungs and possibly to my brain within a year.

Symptoms
Breast lump

Tests

- ultrasound
- mammogram
- CT scan
- histology report
- blood tests

My diagnosis
Invasive ductal breast carcinoma
Stage 2a (T1N1M0)
Grade 3
Triple positive (ER+; PR+; HER2+)

My prognosis
4 yr survival with treatment
OS: 93%   DFS: 86%
Without treatment: OS: 15%
Treatment

- Surgery
- ACT+ H (adriamycin, cyclophosphamide, paclitaxel + herceptin)
- Tamoxifen (5 yr) + Zoladex (2 yr)
- Radiotherapy

Linda's Alignment Template

WHY	NOW		FUTURE HEALTH RISKS
Causes/Risks	**Medical Tests**	**Diagnosis**	**Prognosis**
Environmental chemicals? Genetic predisposition Oestrogen dominance Late first pregnancy (34 yr) Egg harvesting drugs Being overweight Low physical activity Vitamin D deficiency High fat diet High protein diet Alcohol Folic acid deficiency Dietary iodine deficiency	Blood test Ultrasound Mammogram Histology CT scan Surgical report	Invasive ductal breast carcinoma Stage 2a (T1N1M0) Grade 3 Triple positive: ER+ PR+ HER2+	4 yr survival rates *With treatment:* OS: 93% DFS: 86% *Without treatment:* OS: 15% ▸ Metastases to bones, lungs & brain
	End Point	▸ To be in remission for as long as possible (disease-free) ▸ To mitigate any long-term risks of treatment ▸ To preserve fertility	

Linda's End Point

*L*inda has been told that there is no cure for her cancer but that good overall survival rates are possible, particularly due to the availability of targeted treatments, such as Tamoxifen and Herceptin. She did her research and found that there were additional risk factors with the recommended chemotherapy (ACT) combined with herceptin (H) that she wanted to explore.

Linda also did a search on risk factors for breast cancer and found that there were some she couldn't change (genetic predisposition being one, as she had a family history of breast cancer) but others she could change to improve her outcome, such as ensuring nutrient status (vitamin D and iodine), watching her weight, doing regular exercise, and avoiding alcohol, high dietary protein and fat.

Linda's "in principle" end point was to secure long-term remission and mitigate the health risks associated with the treatment. She also wanted to be able to have another baby in the future even though she knew that this could be a risk factor for recurrence. Linda's specific goals focused solely on reduction of the tumoural mass, inhibition of the metastatic potential and to ensure that she was in the percentage that lived the longest, disease-free, by doing whatever she could to make the treatment as effective as possible whilst increasing her capacity for full recovery.

END POINT

Long-term remission

Mitigate long-term risks of treatment

Preserve fertility

SPECIFIC GOALS

remove tumour

reduce potential for metastases

improve response to treatment

reduce side-effects of treatment

ensure capacity to have future children

ensure good recovery potential

Group 1:

Linda is looking for long-term *remission.*

Group 2:

Linda is happy to take conventional and alternative treatments.

Group 3:

Her biggest health risks (aside from the potential rapid spread of her disease) are toxicity from the treatment, including permanent heart damage and leukaemia; also infertility.

Group 4:

Her main objective is to get through treatment and ensure a good recovery potential.

Time frame: She needs to act immediately as the cancer is aggressive, and she needs to monitor to make sure the treatment is working.

End Point	▸ To be in remission for as long as possible (disease-free)	
	▸ To mitigate any long-term risks of treatment	
	▸ To preserve fertility	
Symptoms &/or diagnostics	**Prioritized list of Goals/measurables**	**End point alignment**
	remove tumours	remission, disease-free
	reduce potential for metastases	remission, disease-free
	ensure future capacity to have more children	preserve fertility
	improve my response to treatment	reduce long-term risks increase remission/disease-free survival
	reduce side-effects of treatment	reduce long-term risks
	ensure good recovery potential	reduce long-term risks

Linda's Summary

❝I am 35 years old and have recently been diagnosed with Stage 2, triple positive invasive ductal carcinoma with lymph node involvement. I have had a lumpectomy and axillary clearance and I am about to embark on chemotherapy followed by radiotherapy and take the drugs Herceptin and Tamoxifen, and possibly Zoladex. I am looking to improve my response to treatment for long-term remission, raise my general health and healing potential, and reduce the side-effects & risks of treatment.

Do you have experience and success in treating people like me to improve their outcome and, if so, how can you specifically help me? ❞

Linda's Journey Road Map

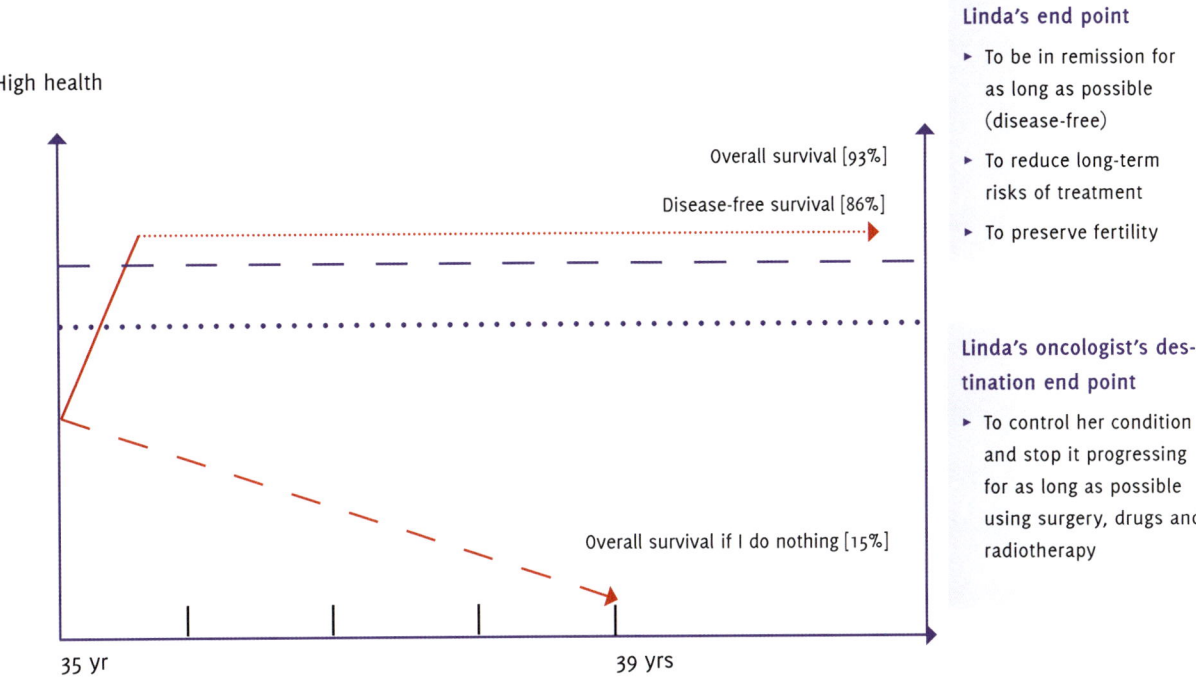

High health

Overall survival [93%]

Disease-free survival [86%]

Overall survival if I do nothing [15%]

35 yr

39 yrs

Linda's end point

- ▶ To be in remission for as long as possible (disease-free)
- ▶ To reduce long-term risks of treatment
- ▶ To preserve fertility

Linda's oncologist's destination end point

- ▶ To control her condition and stop it progressing for as long as possible using surgery, drugs and radiotherapy

Linda underwent surgery and axillary clearance, where 3 of the 36 axillary lymph nodes were infected. Her oncologist has recommended chemotherapy and favours the ACT+H regime. This means that Linda will undergo 6 cycles of adriamycin and cyclophosphamide over a 5 month period, and then have 12 weeks of Taxol (one treatment/week), followed by 5 weeks of radiotherapy. She would start her on Herceptin at the same time as the Taxol which would be taken for a year, and she would also be started on Tamoxifen to be taken over a five year period along with Zoladex for 2 years which will achieve a chemical menopause. The 4 year study that Linda is provided with indicates a 4 year 93% overall survival and an 86% disease-free survival on this treatment. Her oncologist tells her that if she does nothing then she has only a 15% chance of surviving 4 years.

Linda's odds of being in the 86% disease-free survival group at 4 years are pretty good, so she draws up her journey road map with her own end point closely aligned to her oncologist's. The only aspect Linda is unsure about is the recommended chemotherapy regime (ACT-H) which may have inherent risks for her as there is a history of congestive heart disease in her family.

Linda did some further research into her chemotherapy options and found that she could opt for a lesser regime, TC+H (Doxotaxel + carboplatin + Herceptin) with almost equivalent results to the ACT+H regimen and far fewer risks.

She found a study comparing a nonanthracycline regimen (Doxotaxel + carboplatin) + herceptin (TC+H) against an anthracycline (adriamycin) regimen + herceptin (ACT+H). In the ACT+H group there was only a 3% absolute DFS benefit and a 1% absolute OS benefit. But she found that women who received ACT+H were 5 times more likely to experience congestive heart failure and twice as likely to experience sustained asymptomatic cardiac dysfunction. Acute toxicities also occurred on this regimen which included nausea, diarrhoea, vomiting, neuropathy, fatigue and suppression of the immune system. In this study 7 women taking anthracycline developed acute leukemia, and 1 woman in the non-Adriamycin arm developed an acute leukemia after receiving anthracyline outside the study.

When Linda factored in the risks for the ACT+H group (cardiotoxicity and secondary leukaemia [1.6%]), the OS and DFS benefits did not look so attractive, particularly in light of her own risk factors.

Linda spoke about her concerns and findings with her oncologist at her next appointment and was met with a frosty response. Not only that, when she approached the subject of adding alternative treatments, such as dietary changes, supplements (including antioxidants) and herbs, her oncologist told her that diet would make no difference and that she must not, under any circumstances, add antioxidants or herbs as these could undermine the chemotherapy's capacity to work and reduce the survival odds.

Linda was very worried about the advice as she had read a great deal about the benefits of antioxidants and certain herbs in the fight against cancer. When she queried her oncologist's advice, she was told that there were no specific studies to support her recommendations, but that this was the current medical stance based on the hypothesis that chemotherapy and radiotherapy worked via the amount of free radicals generated and that if you "mopped them up with antioxidants" then it would inhibit the treatment's killing capacity.

Comparison between survival rates for stage 2 cancer treated with ACT+H or TC+H

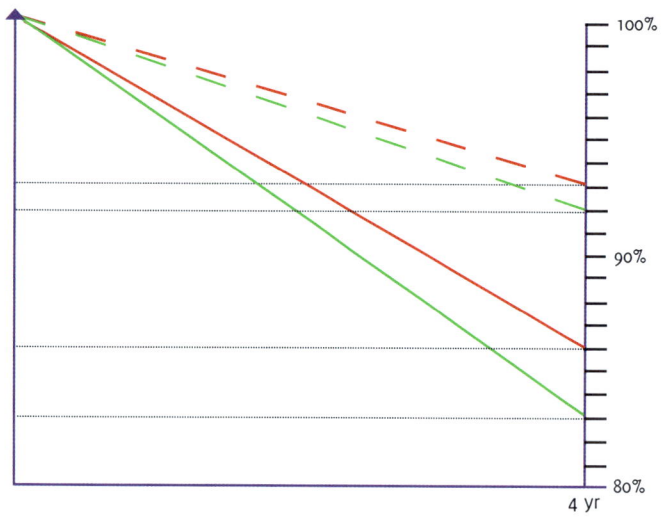

ACT+ H   (adriamycin, cyclophosphamide, paclitaxel + herceptin)

— →   Overall survival (93%)

——→   Disease-free survival (86%)

TC + H (doxotaxel, carboplatin + herceptin)

— →   Overall survival (92%)

——→   Disease-free survival (83%)

Linda's Therapy Alignment Template

THERAPY	GP	Diet therapy	IVF	Surgery	Oncology	Radiology	TCM	Orthomolecular (IV vit C)
Linda's end point								
To be in remission for as long as possible	x	?	x	✓	✓	✓	?	?
To mitigate any long-term risks of treatment	x	?	x	x	x	x	?	?
To preserve fertility	x	x	✓	x	x	x	x	x
List of prioritized goals								
remove tumour	x	x	x	✓	x	x	x	x
reduce potential for metastases	x	?	x	✓	✓	✓	✓	?
ensure future capacity to have more children	x	?	✓	x	x	x	?	x
improve my response to treatment	x	✓	x	x	x	x	✓	?
reduce side-effects of treatment	x	?	x	x	x	x	✓	?
ensure good recovery potential	x	✓	x	x	x	x	✓	?
Tests for monitoring								
Blood tests	✓			✓	✓			
Scans	✓			✓	✓	✓		

Linda places all the various therapies that she will use on her journey and speaks with various practitioners about what they can offer her to help her get to her end point. She also decides to seek help with counselling, meditation and yoga to help cope with the ordeal even though they may not offer a measurable value in terms of specific improvements. She has already had an egg collection, but has still entered this into her alignment template.

Linda's Therapy Alignment Rating Template

Therapy	What is it?	What is its end point? *in relation to my condition*	How does this align to my end point?	Rating
Oncology/ radiology/ surgery	Address cancer using medical treatment speciality (drugs, radiotherapy, surgery); offers medical tests for diagnosis and monitoring	Control condition/increase OS and DFS; &/or alleviate symptoms and rectify abnormal test results with drugs	Offers 4 yr 93% overall survival or 86% disease-free survival	9
General Medicine	Address conditions using drugs; offers medical tests for diagnosis and monitoring; offers referral	Control condition &/or alleviate symptoms/side effects of treatment, rectify abnormal test results with drugs; monitor my condition	Monitor my condition Order tests Refer if condition relapses	6
Diet therapy	Advise, treat with natural products & diet	Improve my general health and support healing	May help keep me in remission for longer May support my fertility	8
TCM herbs	A method using herbs to resolve patterns of disharmony that underpin disease	To improve the functioning of the body and to support healing, help with side-effects of treatment	May help keep me in remission for longer May support my fertility	7
Orthomolecular therapy (IV vit C)	A method to prevent or treat chronic conditions using megadoses of nutrients	To control disease progression & manage symptoms	May help keep me in remission for longer	5

Linda's condition:

▸   Health Risks: short time frame as cancer is aggressive and has already metastasized

▸   Future fertility is an issue as she would like more children

Linda's destination end points:

▸   be in remission for as long as possible

▸   mitigate any long-term health risks from treatment

▸   preserve fertility

Scoring rationale:

Linda has given the top score to her medical team as she realizes that no-one can promise that they can shrink her tumours and inhibit metastasis within a short time frame. As her cancer is aggressive and is already at stage 2, she feels that she doesn't have time to waste. Linda decides to follow the advice of a dietary therapist, who has expertise in treating cancer patients, as she says that she can improve the prognosis and help her body handle the chemotherapy better. Linda is contemplating taking high dose IV vitamin C and B vitamins as a preventive measure but she can't find enough information as to how much value this treatment would offer in addition to what she is already doing - and it's expensive. A TCM herbalist has indicated that she can support Linda through the chemotherapy and alleviate some of the side-effects - but again this will be an added expense, involves weekly travelling and also boiling up the herbs on a daily basis. Based on lifestyle criteria Linda decides against this treatment even though it scores quite highly. No-one claims that they can mitigate the health risks of the ACT+H chemotherapy regime. Linda wants to keep her GP in the loop as he will be her first point of call.

Linda's SWOT analysis comparing the two chemotherapy regimes

STRENGTHS	WEAKNESSES	OPPORTUNITIES	THREATS
Benefits of treatment according to my specialist	Risks or weaknesses of treatment according to my specialist	By having either treatments:	For the ACT+H regime:
▸ ACT+H regime has a OS 1% benefit and DFS 3% benefit over the TC+H regime	▸ The treatment is not a cure and eventual relapses are common	▸ I will be able to continue in my day to day life, watch my kids grow up, work and have quality of life for at least 7 years;	▸ There is a 1.6% chance that I could get secondary leukaemia cancer within a 10 year time frame.
▸ The chemo will mop up occult disease in the rest of my body	▸ 2-3% develop symptomatic congestive heart failure on the ACT+H treatment	▸ I will not need to travel and can stay at home; and	▸ I may feel much worse than I am now with poor quality of life if I suffer the cardiotoxic effects of congestive heart disease which may require long-term medications.
▸ Targeted radiotherapy to the breast area will mop up any remaining cancer cells in this area	▸ 7-17% develop asymptomatic decline in left ventricular ejection fraction on the ACT+H treatment	▸ The government will fund this treatment.	▸ There is a 14% chance that I may relapse and I may need more chemotherapy and the cancer will be more resistant to treatment the more chemo I have now.
	▸ There is a 1.6% risk of secondary leukaemia which can appear within 10 years on the ACT+H treatment		
	▸ There is an increased risk of chest wall metastases and lung metastases with radiotherapy		

Linda decided that the marginal overall survival and disease-free survival benefit for the ACT+H did not outweigh the negatives. The rough equivalence of both trial outcomes persuaded her to go with the lesser chemotherapy (TC+H), and she felt that if the disease did relapse then there may be less chance of resistance to the chemotherapy that she hadn't yet tried. Speaking with various practitioners none could claim that they could mitigate the risks of this treatment, and given her family history of congestive heart disease she felt it was an unnecessary risk.

Linda's Treatment Alignment Template

	Treatment	Surgery	Chemo-therapy	Radio-therapy	Herc-eptin	Tamox-ifen	Zoladex	Diet	IV vit C	Curc-umin
Linda's end point	To be in remission for as long as possible	√	√	√	√	√	√	√	?	√
	To mitigate any long-term risks of treatment	×	×	×	×	×	×	?	?	×
	To preserve fertility	×	×	×	×	×	×	?	×	×
List of prioritized goals	remove tumour	√	×	×	×	×	×	×	×	×
	reduce potential for metastases	√	√	√	√	√	√	√	?	√
	ensure future capacity to have more children	×	×	×	×	×	×	√	×	×
	improve my response to first line treatment	×	×	×	√	√	√	√	?	√
	reduce side-effects of first line treatment	×	×	×	×	×	×	?	?	×
	ensure good recovery potential	×	×	×	×	×	×	√	?	×
Tests for monitoring	Blood tests	√	√	√	√	√	√	×	×	×
	Scans	√	√	√	√	√	√	×	×	×

Once Linda had spoken with all her potential practitioners and determined which of her aspirational end points and goals they could help with she then went on to look at each treatment they were proposing and how it would work specifically in her case. She found that very few promises (if any) could be made other than the claims supported by clinical trials for the drugs that were being proposed. However, the dietary therapist was able to supply her with evidence of how her program worked and what she could expect and she did find some trials which had used curcumin as an adjunct in the type of chemotherapy she was favouring (TC+H) to good effect. She also qualified with each practitioner how they would monitor her progress and she found that the only tests that would give measurable input were blood tests and scans. She identified which test results should be monitored so that she could keep her eye on specific markers to make sure that she was heading in the right direction.

Linda's Treatment Alignment Rating Template

Treatment	What will the treatment do?	How will it help me get to my end point?	What is used to measure outcome?	Rating
Surgery	Removes tumour tissue and reduces risk of metastases	Improves overall and disease-free survival	• Objective: blood tests, scan	10
Chemo-therapy	Gets rid of any cancer cells that may be left behind after surgery, or distant metastases that haven't been identified and to reduce the risk of the cancer coming back.	Improves overall and disease-free survival	• Objective: blood tests, scan	9
Radio-therapy	Kills any remaining cancer cells in the local area.	Improves overall and disease-free survival	• Objective: scan	9
Herceptin	Stops breast cancer cells from growing and multiplying by binding to the HER2 proteins; also triggers the immune system to attack the cancerous cells.	Improves overall and disease-free survival	• Objective: scan	10
Tamoxifen	Blocks oestrogen receptors on breast cells inhibiting the stimulatory effects of oestrogen and stops the cancer from growing. Helps prevent local recurrence in the breast and also reduces risk of developing cancer in the other breast.	Improves overall and disease-free survival	• Objective: scans, blood tests	10
Zoladex	Desensitizes the pituitary gland which stops stimulating the ovaries and stops ovarian production of oestrogen and progesterone; mitigates the negative effects of Tamoxifen on the ovaries.	Improves overall and disease-free survival	• Objective: scan, blood tests	10
Diet Therapy	Helps rebuild my healing potential and to detoxify drugs and other waste products.	May improve overall and disease-free survival. Support general health and immune system. May support my fertility	• Objective: scan, blood tests • Subjective: feeling better, more energy, less symptoms	9
Curcumin	Increases the efficacy of chemotherapy and radiotherapy by sensitizing the cancer cells to these treatments; inhibits breast cancer cell proliferation.	May improve overall and disease-free survival	• Objective: scan, blood tests	7
IV vit C	high dose vitamin C is toxic to tumor cells; it boosts immunity; it can stimulate collagen formation to help wall off the tumor and inhibit metastases.	May improve overall and disease-free survival may support immune system	• Subjective: how do I feel	5

Scoring rationale:

Linda has given the top score to surgery and the targeted treatments as she has read many studies and has seen the contribution these treatments make to both overall survival and disease-free survival. Linda was concerned with her oncologist's advice on using antioxidants and did some further research (http://www.canceractive.com/cancer-active-page-link.aspx?n=470) into vitamin C and cancer. She decided to follow her oncologist's advice and not take the IV vitamin C with the chemotherapy, but she did decide to take therapeutic amounts of curcumin which have been shown to increase the response to both chemotherapy and radiotherapy. Diet therapy also scores highly as, contrary to the advice that diet won't make any difference, she feels that any health outcome is based not just on the treatment itself but also on how well the patient responds to treatment, and she figures that the stronger and healthier she can be (and also if she can get rid of the toxins from the drugs) then this will allow her to recover more completely.

Linda's Therapy & Treatment End Point Alignment

End point				
To be in remission for as long as possible (disease-free)				
To mitigate any long-term risks of treatment				
To preserve fertility				
Prioritized list of Goals/measurables	**End point alignment**	**Therapy**	**Treatment**	**Tests**
remove tumours	remission, disease-free	surgery, oncology, radiology	surgery, drugs, radiotherapy	blood test, scan
reduce potential for metastastases	remission, disease-free	oncology, radiology	drugs, radiotherapy, curcumin	blood test, scan
ensure future capacity to have more children	preserve fertility	IVF clinic	drugs	
improve my response to treatment	reduce long-term risks / remission, disease-free	Diet therapy / Herbal medicine	supplements, diet, curcumin	blood test, scan
reduce side-effects of treatment	reduce long-term risks	Diet therapy, Orthomolecular	diet, supplements, curcumin	
ensure good recovery potential	reduce long-term risks	Diet therapy	diet, supplements	

About Kathryn ....

Kathryn has been supporting, treating and managing patients from all over the world for almost 30 years, and for those who cannot travel she offers telephone and skype consultations.

Kathryn helps many patients with chronic disease and cancer who are trying to juggle a combination of conventional and alternative treatments. Invariably there is no-one at the helm and it is a tough call for the patient to work out which combinations of treatments will give the best outcome. By travelling with clients on their journey, monitoring their progress and helping them to navigate the health system, Kathryn endeavours to make sure they get the best clinical outcome possible.

Kathryn holds qualifications as a Dietary Therapist, a Naturopath and a Gerson Therapist, and has 30 years of experience in the field of dietary healing where she has witnessed the profound healing and cure that can occur through the correct application of diet. She also held a position on the Board of the Gerson Institute and was instrumental in developing their practitioner training program, undertaking the training of practitioners in the US, the UK, Germany and Australia. Her publication *Nutritional Healing, a patient management handbook*, described by Charlotte Gerson as "the 'bible' of the nutritional healer of the future" was written for both patients and practitioners following the Gerson Therapy.

Kathryn also mentors practitioners from around the world with difficult cases and currently runs courses for professionals, health advocates and members of the public. She has several publications amongst which is the widely acclaimed book *Dietary Healing, the complete detox program* ISBN 9780980376289

Please visit www.kathrynalexander.com.au for more information and free resources.

Kathryn lives and works from home in the Sunshine Coast, Australia.

More help for you ....

Consultations: Kathryn offers consultations in person, by skype or phone

Courses: Kathryn offers a range of courses for both professionals and members of the public which include:

- managing your own dietary healing and detoxification program, or that of clients;
- practitioner training in the management of chronic disease; and
- patient advocacy, using the Smart Patient Journey Road Map, navigating the system, making informed choices and monitoring.

Publications:

- Dietary Healing, the complete detox program (printed edition: ISBN 9780980376289; ebook: ISBN 9780980376265)
- Nutritional healing, a patient-management handbook (ebook: ISBN 9780980376241)
- Fundamentals of Cellular Cleansing, parts 1 & 2 (audio visual)
- The principles of detoxification (audio: ISBN 9780980376258)

Made in the USA
Charleston, SC
08 August 2014